Artificial Intell
in Health Care

The Hope, the Hype, the Promise, the Peril

Michael Matheny,
Sonoo Thadaney Israni, Mahnoor Ahmed,
and **Danielle Whicher,** *Editors*

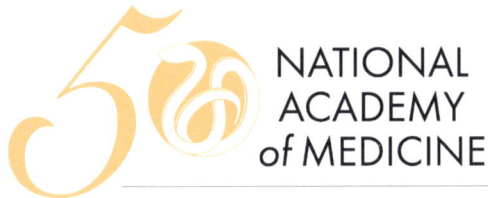

**NATIONAL
ACADEMY
of MEDICINE**

WASHINGTON, DC
NAM.EDU

NATIONAL ACADEMY OF MEDICINE   500 Fifth Street, NW   Washington, DC 20001

This publication has undergone peer review according to procedures established by the National Academy of Medicine (NAM). Publication by the NAM signifies that it is the product of a carefully considered process and is a contribution worthy of public attention, but does not constitute endorsement of conclusions and recommendations by the NAM. The views presented in this publication are those of individual contributors and do not represent formal consensus positions of the authors' organizations; the NAM; or the National Academies of Sciences, Engineering, and Medicine.

International Standard Book Number-13: 978-1-947103-17-7
Library of Congress Control Number: 2020938860

Printed in the United States of America

Suggested citation: Matheny, M., S. Thadaney Israni, M. Ahmed, and D. Whicher, Editors. 2022. *Artificial Intelligence in Health Care: The Hope, the Hype, the Promise, the Peril.* Washington, DC: National Academy of Medicine.

"Knowing is not enough; we must apply.
Willing is not enough; we must do."
—GOETHE

LEADERSHIP
INNOVATION
IMPACT

for a healthier future

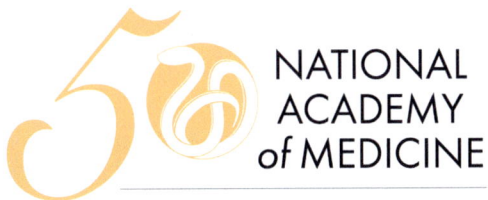

ABOUT THE NATIONAL ACADEMY OF MEDICINE

The **National Academy of Medicine** is one of three Academies constituting the National Academies of Sciences, Engineering, and Medicine (the National Academies). The National Academies provide independent, objective analysis and advice to the nation and conduct other activities to solve complex problems and inform public policy decisions. The National Academies also encourage education and research, recognize outstanding contributions to knowledge, and increase public understanding in matters of science, engineering, and medicine.

The **National Academy of Sciences** was established in 1863 by an Act of Congress, signed by President Lincoln, as a private, nongovernmental institution to advise the nation on issues related to science and technology. Members are elected by their peers for outstanding contributions to research. Dr. Marcia McNutt is president.

The **National Academy of Engineering** was established in 1964 under the charter of the National Academy of Sciences to bring the practices of engineering to advising the nation. Members are elected by their peers for extraordinary contributions to engineering. Dr. John L. Anderson is president.

The **National Academy of Medicine** (formerly the Institute of Medicine) was established in 1970 under the charter of the National Academy of Sciences to advise the nation on issues of health, health care, and biomedical science and technology. Members are elected by their peers for distinguished contributions to medicine and health. Dr. Victor J. Dzau is president.

Learn more about the National Academy of Medicine at NAM.edu.

AUTHORS

MICHAEL MATHENY (*Co-Chair*), Vanderbilt University Medical Center and the Department of Veterans Affairs

SONOO THADANEY ISRANI (*Co-Chair*), Stanford University

ANDREW AUERBACH, University of California, San Francisco

ANDREW BEAM, Harvard University

PAUL BLEICHER, OptumLabs

WENDY CHAPMAN, University of Melbourne

JONATHAN CHEN, Stanford University

GUILHERME DEL FIOL, University of Utah

HOSSEIN ESTIRI, Harvard Medical School

JAMES FACKLER, Johns Hopkins School of Medicine

STEPHAN FIHN, University of Washington

ANNA GOLDENBERG, University of Toronto

SETH HAIN, Epic

JAIMEE HEFFNER, Fred Hutchinson Cancer Research Center

EDMUND JACKSON, Hospital Corporation of America

JEFFREY KLANN, Harvard Medical School and Massachusetts General Hospital

RITA KUKAFKA, Columbia University

HONGFANG LIU, Mayo Clinic

DOUGLAS McNAIR, Bill & Melinda Gates Foundation

ENEIDA MENDONÇA, Regenstrief Institute

JONI PIERCE, University of Utah

W. NICHOLSON PRICE II, University of Michigan

JOACHIM ROSKI, Booz Allen Hamilton

SUCHI SARIA, Johns Hopkins University

NIGAM SHAH, Stanford University

RANAK TRIVEDI, Stanford University

JENNA WIENS, University of Michigan

NAM Staff

Development of this publication was facilitated by contributions of the following NAM staff, under the guidance of J. Michael McGinnis, Leonard D. Schaeffer Executive Officer and Executive Director of the Leadership Consortium for a Value & Science-Driven Health System:

DANIELLE WHICHER, Senior Program Officer (until September 2019)

MAHNOOR AHMED, Associate Program Officer

JESSICA BROWN, Executive Assistant to the Executive Officer (until September 2019)

FASIKA GEBRU, Senior Program Assistant

JENNA OGILVIE, Deputy Director of Communications

REVIEWERS

This Special Publication was reviewed in draft form by individuals chosen for their diverse perspectives and technical expertise, in accordance with review procedures established by the National Academy of Medicine (NAM). We wish to thank the following individuals for their contributions:

PAT BAIRD, Philips

SANJAY BASU, Harvard Medical School

SARA BURROUS, Washington University in St. Louis

KEVIN JOHNSON, Vanderbilt University Medical Center

SALLY OKUN, PatientsLikeMe

J. MARC OVERHAGE, Cerner Corporation

JACK RESNECK, JR., American Medical Association

SARA ROSENBAUM, The George Washington University

PAUL TANG, IBM Watson Health

TIMOTHY M. PERSONS, Chief Scientist and Managing Director, Science, Technology Assessment, and Analytics, U.S. Government Accountability Office *(NOTE: Dr. Persons provided only editorial comments and technical advice on the description of the artificial intelligence technology described in the publication. Dr. Persons did not comment on any policy-related recommendations and did not review or comment on any of the legal content in the publication.)*

The reviewers listed above provided many constructive comments and suggestions, but they were not asked to endorse the content of the publication, and did not see the final draft before it was published. Review of this publication was overseen by **DANIELLE WHICHER,** Senior Program Officer, NAM; **MAHNOOR AHMED,** Associate Program Officer, NAM; and **J. MICHAEL McGINNIS,** Leonard D. Schaeffer Executive Officer, NAM. Responsibility for the final content of this publication rests with the editors and the NAM.

FOREWORD

In 2006, the National Academy of Medicine (NAM) established the Roundtable on Evidence-Based Medicine for the purpose of providing a trusted venue for national leaders in health and health care to work cooperatively toward their common commitment to effective, innovative care that consistently generates value for patients and society. The goal of advancing a "Learning Health System" quickly emerged and was defined as "a system in which science, informatics, incentives, and culture are aligned for continuous improvement and innovation, with best practices seamlessly embedded in the delivery process and new knowledge captured as an integral by-product of the delivery experience."[1]

To advance this goal, and in recognition of the increasingly essential role that digital health innovations in data and analytics contribute to achieving this goal, the *Digital Health Learning Collaborative* was established. Over the life of the collaborative, the extraordinary preventive and clinical medical care implications of rapid innovations in artificial intelligence (AI) and machine learning emerged as essential considerations for the consortium. The publication you are now reading responds to the need for physicians, nurses and other clinicians, data scientists, health care administrators, public health officials, policy makers, regulators, purchasers of health care services, and patients to understand the basic concepts, current state of the art, and future implications of the revolution in AI and machine learning. We believe that this publication will be relevant to those seeking practical, relevant, understandable, and useful information about key definitions, concepts, applicability, pitfalls, rate-limiting steps, and future trends in this increasingly important area.

Michael Matheny, M.D., M.S., M.P.H., and Sonoo Thadaney Israni, M.B.A., have assembled a stellar team of contributors, all of whom enjoy wide respect in their fields. Together, in this well-edited volume that has benefitted from the thorough review process ingrained in the NAM's culture, they present expert,

---

[1] See https://nam.edu/wp-content/uploads/2015/07/LearningHealthSystem_28jul15.pdf.

understandable, comprehensive, and practical insights on topic areas that include the historical development of the field; lessons learned from other industries; how massive amounts of data from a variety of sources can be appropriately analyzed and integrated into clinical care; how innovations can be used to facilitate population health models and social determinants of health interventions; the opportunities to equitably and inclusively advance precision medicine; the applicability for health care organizations and businesses to reduce the cost of care delivery; opportunities to enhance interactions between health care professionals and patients, families, and caregivers; and the role of legal statutes that inform the uptake of AI in health care.

As the co-chairs of the *Digital Health Learning Collaborative*, we are excited by the progress being demonstrated in realizing a virtuous cycle in which the data inevitably produced by every patient encounter might be captured into a "collective memory" of health services to be used to inform and improve the subsequent care of the individual patient and the health system more generally. Enormous datasets are increasingly generated not only in the formal health care setting, but also from medical and consumer devices, wearables, and patient-reported outcomes, as well as environmental, community, and public health sources. They include structured (or mathematically operable) data as well as text, images, and sounds. The landscape also includes data "mash-ups" from commercial, legal, and online social records.

AI has been the tool envisioned to offer the most promise in harvesting knowledge from that collective memory, and as this volume demonstrates, some of that promise is being realized. Among the most important of these promises in the near term is the opportunity to assuage the frustration of health care providers who have been clicking away on electronic health records with modest benefit beyond increased data transportability and legibility. Our hope is that AI will be the "payback" for the investment in both the implementation of electronic health records and the cumbersomeness of their use by facilitating tasks that every clinician, patient, and family would want, but are impossible to do without electronic assistance—such as monitoring a patient for emergent sepsis $24 \times 7 \times 365$ and providing timelier therapy for a condition in which diagnostic delay correlates with increased risk of death.

However, we also appreciate that AI alone cannot cure health care's ills and that new technologies bring novel and potentially under-appreciated challenges. For example, if a machine learning algorithm is trained with data containing a systematic bias, then that bias may be interpreted as normative, exacerbating rather than resolving disparities and inequities in care. Similarly, association of data does not prove causality, and it may not even be explanatory, suggesting that a simultaneous revolution in research methods is also necessary. Finally, the mere existence of substantial and sensitive data assets raises concerns about privacy and security. Aspiring to the promise of AI requires both continuing innovation and attention to the potential perils.

In our opinion, this publication presents a sober and balanced celebration of accomplishments, possibilities, and pitfalls. We commend Drs. Michael McGinnis and Danielle Whicher for their thoughtful sponsorship of the NAM Consortium and *Digital Health Learning Collaborative*, Dr. Matheny and Mrs. Thadaney Israni for their leadership in producing this volume, and to all the contributors who have produced an exceptional resource with practical relevance to a wide array of key stakeholders.

Jonathan B. Perlin, M.D., Ph.D., MACP

Reed V. Tuckson, M.D., FACP
Co-Chairs, Digital Learning Collaborative, Consortium on Value and
Science-Driven Health Care, National Academy of Medicine

CONTENTS

BOXES, FIGURES, AND TABLES

BOXES

FIGURES

TABLES

ACRONYMS AND ABBREVIATIONS

ACM	Association of Computing Machinery
AI	artificial intelligence
AMA	American Medical Association
API	application programming interface
ATM	automated teller machine
AUROC	area under the ROC curve
BBC	British Broadcasting Corporation
CDC	Centers for Disease Control and Prevention
CDM	common data model
CDS	clinical decision support
CGMP	Current Good Manufacturing Process
CLIA	Clinical Laboratory Improvement Amendments
CMS	Centers for Medicare & Medicaid Services
CONSORT	Consolidated Standards of Reporting Trials
CPIC	Clinical Pharmacogenetics Implementation Consortium
CPU	central processing unit
DARPA	Defense Advanced Research Projects Agency
DHLC	Digital Health Learning Collaborative
DOJ	U.S. Department of Justice
ECA	embodied conversational agent
ECG	electrocardiogram
EHR	electronic health record
EU	European Union

FAIR	findability, accessibility, interoperability, and reusability
FDA	U.S. Food and Drug Administration
FDCA	Federal Food, Drug, and Cosmetic Act
FHIR	Fast Healthcare Interoperability Resource
fRamily	friends and family unpaid caregivers
FTC	Federal Trade Commission
FTCA	Federal Trade Commission Act
GDPR	General Data Protection Regulation
GPS	global positioning system
GPU	graphics processing unit
HAZOP	hazard and operability study
HHS	U.S. Department of Health and Human Services
HIE	health information exchange
HIPAA	Health Insurance Portability and Accountability Act
HITECH Act	Health Information Technology for Economic and Clinical Health Act
HIV	human immunodeficiency virus
i2b2	Informatics for Integrating Biology & the Bedside
ICD-10	*International Classification of Diseases, 10th Revision*
IEEE	Institute of Electrical and Electronics Engineers
IOM	Institute of Medicine
IoT	Internet of Things
IMDRF	International Medical Device Regulators Forum
IP	intellectual property
IT	information technology
IVD	in vitro diagnostic device
IVDMIA	in vitro diagnostic multivariate index assay
JITAI	just-in-time adaptive intervention
LDT	laboratory-developed test
Leadership Consortium	National Academy of Medicine Leadership Consortium: Collaboration for a Value & Science-Driven Learning Health System
LHS	learning health system
LOINC	Logical Observational Identifiers Names and Codes

MIT	Massachusetts Institute of Technology
NAM	National Academy of Medicine
NAS	National Academy of Sciences
NeurIPS	Conference on Neural Information Processing Systems
NHTSA	National Highway Traffic Safety Administration
NIH	National Institutes of Health
NITRC	Neuroimaging Informatics Tools and Resources Clearinghouse
NLP	natural language processing
NNH	number needed to harm
NNT	number needed to treat
NPV	negative predictive value
NRC	National Research Council
NSTC	National Science and Technology Council
OHDSI	Observational Health Data Sciences and Informatics
OHRP	Office for Human Research Protections
OMOP	Observational Medical Outcomes Partnership
ONC	The Office of the National Coordinator for Health Information Technology
PARiHS	Promoting Action on Research Implementation in Health Services
PCORnet	Patient-Centered Clinical Research Network
PDSA	plan-do-study-act
PFS	physician fee schedule
PHI	protected health information
PPV	positive predictive value
PR	precision-recall
Pre-Cert	Digital Health Software Precertification Program
QI	quality improvement
QMS	quality management system
R&D	research and development
ROC	receiver operating characteristic
RWD	real-world data
RWE	real-world evidence

SaMD   software as a medical device
SDLC   software development life cycle
SDoH   social determinants of health
SMART   Substitutable Medical Apps, Reusable Technology
STARD   Standards for Reporting of Diagnostic Accuracy Studies

TPR   true positive rate
TPU   tensor processing unit

UDN   Undiagnosed Diseases Network

WEIRD   Western, educated, industrialized, rich, and democratic

SUMMARY

The emergence of artificial intelligence (AI) as a tool for better health care offers unprecedented opportunities to improve patient and clinical team outcomes, reduce costs, and impact population health. Examples include but are not limited to automation; providing patients, "fRamily" (friends, family, and unpaid caregivers), and health professionals with an understandable synthesis of complex health information; and recommendations and visualization of information for shared decision making.

While there have been a number of promising examples of AI applications in health care, we believe it is imperative to proceed with caution, else we may end up with user disillusionment and another AI winter, and/or further exacerbate existing health- and technology-driven disparities. This Special Publication, *Artificial Intelligence in Health Care: The Hope, the Hype, the Promise, the Peril* synthesizes current knowledge to offer a reference document for relevant health care stakeholders such as AI model developers, clinical implementers, clinicians and patients, regulators, and policy makers, to name a few. It outlines the current and near-term AI solutions; highlights the challenges, limitations, and best practices for AI development, adoption, and maintenance; offers an overview of the legal and regulatory landscape for AI tools designed for health care application; prioritizes the need for equity, inclusion, and a human rights lens for this work; and outlines key considerations for moving forward. The major theses are summarized in the section below.

POPULATION-REPRESENTATIVE DATA ACCESSIBILITY, STANDARDIZATION, AND QUALITY ARE VITAL

AI algorithms must be trained on population-representative data to achieve performance levels necessary for scalable "success." Trends such as the cost for storing and managing data, data collection via electronic health records, and

1

exponential consumer health data generation have created a data-rich health care ecosystem. However, this growth in health care data is hampered by the lack of efficient mechanisms for integrating and merging these data beyond their current silos. While there are multiple frameworks and standards in place to help aggregate and achieve sufficient data volume for AI use of data at rest (such as mature health care common data models) and data in motion (such as Health Level Seven International Fast Healthcare Interoperability Resources [HL7 FHIR]), they need wider adoption to support AI tool development, deployment, and maintenance. There continue to be issues of interoperability and scale of data transfers due to cultural, social, and regulatory reasons. Solutions will require the engagement of all relevant stakeholders. Thus, the wider health care community should continue to advocate for policy, regulatory, and legislative mechanisms that improve equitable, inclusive data collection and aggregation, and transparency around how patient health data may be best utilized to balance financial incentives and the public good.

ETHICAL HEALTH CARE, EQUITY, AND INCLUSIVITY SHOULD BE PRIORITIZED

Fulfilling this aspiration will require ensuring population-representative datasets and giving particular priority to what might be termed a new Quintuple Aim of Equity and Inclusion for health and health care (see Figure S-1). Else, the scaling

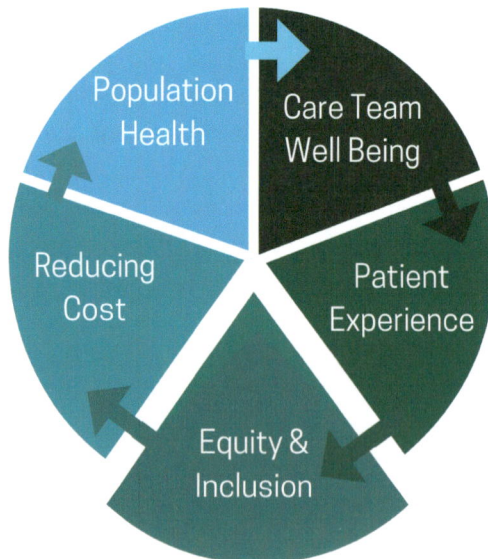

FIGURE S-1 | Advancing to the Quintuple Aim.

possible with AI might further exacerbate the considerable existing inequities in health outcomes at a monumental scale. A single biased human or organizational impact is far less than that of global or national AI.

Prioritizing equity and inclusion should be a clearly stated goal when developing and deploying AI in health care. There are many high-profile examples of biased AI tools that have damaged the public's trust in these systems. It is judicious for developers and implementers to evaluate the suitability of the data used to develop AI tools and unpack the underlying biases in the data, to consider how the tool should be deployed, and to question whether various deployment environments could adversely impact equity and inclusivity. There are widely recognized inequities in health outcomes due to the variety of social determinants of health and perverse incentives in the existing health care system. Unfortunately, consumer-facing technologies have often worsened historical inequities in other fields and are at risk of doing so in health care as well.

THE DIALOGUE AROUND TRANSPARENCY AND TRUST SHOULD CHANGE TO BE DOMAIN- AND USE-CASE DIFFERENTIAL

Transparency is key to building this much needed trust among users and stakeholders, but there are distinct domains with differential needs of transparency. There should be full transparency on the composition, semantics, provenance, and quality of data used to develop AI tools. There also needs to be full transparency and adequate assessment of relevant performance components of AI. However, algorithmic transparency may not be required for all cases. AI developers, implementers, users, and regulators should collaboratively define guidelines for clarifying the level of transparency needed across a spectrum. These are key issues for regulatory agencies and clinical users, and requirements for performance are differential based on risk and intended use. Most importantly, we suggest clear separation of data, algorithmic, and performance reporting in AI dialogue, and the development of guidance in each of these spaces.

NEAR-TERM FOCUS SHOULD BE ON AUGMENTED INTELLIGENCE RATHER THAN FULL AUTOMATION

Some of the AI opportunities include supporting clinicians undertaking tasks currently limited to specialists; filtering out normal or low acuity clinical cases so that specialists can work at the top of their licensure; helping humans address inattention, microaggressions, and fatigue; and improving business process automation. Ensuring human-centered AI tools includes accepting that human override is important for developing user trust because the public has an understandably low tolerance for machine error and that AI tools are being implemented in an environment of inadequate regulation and legislation. The near-term dialogue around AI in health care should focus on promoting, developing, and evaluating tools that support humans rather than attempting to replace them with full automation.

DEVELOP AND DEPLOY APPROPRIATE TRAINING AND EDUCATIONAL PROGRAMS TO SUPPORT HEALTH CARE AI

In order to benefit from, sustain, and nurture AI tools in health care we need a thoughtful, sweeping, and comprehensive expansion of relevant training and educational programs. Given the scale at which health care AI systems could change the medical domain, the educational expansion must be multidisciplinary and engage AI developers, implementers, health care system leadership, frontline clinical teams, ethicists, humanists, and patients and patient caregivers because each brings a core set of much needed requirements and expertise. Health care professional training programs should incorporate core curricula focused on teaching how to appropriately use data science and AI products and services. The needs of practicing health care professionals can be fulfilled via their required continuing education, empowering them to be more informed consumers. Additionally, retraining programs to address a shift in desired skill sets due to increasing levels of AI deployment and the resulting skill and knowledge mismatches will be needed. Last, but not least, consumer health educational programs, at a range of educational levels, to help inform consumers on health care application selection and use are vital.

LEVERAGE EXISTING FRAMEWORKS AND BEST PRACTICES WITHIN THE LEARNING HEALTH CARE SYSTEM, HUMAN FACTORS, AND IMPLEMENTATION SCIENCE

The challenges in operationalizing AI technologies into the health care systems are countless in spite of the fact that this is one of the strongest growth areas in biomedical research and impact. The AI community must develop an integrated best practice framework for implementation and maintenance by incorporating existing best practices of ethical inclusivity, software development, implementation science, and human–computer interaction. This framework should be developed within the context of the learning health care system and be tied to targets and objectives. The cost and burden of implementing AI tools should be weighed against use case needs. AI tools should be pursued where other low-or no-technology solutions will not do as well. Successful AI implementation will need the committed engagement of health care stakeholders—leaders, AI developers, AI implementers, regulators, humanists, patients, and families. Health delivery systems should have a robust and mature underlying information technology (IT) governance strategy in place prior to them embarking on substantial AI deployment and integration. Lastly, national efforts should be deployed to provide capacity for AI deployment in lower resource environments where IT and informatics capacities are less robust. Linked to the prior considerations, this would help lower the entry barrier for adoption of these technologies and help promote greater health care equity. Health care AI could also go beyond the current limited biology-focused research to address patient and communal needs, expanding to meaningful and usable access of social determinants of health and psychosocial risk factors. AI has the potential (with appropriate consent) to link personal and public data for truly personalized health care.

BALANCING DEGREES OF REGULATION AND LEGISLATION OF AI TO PROMOTE INNOVATION, SAFETY, AND TRUST

AI applications have an enormous ability to improve patient outcomes, but they could also pose significant risks in terms of inappropriate patient risk assessment, diagnostic error, treatment recommendations, privacy breaches, and other harms. Regulators should remain flexible, but the potential for lagging legal responses will remain a challenge for AI developers and deployers. In alignment with recent congressional and U.S. Food and Drug Administration developments and guidance, we suggest a graduated approach to the regulation of AI based on the level of patient risk, the level of AI autonomy, and considerations for how static or dynamic certain AI are likely to be. To the extent that machine learning–based models continuously learn from new data, regulators should adopt postmarket surveillance mechanisms to ensure continuing (and ideally improving) high-quality performance. Liability accrued when deploying AI algorithms will continue to be an emerging area as regulators, courts, and the risk-management industries deliberate. Tackling regulation and liability among AI adopters is vital when evaluating the risks and benefits. Regulators should engage stakeholders and experts to continuously evaluate deployed clinical AI for effectiveness and

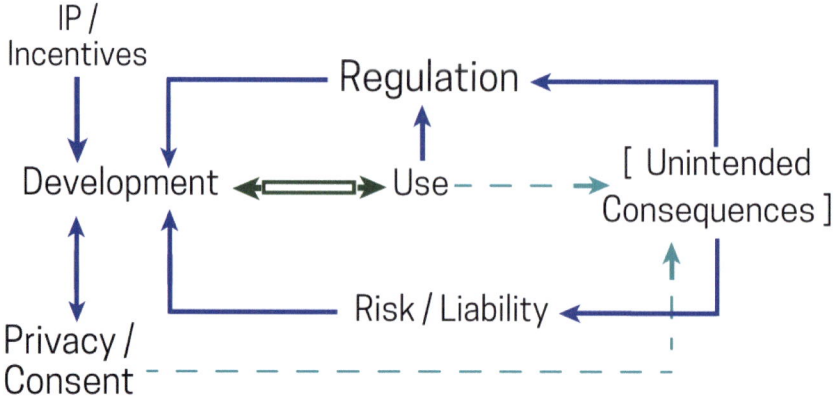

FIGURE S-2 | Appropriately regulating artificial intelligence technologies will require balancing a number of important variables, including intellectual property (IP), concerns around privacy and consent, risks and liability associated with the use of the technologies, and developmental processes.

safety based on real-world data. Throughout that process, transparency can help deliver better-vetted solutions. To enable both AI development and oversight, government agencies should invest in infrastructure that promotes wider, ethical data collection and access to data resources for building AI solutions within a priority of ethical use and data protection (see Figure S-2).

CONCLUSION

AI is poised to make transformative and disruptive advances in health care. It is prudent to balance the need for thoughtful, inclusive health care AI that plans for and actively manages and reduces potential unintended consequences, while not yielding to marketing hype and profit motives. The wisest guidance for AI is to start with real problems in health care, explore the best solutions by engaging relevant stakeholders, frontline users, and patients and their families— including AI and non-AI options—and implement and scale the ones that meet our Quintuple Aim: better health, improved care experience, clinician well-being, lower cost, and health equity throughout the health care system and all forms of health care delivery.

1

ARTIFICIAL INTELLIGENCE IN HEALTH CARE: THE HOPE, THE HYPE, THE PROMISE, THE PERIL

Michael Matheny, Vanderbilt University Medical Center and U.S. Department of Veterans Affairs; Sonoo Thadaney Israni, Stanford University; Danielle Whicher, National Academy of Medicine; and Mahnoor Ahmed, National Academy of Medicine

INTRODUCTION

Health care in the United States, historically focused on encounter-based care and treating illness as it arises rather than preventing it, is now undergoing a sweeping transformation toward a more population health–based approach. This transformation is happening via a series of changes in reimbursement. Among these changes are multiple eras of managed care and capitated population management explorations and increases in reimbursement for value-based care and prevention, both of which attempt to manage the overall health of the patient beyond treatment of illness (ASTHO, 2019; CMS, 2019; Kissam et al., 2019; Mendelson et al., 2017). Even so, U.S. health care expenditures continue to rise without corresponding gains in key health outcomes when compared to many similar countries (see Figure 1-1).

To assess where and how artificial intelligence (AI) may provide opportunities for improvement, it is important to understand the current context of and drivers for change in health care. AI is likely to promote automation and provide context-relevant information synthesis and recommendations (through a variety of tools and in many settings) to patients, "fRamilies" (friends and family unpaid caregivers), and the clinical team. AI developers and stakeholders should prioritize ethical data collection and use, and support data and information visualization through the use of AI (Israni and Verghese, 2019).

Technology innovations and funding are driven by business criteria such as profit, efficiency, and return on investment. It is important to explore how

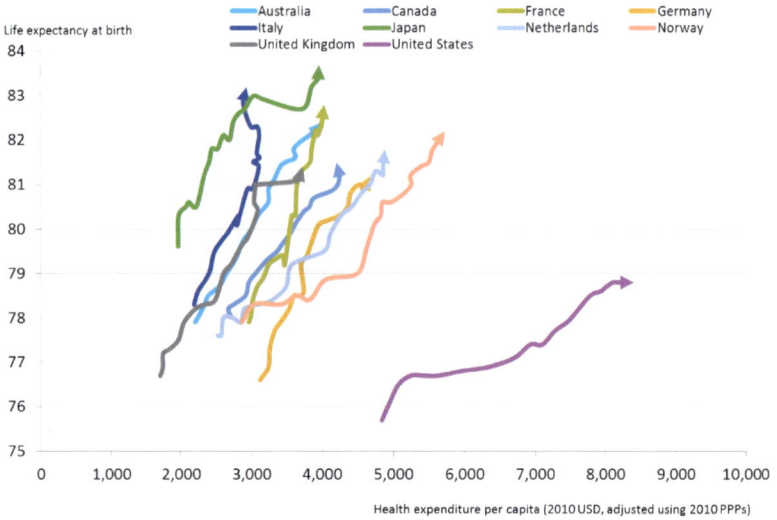

FIGURE 1-1 | Life expectancy gains and increased health spending, selected high-income countries, 1995–2015.
SOURCE: Figure redrawn from OECD, 2017, *Health at a Glance 2017: OECD Indicators*, OECD Publishing, Paris, https://doi.org/10.1787/health_glance-2017-en.

these criteria will influence AI–health care development, evaluation, and implementation. This reality is further challenged by U.S. public and government views of health and health care, which oscillate between health care as social good and health care as economic commodity (Aggarwal et al., 2010; Feldstein, 2012; Rosenthal, 2017). These considerations are likely to drive some clear use cases in health care business operations: AI tools can be used to reduce cost and gain efficiencies through prioritizing human labor focus on more complex tasks; to identify workflow optimization strategies; to reduce medical waste (failure of care delivery, failure of care coordination, overtreatment or low-value care, pricing failure, fraud and abuse, and administrative complexity); and to automate highly repetitive business and workflow processes (Becker's Healthcare, 2018) by using reliably captured and structured data (Bauchner and Fontanarosa, 2019). When implementing these tools, it is critical to be thoughtful, equitable, and inclusive to avoid adverse events and unintended consequences. This requires ensuring that AI tools align with the preferences of users and with end targets of these technologies, and that the tools do not further exacerbate historical inequities in access and outcomes (Baras and Baker, 2019).

Driven by a shift to reimbursement and incentives that support a population health management approach rather than a fee-for-service approach, innovation in AI technologies are likely to improve patient outcomes via applications, workflows, interventions, and support for distributed health care delivery outside a traditional brick and mortar, encounter-based paradigm. The challenges of data accuracy and privacy protection will depend on whether AI technologies are regulated as a medical device or classed as an entertainment application. These consumer-facing tools are likely to support fundamental changes in interactions between health care professionals and patients and their caregivers. Tools such as single-lead electrocardiogram (ECG) surveillance or continuous blood glucose monitors will transform how health data are generated and utilized. They offer the opportunity to incorporate social determinants of health (SDoH) to identify patient populations for target interventions to improve outcomes and reduce health care utilization (Lee and Korba, 2017). Because SDoH interventions are labor-intensive, their scalability is poor. AI may reduce the cost of utilizing SDoH data and provide efficient means of prioritizing scarce clinical resources to impact SDoH (Basu and Narayanaswamy, 2019; Seligman et al., 2017).

All this presumes building solutions for health care challenges that will truly benefit from technological solutions, versus *technochauvinism*—a belief that technology is always the best solution (Broussard, 2018).

These topics are explored through subsequent chapters. This first chapter sets the stage by providing an overview of the development process and structure of this publication; defining key terms and concepts discussed throughout the remaining chapters; and describing several overarching considerations related to AI systems' reliance on data and issues related to trust, equity, and inclusion, which are critical to advancing appropriate use of AI tools in health care settings.

NATIONAL ACADEMY OF MEDICINE

Given the current national focus on AI and its potential utility for improving health and health care in the United States, the National Academy of Medicine (NAM) Leadership Consortium: Collaboration for a Value & Science-Driven Learning Health System (Leadership Consortium)—through its Digital Health Learning Collaborative (DHLC)—brought together experts to explore opportunities, issues, and concerns related to the expanded application of AI in health and health care settings (NAM, 2019a,b).

NAM LEADERSHIP CONSORTIUM: COLLABORATION FOR A VALUE & SCIENCE-DRIVEN LEARNING HEALTH SYSTEM

Broadly, the NAM Leadership Consortium convenes national experts and executive-level leaders from key stakeholder sectors for collaborative activities to foster progress toward a continuously learning health system in which science, informatics, incentives, and culture are aligned for enduring improvement and innovation; best practices are seamlessly embedded in the care process; patients and families are active participants in all elements; and new knowledge is captured as an integral by-product of the care experience. Priorities for achieving this vision include advancing the development of a fully interoperable digital infrastructure, the application of new clinical research approaches, and a culture of transparency on outcomes and cost.

The NAM Leadership Consortium serves as a forum for facilitating collaborative assessment and action around issues central to achieving the vision of a continuously learning health system. To address the challenges of improving both evidence development and evidence application, as well as improving the capacity to advance progress on each of those dimensions, Leadership Consortium members (all leaders in their fields) work with their colleagues to identify the issues not being adequately addressed, the nature of the barriers and possible solutions, and the priorities for action. They then work to marshal the resources of the sectors represented in the Leadership Consortium to work for sustained public–private cooperation for change.

DIGITAL HEALTH LEARNING COLLABORATIVE

The work of the NAM Leadership Consortium falls into four strategic action domains—informatics, evidence, financing, and culture—and each domain has a dedicated innovation collaborative that works to facilitate progress in that area. This Special Publication was developed under the auspices of the DHLC. Co-chaired by Jonathan Perlin from the Hospital Corporation of America and Reed Tuckson from Tuckson Health Connections, the DHLC provides a venue for joint activities that can accelerate progress in the area of health informatics and toward the digital infrastructure necessary for continuous improvement and innovation in health and health care.

PUBLICATION GENESIS

In 2017, the DHLC identified issues around the development, deployment, and use of AI as being of central importance to facilitating continuous improvement and innovation in health and health care. To consider the nature, elements, applications, state of play, key challenges, and implications of AI in health and health care, as well as ways in which the NAM might enhance collaborative progress, the DHLC convened a meeting at the National Academy of Sciences (NAS) building in Washington, DC, on November 30, 2017. Participants included AI experts from across the United States representing different stakeholder groups within the health care ecosystem, including health system representatives; academics; practicing clinicians; representatives from technology companies; electronic health record (EHR) vendors; nonprofit organizations; payer representatives; and representatives from U.S. federal organizations, including the National Institutes of Health, the National Science Foundation, the U.S. Department of Defense, the U.S. Department of Veterans Affairs (VA), and the U.S. Food and Drug Administration. The agenda and participant list for this workshop are included as Appendix B.

Participants generated a list of practical challenges to the advancement and application of AI to improve health and health care (see Table 1-1). To begin to address these challenges, meeting participants recommended that the DHLC establish a working group on AI in health and health care. Formed in February 2018, the working group is co-chaired by Michael Matheny of the Vanderbilt University Medical Center and the VA and Sonoo Thadaney Israni of Stanford University. The group's charge was to accelerate the appropriate development, adoption, and use of valid, reliable, and sustainable AI models for transforming progress in health and health care. To advance this charge, members determined

TABLE 1-1 | Practical Challenges to the Advancement and Application of Artificial Intelligence Tools in Clinical Settings Identified During the November 30, 2017, Digital Health Learning Collaborative Meeting

Challenge	Description
Workflow integration	Understand the technical, cognitive, social, and political factors in play and incentives impacting integration of artificial intelligence (AI) into health care workflows.
Enhanced explainability and interpretability	To promote integration of AI into health care workflows, consider what needs to be explained and approaches for ensuring understanding by all members of the health care team.
Workforce education	Promote educational programs to inform clinicians about AI/machine learning approaches and to develop an adequate workforce.
Oversight and regulation	Consider the appropriate regulatory mechanism for AI/machine learning and approaches for evaluating algorithms and their impact.
Problem identification and prioritization	Catalog the different areas of health care and public health where AI/machine learning could make a difference, focusing on intervention-driven AI.
Clinician and patient engagement	Understand the appropriate approaches for involving consumers and clinicians in AI/machine learning prioritization, development, and integration, and the potential impact of AI/machine learning algorithms on the patient–provider relationship.
Data quality and access	Promote data quality, access, and sharing, as well as the use of both structured and unstructured data and the integration of non-clinical data as critical to developing effective AI tools.

that they would work collaboratively to develop a reference document for model developers, clinical implementers, clinical users, and regulators and policy makers to:

- understand the strengths and limitations of AI;
- promote the use of these methods and technologies within the health care system; and
- highlight areas of future work needed in research, implementation science, and regulatory bodies to facilitate broad use of AI to improve health and health care.

PUBLICATION WORKFLOW

Authors were organized from among the meeting participants along expertise and interest, and each chapter was drafted with guidance from the NAM and the editors, with monthly publication meetings where all authors were invited to participate and update the group. Author biographies can be found in Appendix C.

As an initial step, the authors, the NAM staff, and co-chairs developed the scope and content focus of each of the chapters based on discussion at the initial in-person meeting. Subsequently, the authors for each chapter drafted chapter outlines from this guideline. Outlines were shared with the other authors, the NAM staff, and the working group co-chairs to ensure consistency in the level of detail and formatting. Differences and potential overlap were discussed before the authors proceeded with drafting of each chapter. The working group co-chairs and the NAM staff drafted content for Chapters 1 and 8, and were responsible for managing the monthly meetings and editing the content of all chapters.

After all chapters were drafted, the resulting publication was discussed at a meeting that brought together working group members and external experts at the NAS building in Washington, DC, on January 16, 2019. The goal of the meeting was to receive feedback on the draft publication to improve its utility to the field. Following the meeting, the chapter authors refined and added content to address suggestions from meeting participants. To improve consistency in voice and style across authors, an external editor was hired to review and edit the publication in its entirety before the document was sent out for external review. Finally, 10 external expert reviewers agreed to review the publication and provide critiques and recommendations for further improvement of the content. Working group co-chairs and the NAM staff reviewed all feedback and added recommendations and edits, which were sent to chapter authors for consideration for incorporation. Final edits following chapter author re-submissions were resolved by the co-chairs and the NAM staff. The resulting publication represents the ideas shared at both meetings and the efforts of the working group.

IMPORTANT DEFINITIONS

Throughout the publication, authors use foundational terms and concepts related to AI and its subcomponents. To establish a common understanding, this section describes key definitions for some of these terms and concepts.

U.S. Health Care

This publication relies on preexisting knowledge and a general understanding of the U.S. health care domain. Due to limited space here, a table of key reference materials is included in Appendix A to provide the relevant health care context. This list is a convenient sample of well-regarded reference materials and selected publications written for a general audience. This list is not comprehensive.

Artificial Intelligence

The term "artificial intelligence" (AI) has a range of meanings, from specific forms of AI, such as machine learning, to the hypothetical AI that meets criteria for consciousness and sentience. This publication does not address the hypothetical, as the popular press often does, and focuses instead on the current and near-future uses and applications of AI.

A formal definition of AI starts with the Oxford English Dictionary: "The capacity of computers or other machines to exhibit or simulate intelligent behavior; the field of study concerned with this," or Merriam-Webster online: "1: a branch of computer science dealing with the simulation of intelligent behavior in computers, 2: the capability of a machine to imitate intelligent human behavior." More nuanced definitions of AI might also consider what type of goal the AI is attempting to achieve and how it is pursuing that goal. In general, AI systems range from those that attempt to accurately model human reasoning to solve a problem, to those that ignore human reasoning and exclusively use large volumes of data to generate a framework to answer the question(s) of interest, to those that attempt to incorporate elements of human reasoning but do not require accurate modeling of human processes. Figure 1-2 includes a hierarchical representation of AI technologies (Mills, 2015).

Machine learning is a family of statistical and mathematical modeling techniques that uses a variety of approaches to automatically learn and improve the prediction of a target state, without explicit programming (e.g., Boolean rules)

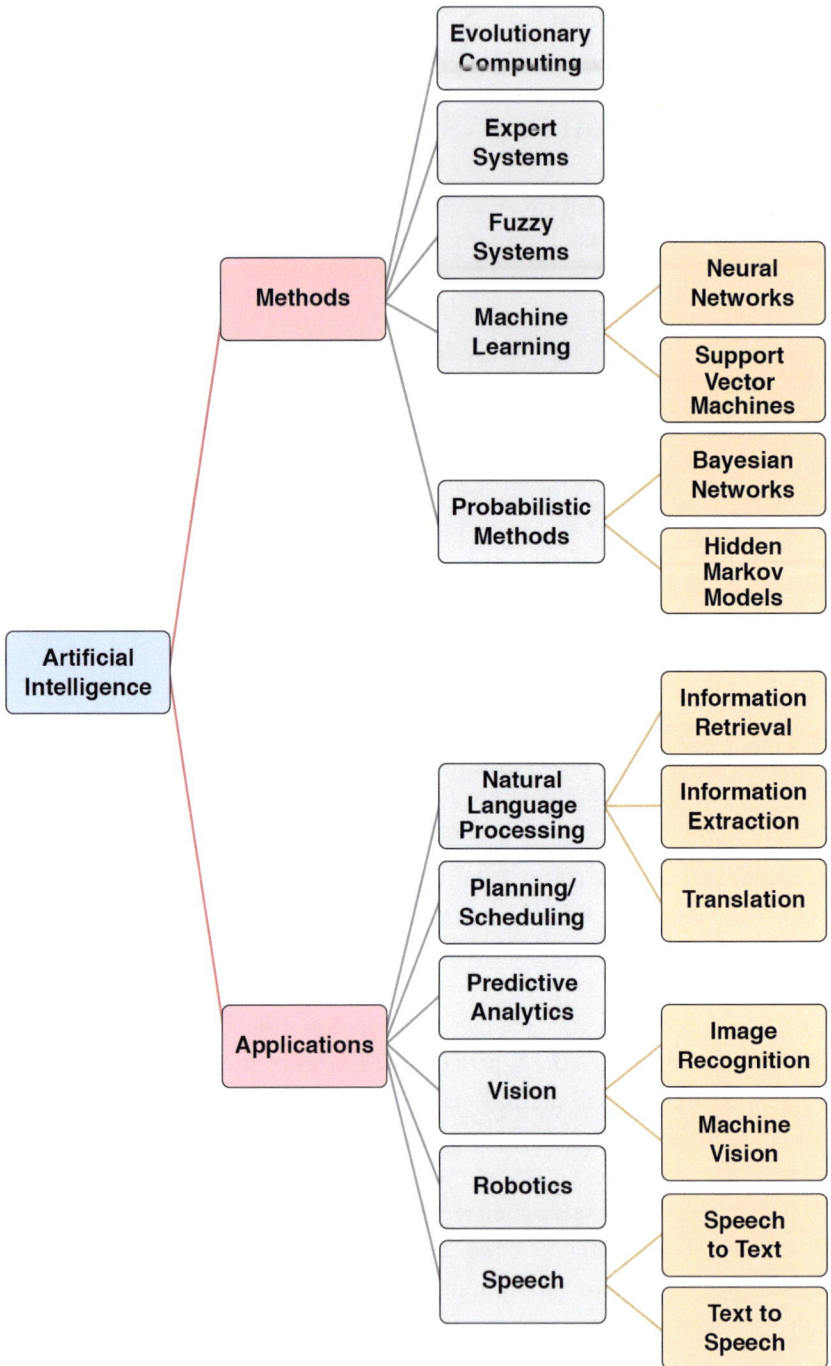

FIGURE 1-2 | A summary of the domains of artificial intelligence.
SOURCE: Adapted with permission from a figure in Mills, M. 2015. Artificial Intelligence in Law—The State of Play in 2015? *Legal IT Insider.* https://www.legaltechnology.com/latest-news/artificial-intelligence-in-law-the-state-of-play-in-2015.

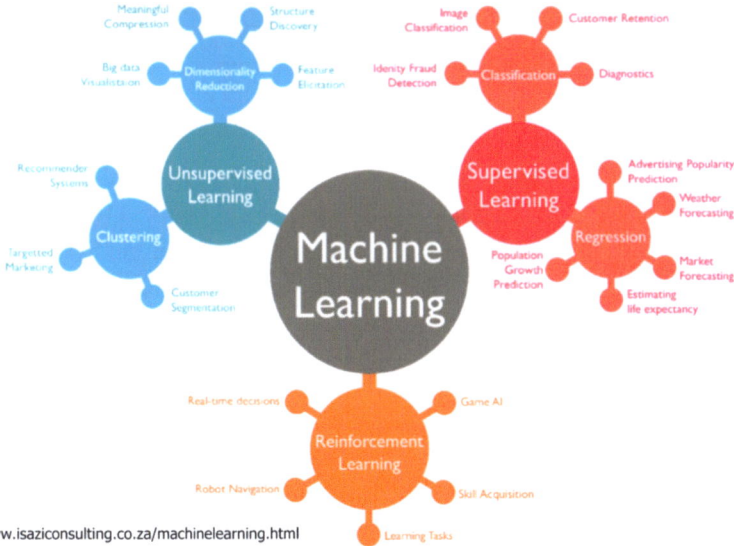

Machine Learning Breakdown

Meaningful Compression
Structure Discovery
Big data Visualization
Dimensionality Reduction
Feature Elicitation
Recommender Systems
Unsupervised Learning
Clustering
Targetted Marketing
Customer Segmentation

Image Classification
Customer Retention
Identity Fraud Detection
Classification
Diagnostics
Supervised Learning
Advertising Popularity Prediction
Weather Forecasting
Regression
Population Growth Prediction
Market Forecasting
Estimating life expectancy

Machine Learning

Real-time decisions
Game AI
Reinforcement Learning
Robot Navigation
Skill Acquisition
Learning Tasks

http://www.isaziconsulting.co.za/machinelearning.html

FIGURE 1-3 | A summary of the most common methods and applications for training machine learning algorithms.
SOURCE: Reprinted with permission from Isazi Consulting, 2015. http://www.isaziconsulting.co.za/machine learning.html.

(Witten et al., 2016). Different methods, such as Bayesian networks, random forests, deep learning, and artificial neural networks use different assumptions and mathematical frameworks for how data are ingested, and learning occurs within the algorithm. Regression analyses, such as linear and logistic regression, are also considered machine learning methods, although many users of these algorithms distinguish them from commonly defined machine learning methods (e.g., random forests, Bayesian networks). The term "machine learning" is widely used by large businesses, but "AI" is more frequently used for marketing purposes. In most cases, "machine learning" is more appropriate. One way to represent machine learning algorithms is to subcategorize them by how they learn inference from the data (as shown in Figure 1-3). The subcategories are *unsupervised learning, supervised learning,* and *reinforcement learning.* These frameworks are discussed in greater detail in Chapter 5.

Natural language processing (NLP) enables computers to understand and organize human languages (Manning and Schütze, 1999). NLP needs to model human reasoning because it considers the meaning behind written and spoken language in a computable, interpretable, and accurate way. NLP has a higher bar than other AI domains because context, interpretation, and nuance add needed information. NLP incorporates rule-based and data-based learning systems, and many of the internal components of NLP systems are themselves machine learning algorithms with pre defined inputs and outputs, sometimes operating under additional constraints. Examples of NLP applications include assessment of cancer disease progression and response to therapy among radiology reports (Kehl et al., 2019), and identification of post-operative complication from routine EHR documentation (Murff et al., 2011).

Speech algorithms digitize audio recordings into computable data elements and convert text into human speech (Chung et al., 2018). This field is closely connected with NLP, with the added complexity of intonation and syllable emphasis impacting meaning. This complicates both inbound and outbound speech interpretation and generation. For examples of how deep learning neural networks have been applied to this field, see a recent systematic review of this topic (Nassif, 2019).

Expert systems are a set of computer algorithms that seek to emulate the decision-making capacity of human experts (Feigenbaum, 1992; Jackson, 1998; Leondes, 2002; Shortliffe and Buchanan, 1975). These systems rely largely on a complex set of Boolean and deterministic rules. An expert system is divided into a knowledge base, which encodes the domain logic, and an inference engine, which applies the knowledge base to data presented to the system to provide recommendations or deduce new facts. Examples of this are some of the clinical decision support tools (Hoffman et al., 2016) being developed within the Clinical Pharmacogenetics Implementation Consortium, which is promoting the use of knowledge bases such as PharmGKB to provide personalized recommendations for medication use in patients based on genetic data results (CPIC, 2019; PharmGKB, 2019).

Automated planning and scheduling systems produce optimized strategies for action sequences (such as clinic scheduling), which are typically executed by intelligent agents in a virtual environment or physical robots designed to automate a task (Ghallab et al., 2004). These systems are defined by complex parameter spaces that require high dimensional calculations.

Computer vision focuses on how algorithms interpret, synthesize, and generate inference from digital images or videos. It seeks to automate or provide human cognitive support for tasks anchored in the human visual system (Sonka et al., 2008). This field leverages multiple disciplines, including geometry, physics, statistics, and learning theory (Forsyth and Ponce, 2003). One example is deploying a computer vision tool in the intensive care unit to monitor patient mobility (Yeung et al., 2019), because patient mobility is key for patient recovery from severe illness and can drive downstream interventions.

AI and Human Intelligence

Combining human intelligence and AI into augmented intelligence focuses on a supportive or assistive role for the algorithms, emphasizing that these technologies are designed to enhance human processing, cognition, and work, rather than replace it. William Ross Ashby originally popularized the term "amplifying intelligence," which transformed into "augmented intelligence" (Ashby, 1964). These terms are gaining popularity because "artificial intelligence" has been burdened with meaning by marketing hype, popular culture, and science fiction—possibly impeding a reasoned and balanced discourse.

AI SYSTEMS RELIANCE ON DATA

Data are critical for delivering evidence-based health care and developing any AI algorithm. Without data, the underlying characteristics of the process and outcomes are unknown. This has been a gap in health care for many years, but key trends (such as commodity wearable technologies) in this domain in the past decade have transformed health care into a heterogeneous data-rich environment (Schulte and Fry, 2019). It is now common in health and health care for massive amounts of data to be generated about an individual from a variety of sources, such as claims data, genetic information, radiology images, intensive care unit surveillance, EHR care documentation, and medical device sensing and surveillance. The reasons for these trends include the scaling of computational capacity through decreases in cost of technology; widespread adoption of EHRs promoted by the Health Information Technology for Economic and Clinical Health (HITECH) Act; precipitous decreases in cost of genetic sample processing (Wetterstrand, 2019); and increasing integration of medical- and consumer-grade sensors. U.S. consumers used approximately 3 petabytes of Internet data every minute of the day in 2018, generating possible health-connected data with each use (DOMO, 2019). There are more than 300,000 health applications in app stores, with more than 200 being added each day and an overall doubling of these applications since 2015 (Aitken et al., 2017).

Data Aggregation

The accumulation of medical and consumer data has resulted in patients, caregivers, and health care professionals being responsible for aggregating, synthesizing, and interpreting data far beyond human cognitive and decision-making capacities. Figure 1-4 predicts the exponential data accumulation and the limits of human cognition for health care decision making (IOM, 2008).

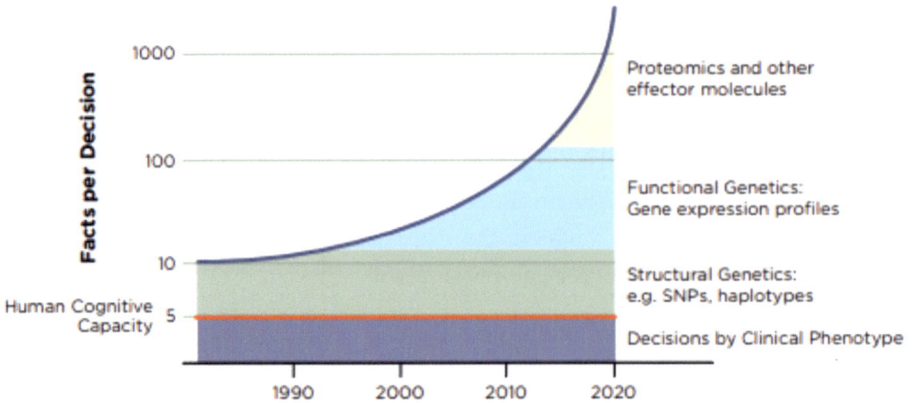

FIGURE 1-4 | Growth in facts affecting provider decisions versus human cognitive capacity.
SOURCES: NRC, 2009; presentation by William Stead at IOM meeting on October 8, 2007, titled "Growth in Facts Affecting Provider Decisions Versus Human Cognitive Capacity."

The growth in data generation and need for data synthesis exceeding human capacity has surpassed prior estimates. This trend most likely underestimates the magnitude of the current data milieu.

AI algorithms require large volumes of training data to achieve performance levels sufficient for "success" (Shrott, 2017; Sun et al., 2017), and there are multiple frameworks and standards in place to promote data aggregation for AI use. These include standardized data representations that both manage data at rest[1] and data in motion.[2] For data at rest, mature common data models (CDMs),[3] such as Observational Medical Outcomes Partnership (OMOP), Informatics for Integrating Biology & the Bedside (i2b2), the Patient-Centered Clinical Research Network (PCORNet), and Sentinel, are increasingly providing a backbone to format, clean, harmonize, and standardize data that can then be used for the training of AI algorithms (Rosenbloom et al., 2017). Some of these CDMs (e.g., OMOP) are also international in focus, which may support compatibility and portability of some AI algorithms across countries. Some health care systems have invested in the infrastructure for developing and maintaining at least one CDM

---

[1] Data at rest: Data stored in a persistent structure, such as a database or in a file system, and not in active use.

[2] Data in motion: Data that are being transported from one computer system to another or between applications in the same computer.

[3] A common data model is a standardized, modular, extensible collection of data schemas that is designed to make it easier to build, use, and analyze data. Data are transformed into the data model from many sources, which allows experts to make informed decisions about data representation, which allows users to easily reuse the data.

through funded initiatives (OHDSI, 2019; Ohno-Machado et al., 2014). Many others have adopted one of these CDMs as a cornerstone of their clinical data warehouse infrastructure to help support operations, quality improvement, and research. This improves the quality and volume of data that are computable and usable for AI in the United States, and promotes transparency and reproducibility (Hripcsak et al., 2015). It is also important for semantic meaning to be mapped to a structured representation, such as Logical Observation Identifiers Names and Codes and *International Classification of Diseases, 10th Revision, Clinical Modification* (ICD-10-CM), as these CDMs leverage these standardized representations.

For data in motion, in order to manage the critical interdigitation with consumers, EHRs, and population health management tools, HL7 FHIR is emerging as an open standard for helping data and AI algorithm outputs flow between applications and to the end user, with many of the large EHR vendors providing support for this standard (Khalilia et al., 2015). Another technology being explored extensively in health care is the use of blockchain to store, transport, and secure patient records (Agbo et al., 2019). Made popular by the bitcoin implementation of this technology, blockchain has a number of benefits, including (1) being immutable and traceable, which allows patients to send records without fear of tampering; (2) securing all records by cryptography; (3) allowing new medical records to be added within the encryption process; and (4) making it possible for patients to get stronger controls over access.

However, there are still many instances where the standardization, interoperability, and scale of data aggregation and transfers are not achieved in practice. Health information exchanges (HIEs), with appropriate permissions, are one method by which data may be aggregated and used for AI algorithm training and validation. Public health agencies and EHRs extensively support data exchange protocols that provide the technical capacity for electronic data sharing. However, because of a variety of barriers, health care professionals and patients are frequently unable to electronically request patient records from an outside facility after care is delivered (Lye et al., 2018; Ross, 2018). Most of today's health data silos and assets reside in individual organizations, and current incentives leave little motivation for much needed collaboration and sharing. A recent review of the legal barriers to the operation and use of HIEs found that legislation in the past 10 years has lowered barriers to use, and points to economic incentives as the most significant current challenge (Mello et al., 2018).

Data access across health care systems, particularly data on staffing, costs and charges, and reimbursements, is critical for private health insurers and the U.S. health care delivery market. But, given the sensitive nature of this information, it is not shared easily or at all. Many institutions, particularly the larger integrated health care delivery networks, are developing internal AI and analytics to help support business decisions; however, in order to effectively influence U.S. health care expenditures, AI algorithms need access to larger and more population-representative data, which is possible through improved data sharing, transparency, and standardization (Green, 2019; Schulte, 2017). The U.S. government has been driving this movement toward access through ongoing efforts to prevent data blocking, and through implementation of a key provision in the 21st Century Cures Act that aims to promote price transparency (ONC, 2019). While further transparency may provide AI with additional opportunities, the U.S. health care system still has a long way to go in addressing the myriad issues preventing widespread data sharing and standardization. This disadvantages U.S. research and innovation when compared to that of other countries.

A key challenge for data integration is the lack of definitive laws and regulations for the secondary use of routinely collected patient health care data. Many of the laws and regulations around data ownership and sharing are country-specific and based on evolving cultural expectations and norms. In 2018, a number of countries promoted personal information protection guidance, moving from laws to specifications. The European Union has rigorous personal privacy prioritizing regulatory infrastructure, detailed in the General Data Protection Regulation that went into effect on May 25, 2019 (European Commission, 2018). In the People's Republic of China (Shi et al., 2019), a non-binding but comprehensive set of guidelines was released in the Personal Information Security Specification. Great Britain's National Health System allows national-level data aggregation for care delivery and research. However, even in more monolithic data environments, reuse of these data for AI is justifiably scrutinized. For instance, in 2018, the British House of Lords report on AI criticized the sharing of identifiable patient data with a profit-motivated Silicon Valley company (House of Lords Select Committee on Artificial Intelligence, 2018, Chapter 2).

Variation in laws and regulations is in part a result of differing and evolving perceptions of appropriate approaches or frameworks for health data ownership, stewardship, and control. There is also a lack of agreement on who should be able to profit from data-sharing activities. In the United States today, health care data that are fully de-identified may be reused for other purposes without explicit consent. However, there is disagreement over what constitutes sufficiently de-identified data, as exemplified by a 2019 lawsuit against a Google–University of Chicago partnership to develop AI tools to predict medical diseases (Wakabayashi, 2019). Patients may not realize that their data could be monetized via AI tools for the financial benefit of various organizations, including the organization that collected the data and the AI developers. If these issues are not sufficiently addressed, we run the risk of an ethical conundrum, where patient-provided data assets are used for monetary gain, without explicit consent or compensation.

This could be similar to Henrietta Lacks's biological tissue story where no consent was obtained to culture her cells (as was the practice in 1951), nor was she or the Lacks family compensated for their monetization (Skloot, 2011). There is a need to address and clarify current regulations, legislation, and patient expectations when patient data are used for building profit-motivated products or for research (refer to Chapter 7).

The lack of national unique patient identifiers in the United States could greatly reduce the error rates of de-duplication during data aggregation. However, there are several probabilistic patient linkage tools that are currently attempting to fill this gap (Kho et al., 2015; Ong et al., 2014, 2017). While there is evidence that AI algorithms can overcome noise from erroneous linkage and duplication of patient records through use of large volumes of data, the extent to which these problems may impact algorithm accuracy and bias remains an open question.

Cloud computing that places physical computational resources in widespread locations, sometimes across international boundaries, is another particularly challenging issue. Cloud computing can result in disastrous cybersecurity breaches as data managers attempt to maintain compliance with many local and national laws, regulations, and legal frameworks (Kommerskollegium, 2012).

Finally, to make AI truly revolutionary, it is critical to consider the power of linking clinical and claims data with data beyond the narrow, traditional care setting by capturing the social determinants of health as well as other patient-generated data. This could include utilizing social media datasets to inform the medical team of the social determinants that operate in each community. It could also include developing publicly available datasets of health-related factors such as neighborhood walkability, food deserts, air quality, aquatic environments, environmental monitoring, and ncw areas not yet explored.

Data Bias

In addition to the issues associated with data aggregation, selecting an appropriate AI training data source is critical because training data influences the output observations, interpretations, and recommendations. If the training data are systematically biased due to, for example, under-representation of individuals of a particular gender, race, age, or sexual orientation, those biases will be modeled, propagated, and scaled in the resulting algorithm. The same is true for human biases (intentional and not) operating in the environment, workflow, and outcomes from which the data were collected. Similarly, social science research subject samples are disproportionately U.S. university undergraduates who are Western, educated, industrialized, rich, and democratic (WEIRD), and this data bias is carried through the behavioral sciences used as the basis for developing algorithms that explain or predict human behaviors (Downey, 2010; Sullivan, 2010).

Bias can also be present in genetic data, where the majority of sequenced DNA comes from people of European descent (Bustamante et al., 2011; Popejoy and Fullerton, 2016; Stanford Engineering, 2019). Training AI from data resources with these biases runs the risk of inaccurately generalizing it to non-representative populations. An apt and provocative term used to describe this training is "weapons of math destruction" (O'Neil, 2017). In her book of the same title, Cathy O'Neil outlines the destruction that biased AI has caused in criminal justice sentencing, human resources and hiring, education, and other systems. If issues of potential biases in training data are not addressed, they further propagate and scale historical inequities and discrimination.

PROMOTING TRUST, EQUITY, AND INCLUSION IN HEALTH CARE AI

Trust, equity, and inclusion need to be prioritized in the health care AI development and deployment processes (Vayena et al., 2018). Throughout this publication, various chapters address topics related to the ethical, equitable, and transparent deployment of AI. In addition, a growing number of codes of ethics, frameworks, and guidelines describe many of the relevant ethical issues (see Table 1-2 for a representative, although not comprehensive, list).

Judy Estrin proposes implementing AI through the lens of human rights values and outlines the anticipated friction, offering thought-provoking questions through which to navigate dilemmas (see Figure 1-5).

Building on the above, we briefly describe several key considerations to ensure the ethical, equitable, and inclusive development and deployment of health care AI.

Diversity in AI Teams

To promote the development of impactful and equitable AI tools, it is important to ensure diversity—of gender, culture, race, age, ability, ethnicity, sexual orientation, socioeconomic status, privilege, etc.—among AI developers. An April 2019 AI Institute Report documents the lack of diversity in the field, describing this as "a moment of reckoning." The report further notes that the "diversity disaster" has led to "flawed systems that exacerbate . . . gender and racial biases" (West et al., 2019). Consider the fact that the "Apple HealthKit, which enabled specialized tracking, such as selenium and copper intake, . . . neglected to include a women's menstrual cycle tracker until iOS 9" (Reiley, 2016). The development team reportedly did not include any women.

TABLE 1-2 | Relevant Ethical Codes, Frameworks, and Guidelines

Guiding Codes and Frameworks	Reference
ACM Code of Ethics and Professional Conduct	Gotterbarn, D. W., B. Brinkman, C. Flick, M. S. Kirkpatrick, K. Miller, K. Vazansky, and M. J. Wolf. 2018. ACM code of ethics and professional conduct. https://www.acm.org/binaries/content/assets/about/acm-code-of-ethics-and-professional-conduct.pdf.
Artificial Intelligence at Google: Our Principles	Google. 2018. Artificial intelligence at Google: Our principles. Google AI. https://ai.google/principles.
Ethical OS: Risk Mitigation Checklist	Institute for the Future and Omidyar Network. 2018. Ethical OS: Risk Mitigation Checklist. https://ethicalos.org/wp-content/uploads/2018/08/EthicalOS_Check-List_080618.pdf.
DeepMind Ethics & Society Team	DeepMind. 2020. DeepMind Ethics & Society Team. https://deepmind.com/about/ethics-and-society.
Partnership on AI Tenets	Partnership on AI. 2018. Partnership on AI tenets. https://www.partnershiponai.org/tenets.
AI Now Report 2018	Whittaker, M., K. Crawford, R. Dobbe, G. Fried, E. Kaziunas, V. Mathur, S. M. West, R. Richardson, J. Schultz, and O. Schwartz. 2018. AI Now Report 2018. AI Now Institute at New York University. https://stanford.app.box.com/s/xmb2cj3e7gsz5vmus0viadt9p3kreekk.
The Trouble with Algorithmic Decisions	Zarsky, T. 2016. The trouble with algorithmic decisions: An analytic road map to examine efficiency and fairness in automated and opaque decision making. Science, Technology, & Human Values 41(1):18–132.
Executive Office of the President	Munoz, C., M. Smith, and D. J. Patil. 2016. Big data: A report on algorithmic systems, opportunity, and civil rights. Executive Office of the President. https://obamawhitehouse.archives.gov/sites/default/files/microsites/ostp/2016_0504_data_discrimination.pdf.
Addressing Ethical Challenges in Machine Learning	Vayena, E., A. Blasimme, and I. G. Cohen. 2018. Machine learning in medicine: Addressing ethical challenges. PLoS Medicine 15(11):e1002689. Figure 1.3.
Do No Harm: A Roadmap for Responsible Machine Learning in Health Care	Wiens, J., S. Saria, M. Sendak, M. Ghassemi, V. X. Liu, F. Doshi-Velez, K. Jung, K. Heller, D. Kale, M. Saeed, P. N. Ossorio, S. Thadaney-Israni, and A. Goldenberg. 2019. Do no harm: A roadmap for responsible machine learning for health care. Nature Medicine 25(9):1337–1340.

In addition, it is imperative that AI development and validation teams include end-user representatives who are likely to be most familiar with the issues associated with frontline implementation and who are knowledgeable about potential biases that may be incorporated into the data.

When developing, validating, and implementing AI tools that aim to promote behavior change to address chronic conditions such as obesity, heart disease, and diabetes, it is critical to engage behavioral scientists to ensure the tools account for behavioral theory and principles to promote change (see Chapter 6 for additional information on AI implementation). AI products that rely too heavily on reminders

Implementing AI through the lens of Human Rights Values requires some 'friction'
Source: Judy Estrin, Technology Pioneer, Entrepreneur, and CEO, JLABS, LLC

What do we value?

How are we each responsible?

We can, but should we?

What does Human Centered mean? To humans, for humans, by humans?

How do we define progress, quality of life, well-being?

"Who knows, who decides, who decides who decides?"
- Shoshana Zuboff, The Age of Surveillance Capitalism

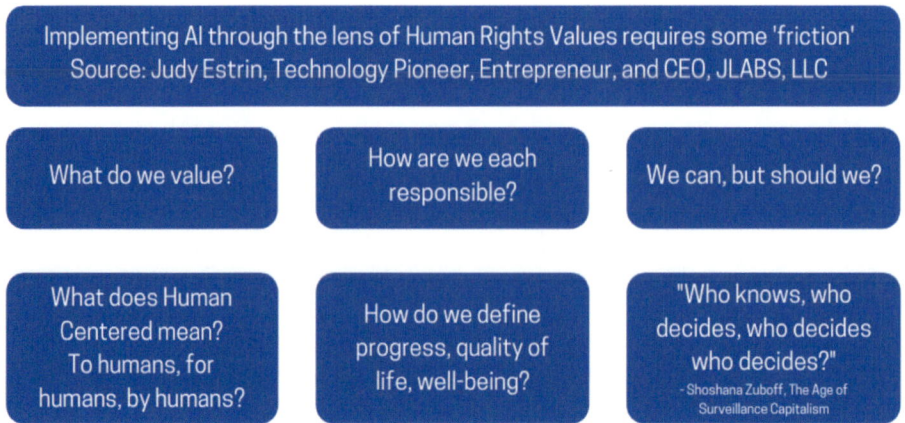

FIGURE 1-5 | Framework for implementing artificial intelligence through the lens of human rights values.
SOURCE: Reprinted with permission from Judy Estrin. Based on a slide Estrin shared at The Future of Human-Centered AI: Governance Innovation and Protection of Human Rights Conference, Stanford University, April 16, 2019.

(e.g., "Remember to exercise 30 minutes today!") and positive reinforcement through social approval (e.g., "Good job!" or "You did it!") to effect change are unlikely to be successful. Decades of research show that behavioral change requires knowledge of the impact of health behaviors as well as a willingness to forgo short-term, concrete reinforcements (e.g., calorie-dense foods) in order to achieve longer-term, more abstract goals (e.g., "healthy weight"). This rich area of research stretches from early conceptual paradigms (Abraham and Sheeran, 2007; Prochaska and Velicer, 1997; Rosenstock, 1974) to more recent literature that have applied behavioral principles in developing digital tools to prevent and manage chronic illnesses in the short and long term (Sepah et al., 2017). The recent melding of behavioral science with digital tools is especially exciting, resulting in companies such as Omada Health, Vida Health, and Livingo, who are deploying digital tools to enhance physical and mental health.

AI-powered platforms make it easier to fractionalize and link users and providers, creating a new "uberization"[4] in health care and a gig economy (Parikh, 2017) in which on-demand workers and contractors take on the risk of erratic employment and the financial risk of health insurance costs. This includes Uber and Lyft drivers, Task Rabbit temporary workers, nurses, physician assistants, and even physicians. Health care and education experienced the fastest growth of gig workers over the past decade, and the continuing trend forces questions related to a moral economy that explores the future of work and workers, guest workers,

---

[4] According to the online Cambridge Dictionary, uberization is the act or process of changing the market for a service by introducing a different way of buying or using it, especially using mobile technology.

and more[5] (British Medical Association, 2018). Many of these on-demand workers also have personal health issues that impact their lives (Bajwa et al., 2018). Thus, it is judicious to involve political and social scientists to examine and plan for the societal impacts of AI in health care.

Problem Identification and Equitable Implementation

Health care AI tools have the capability to impact trust in the health care system on a national scale, especially if these tools lead to worse outcomes for some patients or result in increasing inequities. Ensuring that these tools address, or at least do not exacerbate, existing inequities will require thoughtful prioritization of a national agenda that is not driven purely by profit, but instead by an understanding of the important drivers of health care costs, quality, and access.

As a starting point, system leaders must identify key areas in which there are known needs where AI tools can be helpful, where they can help address existing inequities, and where implementation will result in improved outcomes for all patients. These areas must also have an organizational structure in place that addresses other ethical issues, such as patient–provider relationships, patient privacy, transparency, notification, and consent, as well as technical development, validation, implementation, and maintenance of AI tools within an ever evolving learning health care system.

The implementation of health care AI tools requires that information technologists, data scientists, ethicists and lawyers, clinicians, patients, and clinical teams and organizations collaborate and prioritize governance structures and processes. These teams will need a macro understanding of the data flows, transformations, incentives, levers, and frameworks for algorithm development and validation, as well as knowledge of ongoing changes required post-implementation (see Chapter 5).

When developing and implementing those tools, it may be tempting to ignore or delay the considerations of the needed legal and ethical organizational structure to govern privacy, transparency, and consent. However, there are substantial risks in disregarding these considerations, as witnessed in data uses and breaches, inappropriate results derived from training data, and algorithms that reproduce and scale prejudice via the underlying historically biased data (O'Neil, 2017). There must also be an understanding of the ethical, legal, and regulatory structures that are relevant to the approval, use, and deployment of AI tools, without which there will be liability exposure, unintended consequences, and limitations (see Chapter 7).

---

[5] A 2018 survey showed that 7.7 percent of UK medical workers who are EU citizens would leave the United Kingdom for other regions if the United Kingdom withdrew from the European Union, as it did in 2019.

There are substantial infrastructure costs for internally developed AI health care solutions, and these will likely deter smaller health care delivery systems from being early adopters. Deploying AI tools requires careful evaluation of performance and maintenance. If health care AI tools are effective for cost reduction, patient satisfaction, and patient outcomes, and are implemented as a competitive edge, it could leave resource-constrained systems that do not deploy these tools at a disadvantage. Thus, clear guidance is needed on best practices for assessing and interpreting the opportunities and costs of implementing AI tools. Best practices should be driven by an implementation science research agenda and should engage stakeholders to lower the cost and complexity of AI technologies. This is particularly important for smaller health care systems, many of which are in rural and resource-constrained environments.

Post-implementation, the health care systems and stakeholders will need to carefully monitor the impact of AI tools to ensure that they meet intended goals and do not exacerbate inequities.

Impact of AI on the Patient–Provider Relationship

The well-intentioned introduction of EHRs and the HITECH Act incentives contributed to converting physicians into data-entry clerks, worsening physician burnout, and reducing patient satisfaction (Verghese, 2018). To ensure health care AI tools do not worsen that burden, a fundamental issue is the potential impact of AI on the patient–provider relationship. This could include further degradation of empathic interactions as well as a mismatch between existent and needed skills in the workforce. Throughout this publication, we emphasize the power of AI to augment rather than replace human intelligence, because

> the desirable attributes of humans who choose the path of caring for others include, in addition to scientific knowledge, the capacity to love, to have empathy, to care and express caring, to be generous, to be brave in advocating for others, to do no harm, and to work for the greater good and advocate for justice. How might AI help clinicians nurture and protect these qualities? This type of challenge is rarely discussed or considered at conferences on AI and medicine, perhaps because it is viewed as messy and hard to define. But, if the goal is for AI to emulate the best qualities of human intelligence, it is precisely the territory that cannot be avoided. (Israni and Verghese, 2019)

As discussed in Chapter 4, the U.S. health care system can draw important lessons from the aviation industry, the history of which includes many examples of automation addressing small challenges, but also occasionally creating extraordinary disasters. The 2009 plane crash of an Air France flight from Rio to Paris showed the potential

> unintended consequence of designing airplanes that anyone can fly: anyone can take you up on the offer. Beyond the degradation of basic skills of people who may once have been competent pilots, the fourth-generation jets have enabled people who probably never had the skills to begin with and should not have been in the cockpit. As a result, the mental makeup of airline pilots has changed. (Langewiesche, 2014)

More recently, disasters with Boeing's 737 Max caused by software issues offer another caution: Competent pilots' complaints about next-generation planes were not given sufficient review (Sharpe and Robison, 2019).

Finally, just because technology makes it possible to deploy a particular solution, it may still not be appropriate to do so. Recently, a doctor in California used a robot with a video-link screen in order to tell a patient that he was going to die. After a social media and public relations disaster, the hospital apologized, stating, "We don't support or encourage the use of technology to replace the personal interactions between our patients and their care teams—we understand how important this is for all concerned, and regret that we fell short of the family's expectations" (BBC News, 2019). Technochauvinism in AI will only further complicate an already complex and overburdened health care system.

In summary, health care is a complex field that incorporates genetics, physiology, pharmacology, biology, and other related sciences with the social, human, and cultural experience of managing health. Health care is both a science and an art, and challenges the notion that simple and elegant formulas will be able to explain significant portions of health care delivery and outcomes (Toon, 2012).

PUBLICATION ORGANIZATION

This publication is structured around several distinct topic areas, each covered in a separate chapter and independently authored by the listed expert team. Figure 1-6 shows the relationship of the chapters.

Each chapter is intended to stand alone and represents the views of its authors. In order to allow readers to read each chapter independently there is some redundancy in the material, with relevant references to other chapters where appropriate. Each chapter initially summarizes the key content of the chapter and concludes with a set of key considerations for improving the development, adoption, and use of AI in health care.

Chapter 2 examines the history of AI, using examples from other industries, and summarizes the growth, maturity, and adoption of AI in health care. The

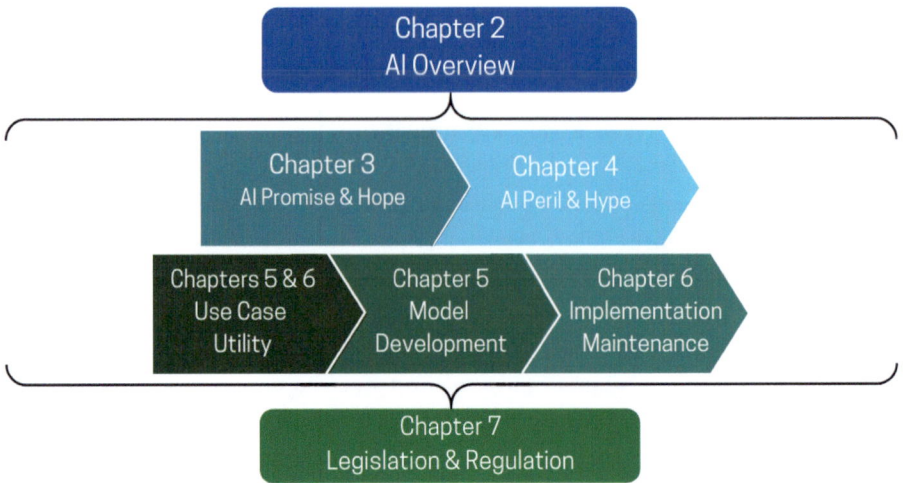

FIGURE 1-6 | Chapter relationship.

chapter also describes the central importance of AI to the realization of the learning health care system.

Chapter 3 describes the potential utility of AI for improving health care delivery and discusses the near-term opportunities and potential gains from the use of AI in health care settings. The chapter also explores the promise of AI by key stakeholder groups, including patients and families, the clinical care team, population and public health program managers, health care business and administrative professionals, and research and development professionals.

Chapter 4 considers some of the unintended consequences of AI in health care work processes, culture, equity, patient–provider relationships, and workforce composition and skills, and offers approaches for mitigating the risks.

Chapter 5 covers the technical processes and best practices for developing and validating AI models, including choices related to data, variables, model complexity, learning approach, set up, and the selection of metrics for model performance.

Chapter 6 considers the key issues and best practices for deploying AI models in clinical settings, including the software development process, the integration of models in health care settings, the application of implementation science, and approaches for model maintenance and surveillance over time.

Chapter 7 summarizes key laws applicable to AI that may be applied in health care, describes the regulatory requirements imposed on AI systems designed for health care applications, and discusses legal and policy issues related to privacy and patient data.

The final chapter builds on and summarizes key themes across the publication and describes critical next steps for moving the field forward equitably and responsibly.

REFERENCES

Abraham, C., and P. Sheeran. 2007. The health belief model. In *Cambridge handbook of psychology, health and medicine*, edited by S. Ayers, A. Baum, C. McManus, S. Newman, K. Wallston, J. Weinman, and R. West, 2nd ed., pp. 97–102. Cambridge, UK: Cambridge University Press.

Agbo, C. C., Q. H. Mahmoud, and J. M. Eklund. 2019. Blockchain technology in healthcare: A systematic review. *Healthcare* 7(2):E56.

Aggarwal, N. K., M. Rowe, and M. A. Sernyak. 2010. Is health care a right or a commodity? Implementing mental health reform in a recession. *Psychiatric Services* 61(11):1144–1145.

Aitken, M., B. Clancy, and D. Nass. 2017. *The growing value of digital health: Evidence and impact on human health and the healthcare system.* https://www.iqvia.com/institute/reports/the-growing-value-of-digital-health (accessed May 12, 2020).

Ashby, W. R. 1964. *An introduction to cybernetics.* London: Methuen and Co. Ltd.

ASTHO (Association of State and Territorial Health Officials). 2019. *Medicaid and public health partnership learning series.* http://www.astho.org/Health-Systems-Transformation/Medicaid-and-Public-Health-Partnerships/Learning-Series/Managed-Care (accessed May 12, 2020).

Bajwa, U., D. Gastaldo, E. D. Ruggiero, and L. Knorr. 2018. The health of workers in the global gig economy. *Global Health* 14(1):124.

Baras, J. D., and L. C. Baker. 2009. Magnetic resonance imaging and low back pain care for Medicare patients. *Health Affairs (Millwood)* 28(6):w1133–w1140.

Basu, S., and R. Narayanaswamy. 2019. A prediction model for uncontrolled type 2 diabetes mellitus incorporating area-level social determinants of health. *Medical Care* 57(8):592–600.

Bauchner, H., and P. B. Fontanarosa. 2019. Waste in the US health care system. *JAMA* 322(15):1463–1464.

BBC News. 2019. *Man told he's going to die by doctor on video-link robot.* March 9. https://www.bbc.com/news/world-us-canada-47510038 (accessed May 12, 2020).

Becker's Healthcare. 2018. *AI with an ROI: Why revenue cycle automation may be the most practical use of AI.* https://www.beckershospitalreview.com/artificial-intelligence/ai-with-an-roi-why-revenue-cycle-automation-may-be-the-most-practical-use-of-ai.html (accessed May 12, 2020).

British Medical Association. 2018. *Almost a fifth of EU doctors have made plans to leave UK following Brexit vote.* December 6. https://psmag.com/series/the-future-of-work-and-workers (accessed May 12, 2020).

Broussard, M. 2018. *Artificial unintelligence: How computers misunderstand the world.* Cambridge, MA: MIT Press.

Bustamante, C. D., F. M. De La Vega, and E. G. Burchard. 2011. Genomics for the world. *Nature* 475:163–165.

Chung, Y. A., Y. Wang, W. N. Hsu, Y. Zhang, and R. Skerry-Ryan. 2018. *Semi-supervised training for improving data efficiency in end-to-end speech synthesis.* arXiv.org.

CMS (Centers for Medicare & Medicaid Services). 2019. Medicare and Medicaid Programs; Patient Protection and Affordable Care Act; Interoperability and Patient Access for Medicare Advantage Organization and Medicaid Managed Care Plans, State Medicaid Agencies, CHIP Agencies and CHIP Managed Care Entities, Issuers of Qualified Health Plans in the Federally-Facilitated Exchanges and Health Care Providers. Proposed rule. *Federal Register* 84(42):7610–7680.

CPIC (Clinical Pharmacogenetics Implementation Consortium). 2019. *What is CPIC?* https://cpicpgx.org (accessed May 12, 2020).

DeepMind Ethics and Society. 2019. *DeepMind ethics & society principles.* https://deepmind.com/applied/deepmind-ethics-society/principles (accessed May 12, 2020).

DOMO. 2019. *Data never sleeps 6.0.* https://www.domo.com/learn/data-never-sleeps-6 (accessed May 12, 2020).

Downey, G. 2010. We agree it's WEIRD, but is it WEIRD enough? *Neuroanthropology.* July 10. https://neuroanthropology.net/2010/07/10/we-agree-its-weird-but-is-it-weird-enough (accessed May 12, 2020).

European Commission. 2018. *2018 reform of EU data protection rules.* https://www.tc260.org.cn/upload/2019-02-01/1549013548750042566.pdf (accessed May 12, 2020).

Feigenbaum, E. 1992. Expert systems: Principles and practice. In *The encyclopedia of computer science and engineering.* http://citeseerx.ist.psu.edu/viewdoc/download?doi=10.1.1.34.9207&rep=rep1&type=pdf (accessed May 12, 2020).

Feldstein, P. J. 2012. *Health care economics.* Clifton Park, NY: Cengage Learning.

Forsyth, D. A., and J. Ponce. 2003. *Computer vision: A modern approach.* Upper Saddle River, NJ: Prentice Hall.

Ghallab, M., D. S. Nau, and P. Traverso. 2004. *Automated planning: Theory and practice.* San Francisco, CA: Elsevier.

Google. 2018. *Artificial intelligence at Google: Our principles.* https://ai.google/principles (accessed May 12, 2020).

Gotterbarn, D. W., B. Brinkman, C. Flick, M. S. Kirkpatrick, K. Miller, K. Vazansky, and M. J. Wolf. 2018. *ACM code of ethics and professional conduct.* https://www.acm.org/binaries/content/assets/about/acm-code-of-ethics-and-professional-conduct.pdf (accessed May 12, 2020).

Green, D. 2019. Commentary: Data-sharing can transform care, so let's get connected. *Modern Healthcare.* https://www.modernhealthcare.com/opinion-editorial/commentary-data-sharing-can-transform-care-so-lets-get-connected (accessed May 12, 2020).

Hoffman, J. M., H. M. Dunnenberger, J. K. Hicks, M. W. Carillo, R. R. Freimuth, M. S. Williams, T. E. Klein, and J. F. Peterson. 2016. Developing knowledge resources to support precision medicine: Principles from the Clinical Pharmacogenetics Implementation Consortium (CPIC). *Journal of the American Medical Informatics Association* 23:796–801.

Hripcsak, G., J. D. Duke, N. H. Shah, C. G. Reich, V. Huser, M. J. Schuemie, M. A. Suchard, R. W. Park, I. C. K. Wong, P. R. Rijnbeek, J. van der Lei, N. Pratt, N. Norén, Y-C. Li, P. E. Stang, D. Madigan, and P. B. Ryan. 2015. Observational Health Data Sciences and Informatics (OHDSI): Opportunities for observational researchers. *Studies in Health Technologies and Information* 216:574–578. https://tmu.pure.elsevier.com/en/publications/observational-health-data-sciences-and-informatics-ohdsi-opportun (accessed May 12, 2020).

House of Lords Select Committee on Artificial Intelligence. 2018. *AI in the UK: Ready, willing and able?* House of Lords, April 16.

Institute for the Future and Omidyar Network. 2018. *Ethical OS: Risk mitigation checklist.* https://ethicalos.org/wp-content/uploads/2018/08/EthicalOS_Check-List_080618.pdf (accessed May 12, 2020).

IOM (Institute of Medicine). 2008. *Evidence-based medicine and the changing nature of health care: 2007 IOM annual meeting summary.* Washington, DC: The National Academies Press. https://doi. org/10.17226/12041.

Isazi Consulting. 2015. *What is machine learning?* http://www.isaziconsulting.co.za/machinelearning.html.

Israni, S. T., and A. Verghese. 2019. Humanizing artificial intelligence. *JAMA* 321(1):29–30.

Jackson, P. 1998. *Introduction to expert systems.* Boston, MA: Addison-Wesley Longman Publishing Co., Inc.

Kehl, K. L., H. Elmarakeby, M. Nishino, E. M. Van Allen, E. M. Lepisto, M. J. Hassett, B. E. Johnson, and D. Schrag. 2019. Assessment of deep natural language processing in ascertaining oncologic outcomes from radiology reports. *JAMA Oncology.* Epub ahead of print. doi: 10.1001/jamaoncol.2019.1800.

Khalilia, M., M. Choi, A. Henderson, S. Iyengar, M. Braunstein, and J. Sun. 2015. Clinical predictive modeling development and deployment through FHIR web services. *AMIA Annual Symposium Proceedings* 717–726.

Kho, A. N., J. P. Cashy, K. L. Jackson, A. R. Pah, S. Goel, J. Boehnke, J. E. Humphries, S. D. Kominers, B. N. Hota, S. A. Sims, B. A. Malin, D. D. French, T. L. Walunas,

D. O. Meltzer, E. O. Kaleba, R. C. Jones, and W. L. Galanter. 2015. Design and implementation of a privacy preserving electronic health record linkage tool. *Chicago Journal of the American Medical Informatics Association* 22(5):1072–1080.

Kissam, S. M., H. Beil, C. Cousart, L. M. Greenwald, and J. T. Lloyd. 2019. States encouraging value-based payment: Lessons from CMS's state innovation models initiative. *The Milbank Quarterly* 97(2):506–542.

Kommerskollegium National Board of Trade. 2012. *How borderless is the cloud?* https://www.wto.org/english/tratop_e/serv_e/wkshop_june13_e/how_borderless_cloud_e.pdf (accessed May 12, 2020).

Langewiesche, W. 2014. The human factor. *Vanity Fair.* September. https://www.vanityfair.com/news/business/2014/10/air-france-flight-447-crash (accessed May 12, 2020).

Lee, J., and C. Korba. 2017. Social determinants of health: How are hospitals and health systems investing in and addressing social needs? *Deloitte Center for Health Solutions.* https://www2.deloitte.com/content/dam/Deloitte/us/Documents/life-sciences-health-care/us-lshc-addressing-social-determinants-of-health.pdf (accessed May 12, 2020).

Leondes, C. T. 2002. *Expert systems: The technology of knowledge management and decision making for the 21st century.* San Diego, CA: Academic Press.

Levi, M. 2018 (April). *Towards a new moral economy: A thought piece.* https://casbs.stanford.edu/sites/g/files/sbiybj9596/f/levi-thought-piece-april-20184.pdf.

Lye, C. T., H. P. Forman, R. Gao, J. G. Daniel, A. L. Hsiao, M. K. Mann, D. deBronkart, H. O. Campos, and H. M. Krumholz. 2018. Assessment of US hospital compliance with regulations for patients' requests for medical records. *JAMA Network Open* 1(6):e183014.

Manning, C. D., and H. Schütze. 1999. *Foundations of statistical natural language processing.* Cambridge, MA: MIT Press.

Mello, M. M., J. Adler-Milstein, K. L. Ding, and L. Savage. 2018. Legal barriers to the growth of health information exchange—Boulders or pebbles? *The Milbank Quarterly* 96(1):110–143.

Mendelson, A., K. Kondo, C. Damberg, A. Low, M. Motuapuaka, M. Freeman, M. O'Neil, R. Relevo, and D. Kansagara. 2017. The effects of pay-for performance programs on health, healthcare use, and processes of care: A systematic review. *Annals of Internal Medicine* 166(5):341–355.

Mills, M. 2015. *Artificial intelligence in law—The state of play in 2015?* https://www.legaltechnology.com/latest-news/artificial-intelligence-in-law-the-state-of-play-in-2015 (accessed May 12, 2020).

Munoz, C., M. Smith, and D. J. Patil. 2016. Big data: A report on algorithmic systems, opportunity, and civil rights. *Executive Office of the President.*

https://obamawhitehouse.archives.gov/sites/default/files/microsites/ostp/2016_0504_data_discrimination.pdf (accessed May 12, 2020).

Murff, H. J., F. Fitzhenry, M. E. Matheny, N. Gentry, K. L. Kotter, K. Crimin, R. S. Dittus, A. K. Rosen, P. L. Elkin, S. H. Brown, and T. Speroff. 2011. Automated identification of postoperative complications within an electronic medical record using natural language processing. *JAMA* 306:848–855.

NAM (National Academy of Medicine). 2019a. *Leadership Consortium for a Value & Science-Driven Health System.* https://nam.edu/programs/value-science-driven-health-care (accessed May 12, 2020).

NAM. 2019b. *Digital learning.* https://nam.edu/programs/value-science-driven-health-care/digital-learning (accessed May 12, 2020).

Nassif, A. B., I. Shahin, I. Attilli, M. Azzeh, and K. Shaalan. 2019. Speech recognition using deep neural networks: A systematic review. *IEEE Access* 7:19143–19165. https://ieeexplore.ieee.org/document/8632885.

NRC (National Research Council). 2009. *Computational technology for effective health care: Immediate steps and strategic directions.* Washington, DC: The National Academies Press. https://doi.org/10.17226/12572.

OECD (Organisation for Economic Co-operation and Development). 2017. *Health at a glance 2017.* https://www.oecd-ilibrary.org/content/publication/health_glance-2017-en (accessed May 12, 2020).

OHDSI (Observational Health Data Sciences and Informatics). 2019. Home. https://ohdsi.org (accessed May 12, 2020).

Ohno-Machado, L., Z. Agha, D. S. Bell, L. Dahm, M. E. Day, J. N. Doctor, D. Gabriel, M. K. Kahlon, K. K. Kim, M. Hogarth, M. E. Matheny, D. Meeker, J. R. Nebeker, and pSCANNER team. 2014. pSCANNER: Patient-centered scalable national network for effectiveness research. *Journal of the American Medical Informatics Association* 21(4):621–626.

ONC (The Office of the National Coordinator for Health Information Technology). 2019. 21st Century Cures Act: Interoperability, information blocking, and the ONC Health IT Certification Program. Final Rule. *Federal Register* 84(42):7424.

O'Neil, C. 2017. *Weapons of math destruction: How big data increases inequality and threatens democracy.* New York: Broadway Books.

Ong, T. C., M. V. Mannino, L. M. Schilling, and M. G. Kahn. 2014. Improving record linkage performance in the presence of missing linkage data. *Journal of Biomedical Informatics* 52:43–54.

Ong, T., R. Pradhananga, E. Holve, and M. G. Kahn. 2017. A framework for classification of electronic health data extraction-transformation-loading challenges in data network participation. *Generating Evidence and Methods to Improve Patient Outcomes (eGEMS)* 5(1):10.

Parikh, R. 2017. Should doctors play along with the uberization of health care? *Slate.* https://slate.com/technology/2017/06/should-doctors-play-along-with-the-uberization-of-health-care.html (accessed May 12, 2020).

Partnership on AI. 2018. *Partnership on AI tenets.* https://www.partnershiponai.org/tenets.

Patient-Centered Clinical Research Network. 2019. *Data driven.* https://pcornet.org/data-driven-common-model (accessed May 12, 2020).

PharmGKB. 2019. Home. https://www.pharmgkb.org (accessed May 12, 2020).

Popejoy, A. B., and S. M. Fullerton. 2016. Genomics is failing on diversity. *Nature* 538(7624):161–164.

Prochaska, J. O., and W. F. Velicer. 1997. The transtheoretical model of health behavior change. *American Journal of Health Promotion* 12(1):38–48.

Reiley, C. E. 2016. When bias in product design means life or death. *Medium.* https://medium.com/@robot_MD/when-bias-in-product-design-means-life-or-death-ea3d16e3ddb2 (accessed May 12, 2020).

Rosenbloom, S. T., R. J. Carroll, J. L. Warner, M. E. Matheny, and J. C. Denny. 2017. Representing knowledge consistently across health systems. *Yearbook of Medical Informatics* 26(1):139–147.

Rosenstock, I. 1974. Historical origins of the health belief model. *Health Education & Behavior* 2(4):328–335.

Rosenthal, E. 2017. *An American sickness.* New York: Penguin.

Ross, C. 2018. The government wants to free your health data. Will that unleash innovation? *STAT.* https://www.statnews.com/2018/03/29/government-health-data-innovation (accessed May 12, 2020).

Schulte, D. 2017. *4 ways artificial intelligence can bend health care's cost curve.* https://www.bizjournals.com/bizjournals/how-to/technology/2017/07/4-ways-artificial-intelligencecan-bend-healthcare.html (accessed May 12, 2020).

Schulte, F., and E. Fry. 2019. Death by 1,000 clicks: Where electronic health records went wrong. *Kaiser Health News & Fortune (Joint Collaboration).* https://khn.org/news/death-by-a-thousand-clicks (accessed May 12, 2020).

Seligman, B., S. Tuljapurkar, and D. Rehkopf. 2017. Machine learning approaches to the social determinants of health in the health and retirement study. *SSM-Population Health* 4:95–99.

Sepah, S. C., L. Jiang, R. J. Ellis, K. McDermott, and A. L. Peters. 2017. Engagement and outcomes in a digital Diabetes Prevention Program: 3-year update. *BMJ Open Diabetes Research and Care* 5:e000422. doi: 10.1136/bmjdrc-2017-000422.

Sharpe, A., and P. Robison. 2019. Pilots flagged software problems on Boeing jets besides Max. *Bloomberg.* https://www.bloomberg.com/news/articles/2019-06-27/boeing-pilots-flagged-software-problems-on-jets-besides-the-max (accessed May 12, 2020).

Shi, M., S. Sacks, Q. Chen, and G. Webster. 2019. Translation: China's personal information security specification. *New America.* https://www.newamerica.org/cybersecurity-initiative/digichina/blog/translation-chinas-personal-information-security-specification (accessed May 12, 2020).

Shortliffe, E. H., and B. G. Buchanan. 1975. A model of inexact reasoning in medicine. *Mathematical Biosciences* 23(3–4):351–379. doi: 10.1016/0025-5564(75)90047-4.

Shrott, R. 2017. Deep learning specialization by Andrew Ng—21 lessons learned. *Medium.* https://towardsdatascience.com/deep-learning-specialization-by-andrew-ng-21-lessons-learned-15ffaaef627c (accessed May 12, 2020).

Skloot, R. 2011. *The immortal life of Henrietta Lacks.* New York: Broadway Books.

Sonka, M., V. Hlavac, and R. Boyle. 2008. *Image processing, analysis, and machine vision*, 4th ed. Boston, MA: Cengage Learning.

Stanford Engineering. 2019. *Carlos Bustamante: Genomics has a diversity problem.* https://engineering.stanford.edu/magazine/article/carlos-bustamante-genomics-has-diversity-problem (accessed May 12, 2020).

Sullivan, A. 2010. Western, educated, industrialized, rich, and democratic. *The Daily Dish.* October 4. https://www.theatlantic.com/daily-dish/archive/2010/10/western-educated-industrialized-rich-and-democratic/181667 (accessed May 12, 2020).

Sun, C., A. Shrivastava, S. Singh, and A. Gupta. 2017. *Revisiting unreasonable effectiveness of data in deep learning era.* https://arxiv.org/pdf/1707.02968.pdf (accessed May 12, 2020).

Toon, P. 2012. Health care is both a science and an art. *British Journal of General Practice* 62(601):434.

Vayena, E., A. Blasimme, and I. G. Cohen. 2018. Machine learning in medicine: Addressing ethical challenges. *PLoS Medicine* 15(11):e1002689.

Verghese, A. 2018. How tech can turn doctors into clerical workers. *The New York Times*, May 16. https://www.nytimes.com/interactive/2018/05/16/magazine/health-issuewhat-we-lose-with-data-driven-medicine.html (accessed May 12, 2020).

Wakabayashi, D. 2019. Google and the University of Chicago are sued over data sharing. *The New York Times.* https://www.nytimes.com/2019/06/26/technology/google-university-chicago-data-sharing-lawsuit.html (accessed May 12, 2020).

West, S. M., M. Whittaker, and K. Crawford. 2019. *Gender, race and power in AI*. AI Now Institute. https://ainowinstitute.org/discriminatingsystems.html (accessed May 12, 2020).

Wetterstrand, K. A. 2019. *DNA sequencing costs: Data from the NHGRI Genome Sequencing Program (GSP)*. https://www.genome.gov/sequencingcostsdata (accessed May 12, 2020).

Whittaker, M., K. Crawford, R. Dobbe, G. Fried, E. Kaziunas, V. Mathur, S. M. West, R. Richardson, J. Schultz, and O. Schwartz. 2018. *AI Now report 2018*. AI Now Institute at New York University. https://stanford.app.box.com/s/xmb2cj3e7gsz5vmus0viadt9p3kreekk (accessed May 12, 2020).

Wiens, J., S. Saria, M. Sendak, M. Ghassemi, V. X. Liu, F. Doshi-Velez, K. Jung, K. Heller, D. Kale, M. Saeed, P. N. Ossorio, S. Thadaney-Israni, and A. Goldenberg. 2019. Do no harm: A roadmap for responsible machine learning for health care. *Nature Medicine* 25(9):1137–1340.

Witten, I. H., E. Frank, M. A. Hall, and C. J. Pal. 2016. *Data mining: Practical machine learning tools and techniques*. Burlington, MA: Morgan Kaufmann.

Yeung, S., F. Rinaldo, J. Jopling, B. Liu, R. Mehra, N. L. Downing, M. Guo, G. M. Bianconi, A. Alahi, J. Lee, B. Campbell, K. Deru, W. Beninati, L. Fei-Fei, and A. Milstein. 2019. A computer vision system for deep-learning based detection of patient mobilization activities in the ICU. *NPJ Digital Medicine* 2:11. doi: 10.1038/s41746-019-0087-z.

Zarsky, T. 2016. The trouble with algorithmic decisions: An analytic road map to examine efficiency and fairness in automated and opaque decision making. *Science, Technology, & Human Values* 41(1):118–132. doi: 10.1177/0162243915605575.

Suggested citation for Chapter 1: Matheny, M., S. Thadaney Israni, D. Whicher, and M. Ahmed. 2019. Artificial intelligence in health care: The hope, the hype, the promise, the peril. In *Artificial intelligence in health care: The hope, the hype, the promise, the peril*. Washington, DC: National Academy of Medicine.

2

OVERVIEW OF CURRENT ARTIFICIAL INTELLIGENCE

James Fackler, Johns Hopkins Medicine, and Edmund Jackson, Hospital Corporation of America

INTRODUCTION

This chapter first acknowledges the roots of artificial intelligence (AI). We then briefly touch on areas outside of medicine where AI has had an impact and highlight where lessons from these other industries might cross into health care.

For decades, the attempt to capture knowledge in the form of a book has been challenging, as indicated by the adage "any text is out of date by the time the book is published." However, in 2019, with what has been determined by some analyses as exponential growth in the field of computer science and AI in particular, change is happening at a pace that renders sentences in this chapter out of date almost immediately. To stay current, we can no longer rely on monthly updates from a stored PubMed search. Rather, daily news feeds from sources such as the Association for the Advancement of Artificial Intelligence or arXiv[1] are necessary. As such, this chapter contains references to both historical publications as well as websites and web-based articles.

It is surpassingly difficult to define AI, principally because it has always been loosely spoken of as a set of human-like capabilities that computers seem about ready to replicate. Yesterday's AI is today's commodity computation. Within that caveat, we aligned this chapter with the definition of AI in Chapter 1. A formal definition of AI starts with the Oxford English Dictionary: "The capacity of computers or other machines to exhibit or simulate intelligent behavior; the field of study concerned with this," or Merriam-Webster online: "1: a branch

---

[1] See https://arxiv.org/list/cs.LG/recent.

of computer science dealing with the simulation of intelligent behavior in computers, 2: the capability of a machine to imitate intelligent human behavior."

HISTORICAL PERSPECTIVE

If the term "artificial intelligence" has a birthdate, it is August 31, 1955, when John McCarthy, Marvin L. Minsky, Nathaniel Rochester, and Claude E. Shannon submitted "A Proposal for the Dartmouth Summer Research Project on Artificial Intelligence." The second sentence of the proposal reads, "The study is to proceed on the basis of the conjecture that every aspect of learning or any other feature of intelligence can in principle be so precisely described that a machine can be made to simulate it" (McCarthy et al., 2006). Naturally, the proposal and the resulting conference—the 1956 Dartmouth Summer Research Project on Artificial Intelligence—were the culmination of decades of thought by many others (Buchanan, 2005; Kline, 2011; Turing, 1950; Weiner, 1948). Although the conference produced neither formal collaborations nor tangible outputs, it clearly galvanized the field (Moor, 2006).

Thought leaders in this era saw the future clearly, although optimism was substantially premature. In 1960, J. C. R. Licklider wrote

> The hope is that, in not too many years, human brains and computing machines will be coupled together very tightly, and that the resulting partnership will think as no human brain has ever thought and process data in a way not approached by the information-handling machines we know today. (Licklider, 1960)

Almost 60 years later, we are closer but not there yet.

Two major competing schools of thought developed in approaching AI: (1) symbolic representation and formal logic expressed as expert systems and advanced primarily with Lisp, a family of computer programming languages (and Prolog in Europe) by John McCarthy, and (2) conceptualization and mathematical frameworks for mirroring neurons in the brain, formalized as "perceptrons" by Frank Rosenblatt (1958; see also McCarthy, 1958). The latter was initially known as the connectionist school, but we now know the technique as artificial neural networks. The McCarthy school of formal logic was founded by the technical paper "Programs with Common Sense," in which McCarthy defines and creates the first full AI program: Advice Taker (McCarthy, 1959). The major thrust of the paper is that "in order for a program to be capable of learning something it must first be capable of being told it," and hence the formalization of declarative logic programming. By the 1970s, however, excitement gave way to disappointment because early successes that worked in well-structured narrow problems failed to either generalize to broader problem solving or deliver operationally useful systems. The disillusionment, summarized in the Automatic Language Processing Advisory Committee report (NRC, 1966) and the Lighthill report (Lighthill, 1973), resulted in an "AI Winter" with shuttered projects, evaporation of research funding, and general skepticism about the potential for AI systems (McCarthy, 1974).

Yet, in health care, work continued. Iconic expert systems such as MYCIN (Shortliffe, 1974) and others such as Iliad, Quick Medical Reference, and Internist-1 were developed to assist with clinical diagnosis. AI flowered commercially in the 1980s, becoming a multibillion-dollar industry advising military and commercial interests (Miller et al., 1982; Sumner, 1993). However, all ultimately failed to reach the hype and lofty promises resulting in a second AI Winter from the late 1980s until the late 2000s.[2]

During the AI Winter, the various schools of computer science, probability, mathematics, and AI came together to overcome the initial failures of AI. In particular, techniques from probability and signal processing, such as hidden Markov models, Bayesian networks, stochastic search, and optimization, were incorporated into AI thinking, resulting in a field known as machine learning. The field of machine learning applies the scientific method to representing, understanding, and utilizing datasets, and, as a result, practitioners are known as data scientists. Popular machine learning techniques include random forests, boosting, support vector machines, and artificial neural networks. See Hastie et al. (2001) or Murphy (2013) for thorough reviews; these methods are also discussed in more detail in Chapter 5.

Around 2010, AI began its resurgence to prominence due to the success of machine learning and data science techniques as well as significant increases in computational storage and power. These advances fueled the growth of technology titans such as Google and Amazon.

Most recently, Rosenblatt's ideas laid the groundwork for artificial neural networks, which have come to dominate the field of machine learning thanks to the successes of Geoffrey Hinton's group, and later others, in solving computational problems in training expressive neural networks and the ubiquity of data necessary for robust training (Halevy et al., 2009; Krizhevsky et al., 2012). The resulting systems are called deep learning systems and showed significant performance improvements over prior generations of algorithms for some use cases. It is noteworthy that Hinton was awarded the 2018 Turing Prize alongside Yoshua Bengio and Yann LeCun for their work on deep learning (Metz, 2019).

Modern AI has evolved from an interest in machines that think to ones that sense, think, and act. It is important at this early stage to distinguish narrow from

---

[2] See Newquist (1994) for a thorough review of the birth, development, and decline of early AI.

general AI. The popular conception of AI is of a computer, hyper capable in all domains, such as was seen even decades ago in science fiction with HAL 9000 in *2001: A Space Odyssey* or aboard the *USS Enterprise* in the Star Trek franchise. These are examples of general AIs and, for now, are wholly fictional. There is an active but niche general AI research community represented by Deepmind, Cyc, and OpenAI, among others. Narrow AI, in contrast, is an AI specialized at a single task, such as playing chess, driving a car, or operating a surgical robot. Certain narrow AIs do exist and are discussed in further detail below.

As discussed above and more in Chapter 4, the word overhyped, however, should be mentioned again. The Gartner Hype Cycle is a good place to start understanding the current state of AI in the broad stages of innovation, inflated expectations, disillusionment, enlightenment, and finally productivity (Gartner, Inc., 2018). While we grow out of the AI Winter, it is crucial that we maintain this perspective. Research publications and marketing claims should not overstate utility. Cautious optimism is crucial (Frohlich et al., 2018).

AI IN NON-HEALTH CARE INDUSTRIES

There are many industries outside of health care that are further along in their adoption of AI into their workflows. The following section highlights a partial list of those industries and discusses aspects of AI use in these industries to be emulated and avoided.

Users

It is critical to consider AI primarily in terms of its relationship with users, particularly in the health care sector. Considerable concern exists about AIs replacing humans in the workforce once they are able to perform functions that previously required a human (Kolko, 2018; Zhang et al., 2019). However, when examined critically, it is usually the case that computer scientists design AI with human users in mind, and as such, AI usually extends the capacity, capability, and performance of humans, rather than replacing them (Topol, 2019). The self-driving car, our first example below, demonstrates how an AI and human might work together to achieve a goal, which enhances the human experience (Hutson, 2017). In other examples such as legal document review, the AI working with the human reviews more documents at a higher level of precision (Xu and Wang, 2019). This concept of a human and AI team is known in the AI literature as a "centaur" (Case, 2018) and in the anthropology literature as a "cyborg" (Haraway, 2000). To date, most of the focus on the use of AI has been to support physicians. However, patients, caregivers, and allied health clinicians of all types will also be

AI users. In the next sections we examine scenarios in which AI may influence health care. Again, it is important to note that, regardless of how extensive the deployment of the AI systems described below, care must be exercised in their translation into health care.

Automotive

Of all of the industries making headlines with the use of AI, the self-driving car has most significantly captured the public's imagination (Mervis, 2017). In concept, a self-driving car is a motor vehicle that can navigate and drive its occupants without their interaction. Whether this should be the aspirational goal (i.e., "without their interaction") is a subject of debate. For this discussion, it is more important to note that the component technologies have been evolving publicly for some years. Navigation has evolved from humans reading paper maps to satellite-based global positioning system (GPS)-enabled navigation devices, to wireless mobile telecommunications networks that evolved from analog to increasingly broadband digital technologies (2G to 3G to 4G to 5G), and most recently, navigation systems that supplement mapping and simple navigation with real-time, crowd-sourced traffic conditions (Mostafa et al., 2018). In research contexts, ad hoc networks enable motor vehicles to communicate directly with each other about emergent situations and driving conditions (Zongjian et al., 2016).

The achievement of successful self-driving cars has been and continues to be evolutionary. In terms of supporting the act of driving itself, automatic transmissions and anti-lock braking systems were early driver-assistance technologies. More recently, we have seen the development of driver-assistance AI applications that rely on sensing mechanisms such as radar, sonar, lidar, and cameras with signal processing techniques, which enable lane departure warnings, blind spot assistance, following distance alerts, and emergency braking (Sujit, 2015).

This recent use of cameras begins to distinguish AI techniques from the prior signal processing techniques. AI processes video data from the cameras at a level of abstraction comparable to that at which a human comprehends. That is, the machine extracts objects such as humans, cyclists, road signs, other vehicles, lanes, and other relevant factors from the video data and has been programmed to identify and interpret the images in a way that is understandable to a human. This combination of computer vision with reasoning comprises a specialized AI for driving.

However, for all the laudable goals, including improving driving safety, errors remain and sometimes those errors are fatal. This is possibly the single most important lesson that the health care domain can learn from the increasing use of AI in other industries. As reported in the press, the woman killed in spring 2018 as she walked her bicycle across the street was sensed by the onboard devices, but the software incorrectly classified her as an object for which braking was unnecessary. It was also reported that the "backup" driver of this autonomous vehicle was distracted, watching video on a cell phone (Laris, 2018).

The point of the above example is not that AI (in this case a self-driving car) is evil. Rather, we need to understand AI not in isolation but as part of a human–AI "team." Certainly, humans without any AI assistance do far worse; on average in 2017, 16 pedestrians were killed each day in traffic crashes (NHTSA, 2018). Reaching back to the 1960 quote from Licklider, it is important to note that the title of his article was "Man–Computer Symbiosis." In this example, the driver–computer symbiosis failed. Even the conceptualization that the human was considered a backup was wrong. The human is not just an alternative to AI; the human is an integral part of the complete system. For clinicians to effectively manage this symbiosis, they must (1) understand their own weaknesses (e.g., fatigue, biases), (2) understand the limits of the sensors and analytics, and (3) be able to assist or assume complete manual control of the controlled process in time to avoid an unfortunate outcome. AI must be viewed as a team member, not an "add-on" (Johnson and Vera, 2019).

Other examples of AI outside of medicine are outlined below. The theme of symbiosis is ubiquitous.

Professional Services

Although AI is often associated with physical devices and activities, it is actually very well suited to professional activities that rely on reasoning and language. For example, x.ai offers the seemingly mundane but intricate service of coordinating professionals' calendars. This is offered through a chat bot, which exercises not only natural language interpretation and generation but also logical reasoning to perform the scheduling.

In another domain, LawGeex and other vendors offer an AI that performs legal contract review and both discovers and appropriately escalates issues found in contract language. In addition, the AI can propose redline edits in coordination with a lawyer. Such an AI streamlines the review of standard contracts, such as nondisclosure agreements, that consume significant, expensive time with little probable value. As with many AI products, the AI enhances the human's capabilities and effectiveness, rather than operating as an autonomous agent.

Accounting and auditing are beginning to utilize AI for repetitive task automation such as accounts receivable coding and anomaly detection in audits (Amani and Fadlalla, 2017). Once again, the reason for this application of AI is speed and accuracy, when paired with a human.

Engineers and architects have long applied technology to enhance their design, and AI is set to accelerate that trend (Noor, 2017). Unusual AI-generated structural designs are in application today. A well-known example is the partition in the Airbus A320, in which AI algorithms utilized biomimetics to design a material almost half as light and equally as strong as the previous design (Micallef, 2016).

Finance has also been an early adopter of machine learning and AI techniques. The field of quantitative analytics was born in response to the computerization of the major trading exchanges. This has not been a painless process. One of the early "automated" trading strategies, portfolio insurance, is widely believed to have either caused or exacerbated the 1987 stock market crash (Bookstaber, 2007). The failure of Long-Term Capital Management offers another cautionary example (Lowenstein, 2011). This fund pursued highly leveraged arbitrage trades, where the pricing and leverage were algorithmically determined. Unexpected events caused the fund to fail spectacularly, requiring an almost $5 billion bailout from various financial institutions. Despite these setbacks, today all major banks and a tremendous number of hedge funds pursue trading strategies that rely on systematic machine learning or AI techniques. Most visible are the high-frequency trading desks, which rely on AI technologies to place, cancel, and execute orders at a speed as minute as one-hundredth of a microsecond, far faster than a human can think, react, and act (Seth, 2019).

Media

Content recommendation, most often based on an individual's previous choices, is the most widely visible application of AI in media. Large distribution channels such as Netflix and Amazon leverage machine learning algorithms for content recommendation to drive sales and engagement (Yu, 2019). These systems initially relied on algorithms such as collaborative filters to identify customers similar to others in terms of what media they consumed and enjoyed. More recently, deep learning techniques have been found superior for this task (Plummer, 2017). Health care examples are limited (Chen and Altman, 2015).

An interesting development has been that early techniques relied on metadata (descriptive features of media) in order to generate recommendations. More recent techniques utilize AI to generate metadata from the media itself, to personalize the presentations of recommendations, and then create recommendations. For instance, computer vision is used now to index film to identify faces, brands, and locations, which are coupled with human tags to create rich metadata (Yu, 2019).

In the music industry, startups such as Hitwizard and Hyperlive generalize these two ideas to attempt to predict which songs will be popular (Interiano et al., 2018). First, the AI structures the music into features such as loudness, beats per minute, and key, among others. Then, it compares this structured representation of the song to others that have been successful in order to identify similarity, and hence the new song's likelihood of also becoming a hit. The general complaint that all the music on the radio "sounds the same" may be based in part on the need to conform to the styles "approved" by the algorithms.

An emerging AI capability is generative art. Google initially released software called Deep Dream, which was able to create art in the style of famous artists, such as Vincent van Gogh (Mordvintsev et al., 2015). This technique is now used in many cell phone apps, such as Prisma Photo Editor,[3] as "filters" to enhance personal photography.

Another more disturbing use of AI surfaces in the trend known as "deepfakes," technology that enables face and voice swapping in both audio and video recordings (Chesney and Citron, 2018). The deepfake technique can be used to create videos of people saying and doing things that they never did, by swapping their faces, bodies, and other features onto videos of people who did say or do what is portrayed in the video. This initially emerged as fake celebrity pornography, but academics have demonstrated that the technique can also be used to create fake political videos (BBC News, 2017). The potential effect of such technology, when coupled with the virality of social networks, for the dissemination of false content is terrifying. Substantial funding is focused on battling deepfakes (Villasenor, 2019). An ethical, societal, and legal response to this technology has yet to emerge.

Compliance and Security

Security is well suited to the application of AI, because the domain exists to detect the rare exception, and vigilance in this regard is a key strength of all computerized algorithms. One current application of AI in security is automated license plate reading, which relies on basic computer vision (Li et al., 2018). Because license plates conform to strict standards of size, color, shape, and location, the problem is well constrained and thus suitable for early AI.

Predictive policing has captured the public imagination, potentially due to popular representations in science fiction films such as *Minority Report* (Perry et al., 2013). State-of-the-art predictive policing technology identifies areas and times of increased risk of crime rather than identifying the victim or perpetrator (Kim et al., 2018). Police departments typically utilize such tools as part of larger strategies. However, implementations of these technologies can propagate racial, gender, and other kinds of profiling when based on historically biased datasets (Caliskan et al., 2017; Garcia, 2016) (see Chapter 1).

[3] See https://prisma-ai.com.

In the commercial sector, AI is finding increasing application in compliance. AI technologies can read e-mails, chat logs, and AI-transcribed phone calls in order to identify insider trading, theft, or other abuses. Research efforts are under way to identify theft, diversion, and abuse from all manner of dispensing devices.

Note that many of these applications are also controversial for privacy concerns and surveillance capacity and scope, in addition to their potential to propagate racial, gender, and sexual orientation biases (see Chapter 1). Large gaps remain in the goal of aligning population and cultural expectations and preferences with the regulation and legislation of privacy, which is a subject covered in more detail in Chapter 7.

Space Exploration

Space exploration is another area—an unusual and interesting one, at that—in which AI has been employed. One might provocatively claim that there is a planet in our solar system (probably) populated exclusively by robots, and that one of those robots is artificially intelligent. On Mars, NASA has sent robot rovers to explore the surface. In Curiosity, the most recent rover, NASA included a navigation and target acquisition AI called AEGIS (Autonomous Exploration for Gathering Increased Science System) (Chien and Wagstaff, 2017; Francis et al., 2017). This AI allows the rover to autonomously select rocks likely to yield successful observational studies. The necessity for AI derives from the communication latency between an Earth-based controller and the distant rover that can cause inefficiency or danger, such as in response to unexpected volcanic eruptions. The NASA Jet Propulsion Laboratory is currently designing an autonomous AI that will enable a self-sufficient probe to explore the methane subsurface oceans of Titan and Europa (Troesch et al., 2018).

AI BY INDIVIDUAL FUNCTIONS

While the concept of an "intelligent machine" has interested philosophers at least as far back as Descartes, the most popular conception was first proposed by Alan Turing (1950). Turing proposed that the question of a machine's ability to think is not constructive, and instead one ought to test whether or not a machine can perform as well as a human in conversation. This has come to be known as the "Turing test," which still serves as the prototype litmus test for many AI tasks. Indeed, in all AI areas—from specialized reasoning, to speech, to vision—researchers attempt to outperform humans using AI.

Where the preceding section considers the many current applications of AI, in this section we consider the components, or faculties, that comprise an AI system or tool. The core of AI is reasoning, whether that is achieved symbolically, probabilistically, or through mathematical optimization. But before an AI system or tool can reason, a representation of the domain of reasoning must first be made. For instance, to play chess, the computer must somehow hold the current state of the board, the rules of the game, and the desired outcome in its memory. Effectively structuring or representing reality is often the key to AI. A key observation is that these representations are often layered; stated differently, an effective representation comprises a hierarchy of abstractions.

Consider chess again: the base representation is the field and players, the next layer may be particular formations of pieces, the next evolving set plays, and so on. By reasoning at higher and higher levels of abstraction, AIs can achieve effectiveness without requiring true human intelligence. George V. Neville-Neil writes:

> We have had nearly 50 years of human/computer competition in the game of chess but does that mean any of those computers are intelligent? No, it does not—for two reasons. The first is that chess is not a test of intelligence; it is the test of a particular skill—of playing chess. The second reason is that thinking chess was a test of intelligence was based on a false cultural premise that brilliant chess players were brilliant minds, more gifted than those around them. Yes, many intelligent people excel at chess, but chess, or any other single skill, does not denote intelligence. (Neville-Neil, 2017)

Thus, an AI system typically receives input from sensors (afferent systems) and operates in the environment through displays/effectors (efferent systems). These capture reality, represent and reason over it, and then affect reality, respectively. The standard representation of this is a keyboard and mouse as inputs, a central processing unit (CPU) and data storage units for processing, and a monitor for output to a human user. A robot with AI may contain sonar for inputs, a CPU, and motorized wheels for its outputs. More sophisticated AIs, such as a personal assistant, may have to interpret and synthesize data from multiple sensors such as a microphone, a camera, and other data inputs in order to interact with a user through a speaker or screen. As each of the effectors, representations, and AI reasoning systems improves, it becomes more seamless, or human-like, in its capabilities.

AI Technologies

AI in the guise of "the next impossible thing computers will do," almost by definition, occupies the forefront of technology at whatever time it is considered. As a result, AI is often conflated with its enabling technology. For instance, in the

1980s there were hardware machines, called Lisp machines, specifically created to execute the AI algorithms of the day (Phillips, 1999). Today, technologies such as graphics processing units (GPUs), the Internet of Things (IoT), and cloud computing are closely associated with AI, while not being AI in and of themselves. In this section, we briefly review and clarify.

GPUs and, recently, tensor processing units (TPUs) are computer hardware elements specialized to perform mathematical calculations rapidly. They are much like the widely understood CPUs, but rather than being generalized so that they are able to perform any operation, GPUs and TPUs are specialized to perform calculations more useful to machine learning algorithms and hence AI systems. The operations in question are linear algebra operations such as matrix multiplication. The GPUs and TPUs enable AI operations.

IoT is the movement to collect sensor data from all manner of physical devices and make them available on the Internet. Examples abound including lightbulbs, doors, cameras, and cars; theoretically anything that can be manufactured might be included. IoT is associated with AI because the data that flow from these devices comprise the afferent arm of AI systems. As IoT devices proliferate, the range of domains to which AI can be applied expands. In the emergent Internet of Medical Things, patient-generated physiological measurements (e.g., pulse oximeters and sphygmomanometers) are added to the data collected from these "environmental" devices. It will be crucial that we "understand the limitations of these technologies to avoid inappropriate reliance on them for diagnostic purposes" (Deep Blue, 2019; Freedson et al., 2012) and appreciate the social risks potentially created by "intervention-generated inequalities" (Veinot et al., 2018).

Cloud computing abstracts computation by separating the computer services from the proximate need for a physical computer. Large technology companies such as Amazon, Google, Microsoft, and others have assembled vast warehouses filled with computers. These companies sell access to their computers and, more specifically, the services they perform over the Internet, such as databases, queues, and translation. In this new landscape, a user requiring a computer service can obtain that service without owning the computer. The major advantage of this is that it relieves the user of the need to obtain and manage costly and complex infrastructure. Thus, small and relatively technologically unsophisticated users, including individuals and companies, may benefit from advanced technology. Most data now are collected in clouds, which means that the complex computing hardware (such as GPU machines) and services (such as natural language processing [NLP]) needed for AI are easily obtainable. Cloud computing also creates challenges in multinational data storage and other international law complexities, some of which are briefly discussed in Chapter 7.

Reasoning and Learning

Computers are recognized as superior machines for their rigorous logic and expansive calculation capabilities, but the point at which formal logic becomes "thinking" or "intelligence" has proven difficult to pinpoint (Turing, 1950). Expert systems that have been successful in military and industrial settings have captured the imagination of the public with the Deep Blue versus Kasparov chess matches. More recently, Google DeepMind's AlphaGo defeated Lee Sedol at the game Go, using deep learning methods (Wikipedia, 2019a).

Adaptive Learning

A defining feature of a machine learning system is that the programmer does not instruct the computer to perform a specific task but, rather, instructs the computer how to learn a desired task from a provided dataset. Programs such as deep learning, reinforcement learning, gradient boosting, and many others comprise the set of machine learning algorithms. The programmer also provides a set of data and describes a task, such as images of cats and dogs and the task to distinguish the two. The computer then executes the machine learning algorithm upon the provided data, creating a new, derivative program specific to the task at hand. This is called training. That program, usually called the model, is then applied to a real-world problem. In a sense, then, we can say that the computer has created the model.

The machine learning process described above comprises two phases, training and application. Once learning is complete, it is assumed that the model is unchanging. However, an unchanging model is not strictly necessary. A machine learning algorithm can alternatively continue to supplement the original training data with data and performance encountered in application and then retrain itself with the augmented set. Such algorithms are called adaptive because the model adapts over time.

All static models in health care degrade in performance over time as characteristics of the environment and targets change, and this is one of the fundamental distinctions between industrial and health care processes (addressed in more detail in Chapter 6). However, adaptive learning algorithms are one of the family of methods that can adapt to this constantly changing environment, but they create special challenges for regulation, because there is no fixed artifact to certify or approve. To draw a health care analogy, the challenge would be like the U.S. Food and Drug Administration (FDA) attempting to approve a molecule that evolved over time. Although it is possible to certify that an adaptive algorithm performs to specifications at any given moment and that the algorithm by which it learns is sound, it is an open question as to whether the future states of an adaptive algorithm can be known to perform at the same or better specification—that is, whether it can be declared safe. FDA has issued guidance that it will approve adapting devices, but significant challenges remain in this domain. For further discussion of these challenges in the regulatory and legislative context, see Chapter 7.

Reinforcement Learning

Understood best in the setting of video games, where the goal is to finish with the most points, reinforcement learning examines each step and rewards positive choices that the player makes based on the resulting proximity to a target end state. Each additional move performed affects the subsequent behavior of the automated player, known as the agent in reinforcement learning semantics. The agent may learn to avoid certain locations to prevent falls or crashes, touch tokens, or dodge arrows to maximize its score. Reinforcement learning with positive rewards and negative repercussions is how robot vacuum cleaners learn about walls, stairs, and even furniture that moves from time to time (Jonsson, 2019).

Computer Vision

Computer vision is a domain of AI that attempts to replicate the human visual apparatus (see Chapter 1). The machine should be able to segment, identify, and track objects in still and moving images. For example, some automobile camera systems continuously monitor for speed limit signs, extract that information, and display it on the dashboard. More advanced systems can identify other vehicles, pedestrians, and local geographic features. As noted above, combining similar computer vision systems with reasoning systems is necessary for the general problem of autonomous driving.

Language and Conversation

The language and conversation domain of AI can be segmented into the interpretation and generation of spoken and written words (see Chapter 1). Textual chatbots that assist humans in tasks such as purchases and queries is one active frontier. Today, spoken words are mainly encountered in the consumer realm in virtual assistants such as Alexa, Siri, Cortana, and others, such as those embedded in cars. These AI systems typically convert audio data into textual data for processing, apply NLP or natural language understanding for the task at hand, generate a textual response, and then convert that into audio. While full conversations are currently beyond the state of the art, simple intent or question-and-answer tasks are now commercially available.

Touch and Movement

Early applications of the robotics domain of AI appeared in industrial manufacturing, autopilots and autonomous vehicles, and home robots such as the Roomba, with additional research having gone into humanoid and canine-like robots. Making four-legged robots walk, run, and recover from falls, in particular, has been vexing. Building on the adaptive learning discussion above, the use of simulated data to speed robot training, which augments but does not fully replace the engineered control mechanisms, is a recent advance in robotics (Hwangbo, 2019).

Smell and Taste

Electronic noses are still marginal but increasingly useful technology (Athamneh et al., 2008). They couple chemosensors with classification systems in order to detect simple and complex smells. There is not yet significant research into an electronic tongue, although early research similar to that concerning electronic noses exists. Additionally, there is early research on computer generation of taste or digital gustation, similar to the computer generation of speech; however, no applications of this technology are apparent today.

KEY STAKEHOLDERS

It is not too strong to assert that AI is the fruit of U.S. government–funded research, carried out initially by programs such as the Defense Advanced Research Projects Agency (DARPA), which funded academic pioneers at the Massachusetts Institute of Technology (MIT), Stanford University, and Carnegie Mellon University in the 1960s. However, as the utility and impact of these technologies has accelerated, a number of other countries have made significant investments in AI. Furthermore, by providing a constant and deep market for AI technologies through energy, space exploration, and national defense, the governments of the United States, China, the European Union, and other countries have enabled AI to take root and thrive.

United States

The United States has been coordinating strategic research and development (R&D) investment in AI technologies for a number of years. In reaction to the Soviet Union's launch of Sputnik in 1957, the U.S. government founded DARPA, which poured significant funding into computing, resulting in the early advancement of AI as well as the Internet. Most foundational AI technology was supported through DARPA funding, beginning in the 1960s.

In 2016, DARPA's AI R&D plan established a number of strategic categories and aims for federal investment, which included recommendations for developing an implementation framework and workforce for AI R&D. The National Institutes of Health has also articulated strategic goals for AI within its Strategic Plan for Data Science, and the U.S. Department of Health and Human Services in conjunction with the Robert Wood Johnson Foundation commissioned a report on how AI will shape the future of public health, community health, and health care delivery (JASON, 2017; NIH, 2018).

In 2018, DARPA announced "AI Next," a $2 billion program to support the further development of AI. Additionally, under the Trump administration, the National Science and Technology Council established the Select Committee on Artificial Intelligence, which is tasked with publicizing and coordinating federal R&D efforts related to AI (White House Office of Science and Technology Policy, 2018). In February 2019, President Donald Trump issued an Executive Order 13859, "Maintaining American Leadership in Artificial Intelligence," which charged the Select Committee on Artificial Intelligence with the generation of a report and a plan (Trump, 2019). This plan, released in June 2019, outlines the national governmental strategy for AI R&D, which includes a broad scope of seven focus areas to guide interagency collaboration, education and training programs, and directed funding programs (NSTC, 2019).

China

China is a recent but energetic participant in the AI community. In 2017, Chinese inventors filed more AI patents than any other country (World Intellectual Property Organization, 2018). In addition, although the specific amount of government funding that China has allocated for AI research is difficult to know, CBInsights (2018) estimated that China represented 48 percent of global AI research funding in 2018, dwarfing other countries' contributions to the field. The Boston Consulting Group reached similar conclusions, noting that up to 85 percent of Chinese companies have either adopted AI processes or are running pilot initiatives to do so. The report could say the same for just approximately 50 percent of companies in the United States, France, Germany, and Switzerland and 40 percent of companies in Austria and Japan (Duranton et al., 2018).

China has a number of advantages that make AI progress more feasible. Foremost, the government actively supports companies' pushes into AI, pursuing its stated goal of becoming the world leader in the field by 2030 (Mozur, 2017). Additionally, data are more available in China, as there are at least 700 million

Internet-connected smartphone users (Gerbert et al., 2018). Finally, in the health care market in particular, Chinese privacy laws are more lax than in the United States (Simonite, 2019).

European Union and the United Kingdom

In the past decade, Europe has developed a robust AI ecosystem, placing it well within the ranks of the United States and China. With an equal balance of corporate non-R&D and R&D entities, the region is second to the United States for most players in the space (EU Commission Joint Research Centre, 2018). However, unlike the United States and China where government funding has propelled the industry, AI in Europe stems from accelerating investment from private equity and venture capital firms (Ernst and Young, 2019).

To increase global competitiveness there has been a recent uptick of national attention and investment in AI (Ernst and Young, 2019). Several countries, namely Germany and France, have written national AI strategies, although each differs in motivation and approach. Dedicating €3 billion to AI research and development, Germany aims to expand the integration of AI in business processes. Comparatively, the French plan focuses on the potential of AI for defense and security, transportation, and health (Franke and Sartori, 2019).

Ultimately, the European Union sees the strength in advancing its AI agenda through coordination among its member states. In April 2018, 25 EU countries pledged to work together to boost "Europe's technology and industrial capacity in AI" while "addressing socio-economic challenges and ensuring an adequate legal and ethical framework" (European Union Member States Representatives, 2018). Adhering to its commitment to ethics, the European Union released guidelines in April 2019 for the development of trustworthy AI solutions that could foreseeably shape the regulation of AI in the European Union and overseas (EU Commission, 2019).

United Kingdom

It is unsurprising that the United Kingdom leads Europe in AI. As previously discussed, Turing's efforts in the 1950s planted the seeds for the country's leadership in this area, which, for the most part, has been cultivated by the country's thriving startup community (UK House of Commons, Science and Technology Committee, 2016; UK House of Lords, 2018). More recently, the government has engaged in improving the country's AI standing through financial support and the launch of several AI initiatives aimed at exploring and preparing for the sustainable procurement of AI technology. Building on the findings of these initiatives, the United Kingdom in 2018 unveiled its AI Sector Deal, a broad industry plan to stimulate innovation, build digital infrastructure, and develop workforce competency in data science, engineering, and mathematics (UK Government, 2019).

Academic

In the United States, MIT, Stanford, and Carnegie Mellon pioneered AI research in the 1960s, and these, and many others, continue to do so today. Cambridge University in the United Kingdom and Tsinghua University in China also produce leading AI research. Also important was the role of commercially supported research institutes, such as Nokia Bell Labs (formerly Bell Laboratories), which supported much of Claude E. Shannon's pioneering work in digital communications and cryptography, and Xerox PARC, which continues with laboratories such as Microsoft Research and Facebook's Building X (Shannon, 1940; Xerox, 2019). Indeed, there is significant tension between commercial facilities and academic institutions regarding talent (Reuters, 2016). Uber, for instance, at one point recruited almost the entire computer vision faculty of Carnegie Mellon, to the university's consternation.

AI-specific conferences, such as the Conference on Neural Information Processing Systems[4] (NeurIPS), the preeminent academic AI conference, attract thousands of abstract submissions annually. Furthermore, the number of AI submissions to journals and conferences that are not AI specific is increasing annually.

Commercial Sector

Programmers have always developed AI systems in order to achieve specific goals, and this inherent usefulness of the technology has frequently spawned or spun out into commercial activity. This activity has been focused in the technology sector, but a significant development during 2017 and 2018 was the focus on the digital transformation of other industries seeking to lay a foundation so that they might capitalize on the advantages of AI. Health care is one such sector.

In addition to the academic participants in the founding Dartmouth Summer Research Project on Artificial Intelligence, the sole commercial participant was Trenchard More of IBM. Since the 1956 meeting, IBM has maintained an active role in the AI community. In 2011, IBM captured the public imagination by winning *Jeopardy!* with its AI system Watson (Wikipedia, 2019b). Watson has evolved into a commercially available family of products and has also been deployed with variable success in the clinical setting (Freeman, 2017; Herper, 2017).

---

[4] See https://nips.cc.

Many of the most successful technology companies, including Amazon, Facebook, Google, Microsoft, Tesla, and Uber, are deeply reliant on AI within their products and have contributed significantly to its expansion.

In addition to these more established companies, the past 5 years have witnessed something akin to a Cambrian explosion of the number of startups in the AI space. A good, if instantly outdated, reference is CBInsight's AI 100, which lists the 100 most promising startups in the field (CBInsights, 2019).

Professional Societies

In addition, a number of civil and professional societies exist that provide leadership and policy in the AI space. These include, but are not limited to, those listed below.

IEEE (Institute of Electrical and Electronics Engineers) is the professional society for engineers, scientists, and allied professionals, including computer scientists, software developers, information technology professionals, physicists, and medical doctors. IEEE has formed several societies, such as the Signal Processing Society and Computational Intelligence Society, both of which produce publications relating to AI.

The Association for Computing Machinery (ACM) is a professional society for computing educators, researchers, and professionals. A special interest group on AI, known as SIGAI, exists within ACM.

The Electronic Frontier Foundation is a nonprofit agency concerned with digital liberties and rights. It considers AI ethics and laws and aims to protect the rights of users and creators of AI technology.

Notably in health care, the American Medical Association (AMA) passed its first policy recommendation on augmented intelligence in June 2018. The policy states that AMA will "promote [the] development of thoughtfully designed, high-quality, clinically validated health care AI" (AMA, 2018). Furthermore, the AMA *Journal of Ethics* dedicated its February 2019 issue to AI in health care.

Nonprofits

As a reaction to an increasing concentration of AI within the commercial sector, OpenAI was founded as a nonprofit research entity. Along the same vein as the open source movement, which maintains the general availability of software, OpenAI's mission is to promote the accessibility of AI intellectual property to all for the purposes of developing technology that services the public good (OpenAI, 2019).

Public–Private Partnerships

There are other notable public–private partnerships that have recently formed to work in the AI sector to bridge collaboration in these spaces. For example, Partnership for AI is a large consortium of more than 90 for-profit and nonprofit institutions in multiple countries to share best practices and further research in AI, to advance public understanding of AI, and to promote socially benevolent applications in AI (Partnership on AI, 2018). Another example is AINow, which is hosted by New York University but receives funding from a variety of large for-profit and nonprofit institutions interested in AI development.

KEY CONSIDERATIONS

In summary, we would like to highlight key considerations for future AI applications and endeavors, which can be learned by examining AI's history and evaluating AI up to the current era.

- As described in more detail in Chapters 3 and 4, history has shown that AI has gone through multiple cycles of emphasis and disillusionment in use. It is critical that all stakeholders be aware of and actively seek to educate and address public expectations and understanding of AI (and associated technologies) in order to manage hype and establish reasonable expectations, which will enable AI to be applied in effective ways that have reasonable opportunities for sustained success.
- Integration of reinforcement learning into various elements of the health care system will be critical in order to develop a robust, continuously improving health care industry and to show value for the large efforts invested in data collection.
- Support and emphasis for open source and free tools and technologies for use and application of AI will be important to reduce cost and maintain wide use of AI technologies as the domain transitions from exponential growth to a future plateau stage of use.
- The domain needs strong patient and consumer engagement and empowerment to ensure that preferences, concerns, and expectations are transmitted and ethically, morally, and appropriately addressed by AI stakeholder users.
- Large-scale development of AI technologies in industries outside of health care should be carefully examined for opportunities for incorporation of those advances within health care. Evaluation of these technologies should include consideration for whether they could effectively translate to the processes and workflows in health care.

REFERENCES

AMA (American Medical Association). 2018. *AMA passes first policy recommendations on augmented intelligence.* Press release. https://www.ama-assn.org/press-center/press-releases/ama-passes-first-policy-recommendations-augmented-intelligence.

Amani, F. A., and A. M. Fadlalla. 2017. Data mining applications in accounting: A review of the literature and organizing framework. *International Journal of Accounting Information Systems* 24:32–58. https://doi.org/10.1016/j.accinf.2016.12.004.

Athamneh, A. I., B. W. Zoecklein, and K. Mallikarjunan. 2008. Electronic nose evaluation of cabernet sauvignon fruit maturity. *Journal of Wine Research* 19: 69–80.

BBC News. 2017. *Fake Obama created using AI video tool.* https://www.youtube.com/watch?v=AmUC4m6w1wo.

Bookstaber, R. 2007. *A demon of our own design: Markets, hedge funds, and the perils of financial innovation.* New York: John Wiley & Sons.

Buchanan, B. G. 2005. A (very) brief history of artificial intelligence. *AI Magazine* 26(4):53–60.

Caliskan, A., J. J. Bryson, and A. Narayanan. 2017. Semantics derived automatically from language corpora contain human-like biases. *Science* 356:183–186.

Case, N. 2018. How to become a centaur. *MIT Press.* https://doi.org/10.21428/61b2215c.

CBInsights. 2018. *Artificial intelligence trends to watch in 2018.* https://www.cbinsights.com/research/report/artificial-intelligence-trends-2018 (accessed November 5, 2019).

CBInsights. 2019. *AI100: The artificial intelligence startups redefining industries.* https://www.cbinsights.com/research/artificial-intelligence-top-startups.

Chen, J. H., and R. B. Altman. 2015. Data-mining electronic medical records for clinical order recommendations: Wisdom of the crowd or tyranny of the mob? *AMIA Joint Summits on Translational Science Proceedings.* Pp. 435–439. https://www.ncbi.nlm.nih.gov/pmc/articles/PMC4525236.

Chesney, R., and D. K. Citron. 2018. Deep fakes: A looming challenge for privacy, democracy, and national security. *California Law Review* 107. https://dx.doi.org/10.2139/ssrn.3213954.

Chien, S., and K. L. Wagstaff. 2017. Robotic space exploration agents. *Science Robotics* 2(7). https://doi.org/10.1126/scirobotics.aan4831.

Deep Blue. 2019. *IBM's 100 icons of progress.* http://www-03.ibm.com/ibm/history/ibm100/us/en/icons/deepblue.

Duranton, S., J. Erlebach, and M. Pauly. 2018. *Mind the (AI) gap: Leadership makes the difference.* Boston, MA: Boston Consulting Group. https://media-publications.bcg.com/france/Mind-the-(AI)-Gap-Press-deckVF.pdf.

Ernst & Young. 2019. *Artificial intelligence in Europe–Germany: Outlook for 2019 and beyond.* Prepared for Microsoft. https://www.ey.com/Publication/vwLUAssets/ey-artificial-intelligence-in-europe/$FILE/ey-artificial-intelligence-in-europe-germany.pdf.

EU Commission. 2019. *Ethics Guidelines for Trustworthy Artificial Intelligence.* https://ec.europa.eu/digital-single-market/en/news/ethics-guidelines-trustworthy-ai.

European Commission Joint Research Centre. 2018. *Artificial intelligence: A European perspective.* http://publications.jrc.ec.europa.eu/repository/bitstream/JRC113826/ai-flagship-report-online.pdf.

European Union Member States Representatives. 2018. *EU declaration on cooperation on artificial intelligence.* https://ec.europa.eu/jrc/communities/en/node/1286/document/eu-declaration-cooperation-artificial-intelligence.

Francis, R., T. Estlin, G. Doran, S. Johnstone, D. Gaines, V. Verma, M. Burl, J. Frydenvang, S. Montano, R. C. Wiens, S. Schaffer, O. Gasnault, L. DeFlores, D. Blaney, and B. Bornstein. 2017. AEGIS autonomous targeting for ChemCam on Mars Science Laboratory: Deployment and results of initial science team use. *Science Robotics* 2(7). https://doi.org/10.1126/scirobotics.aan4582.

Franke, U., and P. Sartori. 2019. *Machine politics: Europe and the AI revolution.* Policy brief. https://www.ecfr.eu/publications/summary/machine_politics_europe_and_the_ai_revolution.

Freedson, P., H. R. Bowles, R. Troiano, and W. Haskell. 2012. Assessment of physical activity using wearable monitors: Recommendations for monitor calibration and use in the field. *Medicine and Science in Sports and Exercise* 44:S1–S4. https://doi.org/10.1249/MSS.0b013e3182399b7e.

Freeman, D. H. 2017. A reality check for IBM's AI ambitions. *MIT Technology Review.* https://www.technologyreview.com/s/607965/a-reality-check-for-ibms-ai-ambitions.

Frohlich, H., R. Balling, N. Beerenwinkel, O. Kohlbacher, S. Kumar, T. Lengauer, M. H. Maathuis, Y. Moreau, S. A. Murphy, T. M. Przytycka, M. Rebhan, H. Rost, A. Schuppert, M. Schwab, R. Spang, D. Stekhoven, J. Sun, A. Weber, D. Ziemek, and B. Zupan. 2018. From hype to reality: Data science enabling personalized medicine. *BMC Medicine* 16:150.

Garcia, M. 2016. Racist in the machine: The disturbing implications of algorithmic bias. *World Policy Journal* 33:111–117.

Gartner, Inc. 2018. *5 trends emerge in the Gartner Hype Cycle for Emerging Technologies.* SmarterWithGartner. https://www.gartner.com/smarterwithgartner/5-trends-emerge-in-gartner-hype-cycle-for-emerging-technologies-2018.

Gerbert, P., M. Reeves, S. Ransbotham, D. Kiron, and M. Spira. 2018. Global competition with AI in business: How China differs. *MIT Sloan Management Review.* https://sloanreview.mit.edu/article/global-competition-of-ai-in-business-how-china-differs (accessed November 8, 2019).

Halevy, A., P. Norvig, and F. Pereira. 2009. The unreasonable effectiveness of data. *IEEE Intelligent Systems* 24:8–12. https://static.googleusercontent.com/media/research.google.com/en//pubs/archive/35179.pdf.

Haraway, D. 2000. A cyborg manifesto. In *The Cybercultures Reader*, edited by D. Bell and B. Kennedy. London, UK, and New York: Routledge.

Hastie, T., R. Tibshirani, and J. Friedman. 2001. *The elements of statistical learning: Data mining, inference, and prediction.* New York: Springer-Verlag.

Herper, M. 2017. MD Anderson benches IBM Watson in setback for artificial intelligence in medicine. *Forbes.* https://www.forbes.com/sites/matthewherper/2017/02/19/md-anderson-benches-ibm-watson-in-setback-for-artificial-intelligence-in-medicine/#54ada2e83774.

Hutson, M. 2017. A matter of trust. *Science* 358:1375–1377. https://doi.org/10.1126/science.358.6369.1375.

Hwangbo, J., J. Lee, A. Dosovitskiy, D. Bellicoso, V. Tsounis, V. Koltun, and M. Hutter. 2019. Learning agile and dynamic motor skills for legged robots. *Science Robotics* 4:13.

Interiano, M., K. Kazemi, L. Wang, J. Yang, Z. Yu, and N. L. Komarova. 2018. Musical trends and predictability of success in contemporary songs in and out of the top charts. *Royal Society Open Science* 5:171274.

JASON. 2017. *Artificial intelligence for health and health care.* https://www.healthit.gov/sites/default/files/jsr-17-task-002_aiforhealthandhealthcare12122017.pdf.

Johnson, M., and A. H. Vera. 2019. No AI is an island: The case for teaming intelligence. *AI Magazine* 40:17–27.

Jonsson, A. 2019. Deep reinforcement learning in medicine. *Kidney Disease (Basel)* 5(1):18–22.

Kim, S., P. Joshi, P. S. Kalsi, and P. Taheri. 2018. *Crime analysis through machine learning.* 9th Annual Information Technology, Electronics and Mobile Communication Conference, Vancouver.

Kline, R. R. 2011. Cybernetics, automata studies, and the Dartmouth Conference on Artificial Intelligence. *IEEE Annals of the History of Computing* 33(4):5–16.

Kolko, J. 2018. 5 questions we should be asking about automation and jobs. *Harvard Business Review.* https://hbr.org/2018/12/5-questions-we-should-be-asking-about-automation-and-jobs (accessed November 5, 2019).

Krizhevsky, A., I. Sutskever, and G. E. Hinton. 2012. *ImageNet classification with deep convolutional neural networks.* Presented at 25th International Conference on Neural Information Processing Systems. https://papers.nips.cc/paper/4824-imagenet-classification-with-deep-convolutional-neural-networks.pdf (accessed November 8, 2019).

Laris, M. 2018. Raising the bar: Uber details shortcomings in self-driving car that killed pedestrian. *The Washington Post.* https://www.washingtonpost.com/local/trafficandcommuting/raising-the-bar-uber-details-shortcomings-in-self-driving-car-that-killed-pedestrian/2018/11/01/5152bc54-dd42-11e8-b3f0-62607289efee_story.html.

Li, H., P. Wang, M. You, and C. Shenb. 2018. Reading car license plates using deep neural networks. *Image and Vision Computing* 27:14–23.

Licklider, J. C. R. 1960. Man-computer symbiosis. *IRE Transactions on Human Factors in Electronics* 1:4–11.

Lighthill, J. 1973. Artificial intelligence: A general survey. In *Artificial Intelligence: A Paper Symposium.* Science Research Council, UK.

Lowenstein, R. 2011. *When genius failed.* New York: Random House.

McCarthy, J. 1958. *Programs with common sense.* Paper presented at Symposium on Mechanization of Thought Processes at National Physical Laboratory, Teddington, UK.

McCarthy, J. C. 1959. *Programs with common sense.* http://www-formal.stanford.edu/jmc/mcc59/mcc59.html.

McCarthy, J. 1974. Review of "Artificial Intelligence: A General Survey," by Professor Sir James Lighthill. *Artificial Intelligence* 5:317–322.

McCarthy, J., M. L. Minsky, N. Rochester, and C. E. Shannon. 2006. A proposal for the Dartmouth Summer Research Project on Artificial Intelligence, August 31, 1955. *AI Magazine* 27(4):12–14.

Mervis, J. 2017. Not so fast. *Science* 358:1370–1374.

Metz, C. 2019. Turing award won by 3 pioneers in artificial intelligence. *The New York Times.* https://www.nytimes.com/2019/03/27/technology/turing-award-ai.html.

Micallef, K. 2016. Airbus generates bionic design for flights of the future. *Redshift.* https://www-p7.autodesk.com/redshift/bionic-design.

Miller, R. A., H. E. Pople, and J. D. Myers. 1982. Internist-1, an experimental computer-based diagnostic consultant for general internal medicine. *New England Journal of Medicine* 307:468–476.

Moor, J. 2006. The Dartmouth College Artificial Intelligence Conference: The next fifty years. *AI Magazine* 27(4):87–91.

Mordvintsev, A., M. Tyka, and C. Olah. 2015. Deepdream. *GitHub.* https://github. com/google/deepdream.

Mostafa, A. N., C. Pranamesh, S. Anuj, B. G. Stephen, and H. Mingyi. 2018. Evaluating the reliability, coverage, and added value of crowdsourced traffic incident reports from Waze. *Transportation Research Record: Journal of the Transportation Research Board* 2672:34–43.

Mozur, P. 2017. Beijing wants A.I. to be made in China by 2030. *The New York Times.* https://www.nytimes.com/2017/07/20/business/china-artificial-intelligence. html (accessed November 8, 2019).

Murphy, K. P. 2013. *Machine learning: A probabilistic perspective.* Cambridge, MA: MIT Press.

Neville-Neil, G.V. 2017. The chess player who couldn't pass the salt. *Communications of the ACM* 60(4):24–25. https://doi.org/10.1145/3055277.

Newquist, H. P. 1994. *The brain makers: The history of artificial intelligence.* Upper Saddle River, NJ: Prentice Hall.

NHTSA (National Highway Traffic Safety Administration). 2018. *2017 fatal motor vehicle crashes: Overview.* Traffic Safety Facts Research Note DOT HS 812 603. Washington, DC: U.S. Department of Transportation. https:// crashstats.nhtsa.dot.gov/Api/Public/ViewPublication/812603 (accessed November 8, 2019).

NIH (National Institutes of Health). 2018. *NIH strategic plan for data science.* https://datascience.nih.gov/strategicplan (accessed December 7, 2019).

Noor, A. K. 2017. AI and the future of machine design. *Mechanical Engineering* 139(10):38–43.

NRC (National Research Council). 1966. *Language and machines: Computers in translation and linguistics: A report.* Washington, DC: National Academy Press. https://doi.org/10.17226/9547.

NSTC (National Science and Technology Council). 2019. *The national artificial intelligence research and development strategic plan: 2019 update.* https:// www.nitrd.gov/pubs/National-AI-RD-Strategy-2019.pdf (accessed December 13, 2019).

OpenAI. 2019. *OpenAI.* https://openai.com.

Partnership on AI. 2018. *Meet the partners.* https://www.partnershiponai.org/partners.

Perry, W. L., B. McInnis, C. Price, S. Smith, and J. S. Hollywood. 2013. *Predictive policing: The role of crime forecasting in law enforcement operations.* Santa Monica, CA: RAND Corporation. https://www.rand.org/content/dam/rand/pubs/research_reports/RR200/RR233/RAND_RR233.pdf.

Phillips, E. M. 1999. *If it works, it's not AI: A commercial look at artificial intelligence startups.* M.S. thesis, Massachusetts Institute of Technology.

Plummer, L. 2017. This is how Netflix's top-secret recommendation system works. *Wired.* https://www.wired.co.uk/article/how-do-netflixs-algorithms-work-machine-learning-helps-to-predict-what-viewers-will-like.

Reuters. 2016. One year after announcing pact, the Uber-Carnegie Mellon Partnership is stalled. *Fortune.* http://fortune.com/2016/03/21/uber-carnegie-mellon-partnership.

Rosenblatt, F. 1958. The perceptron: A probabilistic model for information storage and organization in the brain. *Psychological Review* 65(6):386–408.

Seth, S. 2019. The world of high-frequency algorithmic trading. *Investopedia.* https://www.investopedia.com/articles/investing/091615/world-high-frequency-algorithmic-trading.asp.

Shannon, C. E. 1940. *A symbolic analysis of relay and switching circuits.* Cambridge, MA: Massachusetts Institute of Technology.

Shortliffe, E. H. 1974. *MYCIN: A rule-based computer program for advising physicians regarding antimicrobial therapy selection.* Palo Alto, CA: Stanford Artificial Intelligence Laboratory, Stanford University.

Simonite, T. 2019. How health care data and lax rules help China prosper in AI. *Wired.* https://www.wired.com/story/health-care-data-lax-rules-help-china-prosper-ai.

Sujit, S. B. 2015. *Effective test strategy for testing automotive software.* International Conference on Industrial Instrumentation and Control, Prune, India. https://www.semanticscholar.org/paper/Effective-test-strategy-for-testing-automotive-Barhate/aeff9109e6214cd4586af032e968c5daabf945d2.

Sumner, W. I. 1993. Review of Iliad and Quick Medical Reference for primary care providers. *Archives of Family Medicine* 2:87–95.

Topol, E. 2019. *Deep medicine: How artificial intelligence can make healthcare human again.* New York: Basic Books.

Troesch, M., S. Chien, Y. Chao, J. Farrara, J. Girton, and J. Dunlap. 2018. Autonomous control of marine floats in the presence of dynamic, uncertain ocean currents. *Robotics and Autonomous Systems* 108:100–114.

Trump, D. 2019. Executive Order 13859: Maintaining American leadership in artificial intelligence. *Federal Register* 84(3967):3967–3972. https://www.federalregister.gov/documents/2019/02/14/2019-02544/maintaining-american-leadership-in-artificial-intelligence.

Turing, A. M. 1950. Computing machinery and intelligence. *Mind* 49:433–460.

UK Government. 2019. *AI sector deal*. Policy paper. https://www.gov.uk/government/publications/artificial-intelligence-sector-deal/ai-sector-deal.

UK House of Commons, Science and Technology Committee. 2016. *Robotics and artificial intelligence*. Fifth Report of Session 2016–17. https://publications.parliament.uk/pa/cm201617/cmselect/cmsctech/145/145.pdf.

UK House of Lords, Select Committee on Artificial Intelligence. 2018. *AI in the UK: Ready, willing and able?* Report of Session 2017–19. https://publications.parliament.uk/pa/ld201719/ldselect/ldai/100/100.pdf.

Veinot, T. C., H. Mitchell, and J. S. Ancker. 2018. Good intentions are not enough: How informatics interventions can worsen inequality. *Journal of the American Medical Informatics Association* 25:1080–1088. https://doi.org/10.1093/jamia/ocy052.

Villasenor, J. 2019. Artificial intelligence, deepfakes, and the uncertain future of truth. *TechTank blog*, Brookings Institution. https://www.brookings.edu/blog/techtank/2019/02/14/artificial-intelligence-deepfakes-and-the-uncertain-future-of-truth.

Weiner, N. 1948. *Cybernetics: Or control and communication in the animal and the machine.* Cambridge, MA: MIT Press.

White House Office of Science and Technology Policy. 2018. *Summary of the 2018 White House summit on artificial intelligence for American industry.* https://www.whitehouse.gov/wp-content/uploads/2018/05/Summary-Report-of-White-House-AI-Summit.pdf.

Wikipedia. 2019a. *AlphaGo versus Lee Sedol.* https://en.wikipedia.org/wiki/AlphaGo_versus_Lee_Sedol.

Wikipedia. 2019b. *Watson (computer).* https://en.wikipedia.org/wiki/Watson (computer).

World Intellectual Property Organization. 2018. *World intellectual property indicators 2018.* https://www.wipo.int/edocs/pubdocs/en/wipo_pub_941_2018.pdf.

Xerox. 2019. *Xerox and PARC define the era of artificial intelligence.* https://www.xerox.com/en-kn/insights/artificial-intelligence-today.

Xu, N., and K. Wang. 2019. Adopting robot lawyer? The extending artificial intelligence robot lawyer technology acceptance model for legal industry by an exploratory study. *Journal of Management & Organization* 1–19. https://doi.org/10.1017/jmo.2018.81.

Yu, A. 2019. How Netflix uses AI, data science, and machine learning—From a product perspective. *Medium*. https://becominghuman.ai/how-netflix-uses-ai-and-machine-learning-a087614630fe.

Zhang, D. D., G. Peng, and Y. O. Yao. 2019. Artificial intelligence or intelligence augmentation? Unravelling the debate through an industry-level analysis. *SSRN*. https://dx.doi.org/10.2139/ssrn.3315946.

Zongjian, H., C. Jiannong, and L. Xuefeng. 2016. *SDVN: Enabling rapid network innovation for heterogeneous vehicular communication*. IEEE Network 30:10–15.

Suggested citation for Chapter 2: Fackler, J., and E. Jackson. 2020. Overview of current artificial intelligence. In *Artificial intelligence in health care: The hope, the hype, the promise, the peril*. Washington, DC: National Academy of Medicine.

3

HOW ARTIFICIAL INTELLIGENCE IS CHANGING HEALTH AND HEALTH CARE

Joachim Roski, Booz Allen Hamilton; Wendy Chapman, University of Melbourne; Jaimee Heffner, Fred Hutchinson Cancer Research Center; Ranak Trivedi, Stanford University; Guilherme Del Fiol, University of Utah; Rita Kukafka, Columbia University; Paul Bleicher, OptumLabs; Hossein Estiri, Harvard Medical School; Jeffrey Klann, Harvard University; and Joni Pierce, University of Utah

INTRODUCTION

This chapter explores the positive, transformative *potential* of artificial intelligence (AI) for health and health care. We discuss possible AI applications for patients and their families; the caregiving team of clinicians, public health professionals, and administrators; and health researchers (Roski et al., 2018). These solutions offer readers a *glimpse* of a possible future. We end by offering perspective about how AI might transform health care and by providing high-level considerations for addressing barriers to that future.

The health care industry has been investing for years in technology solutions, including AI. There have been some promising examples of health care AI solutions, but there are gaps in the evaluation of these tools in the peer-reviewed literature, and so it can be difficult to assess their impact. Also difficult to assess is the impact of combined solutions. Specific technology solutions when coupled may improve positive outcomes synergistically. For example, an AI solution may become exponentially more powerful if it is coupled with augmented reality, virtual reality, faster computing systems, robotics, or the Internet of Things (IoT). It is impossible to predict in advance.

This chapter presents the potential of AI solutions for patients and families, clinical care teams, public health program managers, business administrators, and researchers. Table 3-1 provides examples of the types of applications of AI for

TABLE 3-1 | Examples of Artificial Intelligence Applications for Stakeholder Groups

Use Case or User Group	Category	Examples of Applications	Technology
Patients and families	Health monitoring Benefit/risk assessment Disease prevention and management	• Devices and wearables • Smartphone and tablet apps, websites • Obesity reduction • Diabetes prevention and management • Emotional and mental health support	Machine learning, natural language processing (NLP), speech recognition, chatbots Conversational artificial intelligence (AI), NLP, speech recognition, chatbots
	Medication management	• Medication adherence	Robotic home telehealth
	Rehabilitation	• Stroke rehabilitation using apps and robots	Robotics
Clinician care teams	Early detection, prediction, and diagnostics tools	• Imaging for cardiac arrhythmia detection, retinopathy • Early cancer detection (e.g., melanoma)	Machine learning
	Surgical procedures	• Remote-controlled robotic surgery • AI-supported surgical roadmaps	Robotics, machine learning
	Precision medicine	• Personalized chemotherapy treatment	Supervised machine learning, reinforcement learning
	Patient safety	• Early detection of sepsis	Machine learning
Public health program managers	Identification of individuals at risk Population health	• Suicide risk identification using social media • Eldercare monitoring	Deep learning (convolutional and recurrent neural networks) Deep learning, geospatial pattern mining, machine learning
	Population health	• Air pollution epidemiology • Water microbe detection	Deep learning, geospatial pattern mining, machine learning
Business administrators	*International Classification of Diseases, 10th Revision* coding	• Automatic coding of medical records for reimbursement	Machine learning, NLP
	Fraud detection	• Health care billing fraud • Detection of unlicensed providers	Supervised, unsupervised, and hybrid machine learning
	Cybersecurity	• Protection of personal health information	Machine learning, NLP
	Physician management	• Assessment of physician competence	Machine learning, NLP
Researchers	Genomics Disease prediction Discovery	• Analysis of tumor genomics • Prediction of ovarian cancer • Drug discovery and design	Integrated cognitive computing Neural networks Machine learning, computer-assisted synthesis

these stakeholders. These examples are not exhaustive. The following sections explore the promise of AI in health care in more detail.

AI SOLUTIONS FOR PATIENTS AND FAMILIES

AI could soon play an important role in the self-management of chronic diseases such as cardiovascular diseases, diabetes, and depression. Self-management tasks can range from taking medications, modifying diet, and getting more physically active to care management, wound care, device management, and the delivery of injectables. Self-management can be assisted by AI solutions, including conversational agents, health monitoring and risk prediction tools, personalized adaptive interventions, and technologies to address the needs of individuals with disabilities. We describe these solutions in the following sections.

Conversational Agents

Conversational agents can engage in two-way dialogue with the user via speech recognition, natural language processing (NLP), natural language understanding, and natural language generation (Laranjo et al., 2018). AI is behind many of them. These interfaces may include text-based dialogue, spoken language, or both. They are called, variously, virtual agents, chatbots, or chatterbots. Some conversational agents present a human image (e.g., the image of a nurse or a coach) or nonhuman image (e.g., a robot or an animal) to provide a richer interactive experience. These are called embodied conversational agents (ECAs). These visible characters provide a richer and more convincing interactive experience than non-embodied voice-only agents such as Apple's Siri, Amazon's Alexa, or Microsoft's Cortana. The imagistic entities can communicate nonverbally through hand gestures and facial expressions.

In the "self-management" domain, conversational agents already exist to address depression, smoking cessation, asthma, and diabetes. Although many chatbots and ECAs exist, evaluation of these agents has, unfortunately, been limited (Fitzpatrick et al., 2017).

The future potential for conversational agents in self-management seems high. While simulating a real-world interaction, the agent may assess symptoms, report back on outputs from health monitoring, and recommend a course of action based on these varied inputs. Most adults say they would use an intelligent virtual coach or an intelligent virtual nurse to monitor health and symptoms at home. There is somewhat lower enthusiasm for mental health support delivered via this method (Accenture, 2018).

Social support improves treatment outcomes (Hixson et al., 2015; Wicks et al., 2012). Conversational agents can make use of humans' propensity to treat computers as social agents. Such support could be useful as a means of combating loneliness and isolation (Stahl and Coeckelbergh, 2016; Wetzel, 2018). In other applications, conversational agents can be used to increase the engagement and effectiveness of interventions for health behavior change. Most studies of digital interventions for health behavior change have included support from either professionals or peers. It is worth noting that professionally supported interventions cost two to three times what technology interventions cost. A conversational agent could provide some social support and increased engagement while remaining scalable and cost-effective. Moreover, studies have shown that people tend to be more honest when interacting with technology than with humans (Borzykowski, 2016).

In the next decade, conversational AI will probably become more widely used as an extender of clinician support or as a stopgap where other options are not available (see Chapter 1). Now under development are new conversational AI strategies to infer emotion from voice analysis, computer vision, and other sources. We think it is likely that systems will thus become more conversant in the emotional domain and more effective in their communication.

Health Monitoring and Risk Prediction

AI can use raw data from accelerometers, gyroscopes, microphones, cameras, and other sensors, including smartphones. Machine learning algorithms can be trained to recognize patterns from the raw data inputs and then categorize these patterns as indicators of an individual's behavior and health status. These systems can allow patients to understand and manage their own health and symptoms as well as share data with medical providers.

The current acceptance of wearables, smart devices, and mobile health applications has risen sharply. In just a 4-year period, between 2014 and 2018, the proportion of U.S. adults reporting that they use wearables increased from 9 percent to 33 percent. The use of mobile health apps increased from 16 percent to 48 percent (Accenture, 2018). Consumer interest is high (~50 percent) in using data generated by apps, wearables, and IoT devices to predict health risks (Accenture, 2018). Since 2013, AI startup companies with a focus on health care and wearables have raised $4.3 billion to develop, for example, bras designed for breast cancer risk prediction and smart clothing for cardiac, lung, and movement sensing (Wiggers, 2018).

Timely Personalized Interventions

AI-driven adaptive interventions are called JITAIs, or "just-in-time adaptive interventions." These are learning systems that deliver dynamic, personalized treatment to users over time (Nahum-Shani et al., 2015; Spruijt-Metz and Nilsen, 2014). The JITAI makes decisions about when and how to intervene based on response to prior intervention, as well as on awareness of current context, whether internal (e.g., mood, anxiety, blood pressure) or external (e.g., location, activity). JITAI assistance is provided when users are most in need of it or will be most receptive to it. These systems can also tell a clinician when a problematic pattern is detected. For example, a JITAI might detect when a user is in a risky situation for substance abuse relapse—and deliver an intervention against it.

These interventions rely on sensors, rather than a user's self-report, to detect states of vulnerability or intervention opportunity. This addresses two key self-management challenges: the high user burden of self-monitoring and the limitations of self-awareness. As sensors become more ubiquitous in homes, in smartphones, and on bodies, the data sources for JITAIs are likely to continue expanding. AI can be used to allow connected devices to communicate with one another. (Perhaps a glucometer might receive feedback from refrigerators regarding the frequency and types of food consumed.) Leveraging data from multiple inputs can uniquely enhance AI's ability to provide real-time behavioral management.

Assistance for Individuals with Cognitive Disabilities

According to the Centers for Disease Control and Prevention, 16 million individuals are living with cognitive disability in the United States alone. Age is the single best predictor of cognitive impairments, and an estimated 5 million Americans more than 65 years old have Alzheimer's disease. These numbers are expected to increase due to the growth of an aging population: currently nearly 9 percent of all adults are more than 65 years old, a percentage expected to double by 2050 (CDC, 2018; Family Caregiver Alliance, 2019). Critically, 15.7 million family members provide unpaid care and support to individuals with Alzheimer's disease or other dementias (Alzheimers.net, 2019). The current system of care is unprepared to handle the current or future load of patient needs, or to allow individuals to "age in place" at their current homes rather than relocating to assisted living or nursing home facilities (Family Caregiver Alliance, 2019).

Smart home monitoring and robotics may eventually use AI to address these challenges (Rabbitt et al., 2015). Home monitoring has the potential to increase independence and improve aging at home by monitoring physical space, falls, and amount of time in bed. (Excessive time in bed can be both the cause and outcome of depression, and places the elderly at high risk for bedsores, loss of mobility, and increased mortality.) Currently available social robots such as PARO, Kabochan, and PePeRe provide companionship and stimulation for dementia patients. Recently, the use of robotic pets has been reported to be helpful in reducing agitation in nursing home patients with dementia (Schulman-Marcus et al., 2019; YellRobot, 2018).

For example, PARO is a robot designed to look like a cute, white baby seal that helps calm patients in hospitals and nursing homes. Initial pilot testing of PARO with 30 patient–caregiver dyads showed that PARO improved affect and communication among those dementia patients who interacted with the robot. This benefit was especially seen among those with more cognitive deficits. Larger clinical trials have also demonstrated improvements in patient engagement, although the effects on cognitive symptoms remain ambiguous (Moyle et al., 2017).

Although socially assistive robots are designed primarily for older adult consumers, caregivers also benefit from them because they relieve caregiver burden a bit and thus improve their well-being. As the technology improves, it may be that robots will do increasingly sophisticated tasks. Future applications of robotics are being developed to provide hands-on care. Platforms for smart home monitoring may eventually incorporate caregiver and patient needs in one seamless experience to ensure a family-wide experience rather than individual experiences. Designers of smart home monitoring should consider the ethics of equitable access by designing AI for the elderly, the dependent, and the short- or long-term disabled (Johnson, 2018).

AI SOLUTIONS FOR THE CLINICIAN CARE TEAM

There are two main areas of opportunity for AI in clinical care: (1) enhancing and optimizing care delivery, and (2) improving information management, user experience, and cognitive support in electronic health records (EHRs). Strides have been made in these areas for decades, largely through rule-based, expert-designed applications typically focused on specific clinical areas or problems. AI techniques offer the possibility of improving performance further.

Care Delivery

The amount of relevant data available for patient care is growing and will continue to grow in volume and variety. Data recorded digitally through EHRs only scratch the surface of the types of data that (when appropriately consented) could be leveraged for improving patient care. Clinicians are beginning to have access to data generated from wearable devices, social media, and public health records; to data about consumer spending, grocery purchase nutritional value, and an individual's exposome; and to the many types of -omic data specific to an individual. AI will probably, we think, have a profound effect on the entire clinical care process, including prevention, early detection, risk/benefit identification, diagnosis, prognosis, and personalized treatment.

Prediction, Early Detection, Screening, and Risk Assessment

The area of prediction, early detection, and risk assessment for individuals is one of the most fruitful AI applications (Sennaar, 2018). In this chapter, we discuss examples of such use; Chapters 5 and 6 provide thoughts about external evaluation.

Diagnosis

There are a number of demonstrations of AI in diagnostic imaging. Diagnostic image recognition can differentiate between benign and malignant melanomas, diagnose retinopathy, identify cartilage lesions within the knee joint (Liu et al., 2018), detect lesion-specific ischemia, and predict node status after positive biopsy for breast cancer. Image recognition techniques can differentiate among competing diagnoses, assist in screening patients, and guide clinicians in radiotherapy and surgery planning (Matheson, 2018). Automated image classification may not disrupt medicine as much as the invention of the roentgenogram did, but the roles of radiologists, dermatologists, pathologists, and cardiologists will likely change as AI-enabled diagnostic imaging improves and expands. Combining output from an AI diagnostic imaging prediction with prediction from the physician seems to decrease human error (Wang et al., 2016). Although some believe AI will replace physicians in diagnostic imaging, it is more likely that these techniques will mainly be assistive, sorting and prioritizing images for more immediate review, highlighting important findings that might have been missed, and classifying simple findings so that the humans can spend more time on complex cases (Parakh et al., 2019).

Histopathologic diagnosis has seen similar gains in cancer classification from tissue, in universal microorganism detection from sequencing data, and in analysis of a single drop of body fluid to find evidence of bacteria, viruses, or proteins that could indicate an illness (Best, 2017).

Surgery

AI is becoming more important for surgical decision making. It brings to bear diverse sources of information, including patient risk factors, anatomic information, disease natural history, patient values, and cost, to help physicians and patients make better predictions regarding the consequences of surgical decisions. For instance, a deep learning model was used to predict which individuals with treatment-resistant mesial temporal lobe epilepsy would most likely benefit from surgery (Gelichgerrcht et al., 2018). AI platforms can provide roadmaps to aid the surgical team in the operating room, reducing risk and making surgery safer (Newmarker, 2018). In addition to planning and decision making, AI may be applied to change surgical techniques. Remote-controlled robotic surgery has been shown to improve the safety of interventions where clinicians are exposed to high doses of ionizing radiation and makes surgery possible in anatomic locations not otherwise reachable by human hands (Shen et al., 2018; Zhao et al., 2018). As autonomous robotic surgery improves, it is likely that surgeons will in some cases oversee the movements of robots (Shademan et al., 2016).

Personalized Management and Treatment

Precision medicine allows clinicians to tailor medical treatment to the individual characteristics of each patient. Clinicians are testing whether AI will permit them to personalize chemotherapy dosing and map patient response to a treatment so as to plan future dosing (Poon et al., 2018). AI-driven NLP has been used to identify polyp descriptions in pathology reports that then trigger guideline-based clinical decision support to help clinicians determine the best surveillance intervals for colonoscopy exams (Imler et al., 2014). Other AI tools have helped clinicians select the best treatment options for complex diseases such as cancer (Zauderer et al., 2014).

The case of clinical equipoise—when clinical practice guidelines do not present a clear preference among care treatment options—also has significant potential for AI. Using retrospective data from other patients, AI techniques can predict treatment responses of different combinations of therapies for an individual patient (Brown, 2018). These types of tools may serve to help select a treatment immediately and may also provide new knowledge to future practice guidelines. Possibly useful will be dashboards demonstrating predicted outcomes along with cost of treatment and expected changes based on patient behavior, such as increased exercise. These may provide an excellent platform for shared decision making involving the patient, family, and clinical team. AI could also support a patient-centered medical homes model (Jackson et al., 2013).

As genome-phenome integration is realized, the use of genetic data in AI systems for diagnosis, clinical care, and treatment planning will probably increase. To truly impact routine care, though, genetic datasets will need to better represent the diversity of patient populations (Hindorff et al., 2018).

AI can also be used to find similar cases from patient records in an EHR to support treatment decisions based on previous outcomes (Schuler et al., 2018).

Improving Information Management, User Experience, and Cognitive Support in EHRs

The following sections describe a few areas that could benefit from AI-supported tools integrated with EHR systems, including information management (e.g., clinical documentation, information retrieval), user experience, and cognitive support.

Information Management

EHR systems and regulatory requirements have introduced significant clinical documentation responsibilities to providers, without necessarily supporting patient care decisions (Shanafelt et al., 2016). AI has the potential to improve the way in which clinicians store and retrieve clinical documentation. For example, the role of voice recognition systems in clinical documentation is well known. However, such systems have been used mostly to support clinicians' dictation of narrative reports, such as clinical notes and diagnostic imaging reports (Hammana et al., 2015; Zick and Olsen, 2001). As mentioned previously, AI-enabled conversational and interactive systems (e.g., Amazon's Alexa, Apple's Siri) are now widespread outside of health care. Similar technology could be used in EHR systems to support various information management tasks. For example, clinicians could ask a conversational agent to find specific information in the patient's record (e.g., "Show me the patient's latest HbA1c results"), enter orders, and launch EHR functions. Instead of clicking through multiple screens to find relevant patient information, clinicians could verbally request specific information and post orders while still looking at and talking to the patient or caregivers (Bryant, 2018). In the near future, this technology has the potential to improve the patient–provider relationship by reducing the amount of time clinicians spend focused on a computer screen.

Cognitive Support

AI has the potential to not only improve existing clinical decision support (CDS) modalities but also enable a wide range of innovations with the potential to disrupt patient care. Improved cognitive support functions include smarter CDS alerts and reminders as well as better access to peer-reviewed literature.

Smarter CDS Alerts and Reminders

A core cause for clinicians' dissatisfaction with EHR systems is the high incidence of irrelevant pop-up alerts that disrupt the clinical workflow and contribute to "alert fatigue" (McCoy et al., 2014). This problem is partially caused by the low specificity of alerts, which are frequently based on simple and deterministic handcrafted rules that fail to consider the full clinical context. AI can improve the specificity of alerts and reminders by considering a much larger number of patient and contextual variables (Joffe et al., 2012). It can provide probability thresholds that can be used to prioritize alert presentation and determine alert format in the user interface (Payne et al., 2015). It can also continuously learn from clinicians' past behavior (e.g., by lowering the priority of alerts they usually ignore).

Improved Access to Biomedical Literature to Support Clinical Decision Making

Recent advances in AI show promising applications in clinical knowledge retrieval. For example, mainstream medical knowledge resources are already using machine learning algorithms to rank search results, including algorithms that continuously learn from users' search behavior (Fiorini et al., 2018). AI-enabled clinical knowledge retrieval tools could also be accessed through the same conversational systems that allow clinicians to retrieve patient information from the EHR. Through techniques such as information extraction, NLP, automatic summarization, and deep learning, AI has the potential to transform static narrative articles into patient-specific, interactive visualizations of clinical evidence that could be seamlessly accessed within the EHR. In addition, "living systematic reviews" can continuously update clinical evidence as soon as the results of new clinical trials become available, with EHRs presenting evidence updates that may warrant changes to the treatment of specific patients (Elliott et al., 2014).

AI SOLUTIONS FOR POPULATION/PUBLIC HEALTH PROGRAM MANAGEMENT

Next, we explore AI solutions for population and public health programs. These include solutions that could be implemented by health systems (e.g., accountable care organizations), health plans, or city, county, state, and federal public health departments or agencies. Population health examines the distribution of health outcomes within a population, the range of factors that influence the distribution of health outcomes, and the policies and interventions that affect those factors (Kindig and Stoddart, 2003). Population health programs are often implemented through nontraditional partnerships among different sectors of the community— public health, industry, academia, health care, local government entities, etc. On the other hand, public health is the science of protecting and improving the health of people and their communities (CDC Foundation, 2019). This work is achieved by promoting healthy lifestyles, researching disease and injury prevention, and detecting, preventing, and responding to infectious diseases. Overall, public health is concerned with protecting the health of entire populations. These populations can be as small as a local neighborhood or as big as an entire country or region of the world.

Health Communication and Health Campaigns Enabled by AI

AI can help identify specific demographics or geographical locations where the prevalence of disease or high-risk behaviors exist. Researchers have successfully applied convolutional neural network analytic approaches to quantify associations between the built environment and obesity prevalence. They have shown that physical characteristics of a neighborhood can be associated with variations in obesity prevalence across different neighborhoods (Maharana and Nsoesie, 2018). Shin et al. (2018) applied a machine learning approach that uses both biomarkers and sociomarkers to predict and identify pediatric asthma patients at risk of hospital revisits.

Without knowing specific symptom-related features, the sociomarker-based model correctly predicted two out of three patients at risk. Once identified, population or regions can be targeted with computational health campaigns that blur the distinction between interpersonal and mass influence (Cappella, 2017). However, the risks of machine learning in these contexts have also been described (Cabitza et al., 2017). They include (1) the risk that clinicians become unable to recognize when the algorithms are incorrect, (2) lack of an ability for the algorithms to address the context of care, or (3) the intrinsic lack of reliability of some medical data. However, many of these challenges are not intrinsic to machine learning or AI, but rather represent misuse of the technologies.

Population Health Improvement Through Chronic Disease Management

A spectrum of market-ready AI approaches to support population health programs already exists. They are used in areas of automated retinal screening, clinical decision support, predictive population risk stratification, and patient self-management tools (Contreras and Vehi, 2018; Dankwa-Mullan et al., 2019). Several solutions have received regulatory approval; for example, the U.S. Food and Drug Administration approved Medtronic's Guardian Connect, marking the first AI-powered continuous glucose monitoring system. Crowd-sourced, real-world data on inhaler use, combined with environmental data, led to a policy recommendations model that can be replicated to address many public health challenges by simultaneously guiding individual, clinical, and policy decisions (Barrett et al., 2018).

There is an alternative approach to standard risk prediction models that applies AI tools. For example, predictive models using machine learning algorithms may facilitate recognition of clinically important unanticipated predictor variables that may not have previously been identified by "traditional" research approaches that rely on statistical methods testing a priori hypotheses (Waljee et al., 2014). Enabled by the availability of data from administrative claims and EHRs, machine learning can enable patient-level prediction, which moves beyond average population effects to consider personalized benefits and risks. Large-scale, patient-level prediction models from observational health care data are facilitated by a common data model that enables prediction researchers to work across computer environments. An example can be found from the Observational Health Data Sciences and Informatics collaborative, which has adopted the Observational Medical Outcomes Partnership common data model for patient-level prediction models using observational health care data (Reps et al., 2018).

Another advantage of applying AI approaches to predictive models is the ability not only to predict risk but also the presence or absence of a disease in an individual. As an example, successful use of a memetic pattern-based algorithm approach was demonstrated in a broad risk spectrum of patients undergoing coronary artery disease evaluation and was shown to successfully identify and exclude coronary artery disease in a population instead of just predicting the probability of future events (Zellweger et al., 2018). In addition to helping health care organizations identify individuals with elevated risks of developing chronic conditions early in the disease's progression, this approach may prevent unnecessary diagnostic procedures in patients where procedures may not be warranted and also support better outcomes.

Not all data elements needed to predict chronic disease can be found in administrative records and EHRs. Creating risk scores that include a blend of social, behavioral, and clinical data may help give providers the actionable, 360-degree insight necessary to identify patients in need of proactive, preventive care while meeting reimbursement requirements and improving outcomes (Kasthurirathne et al., 2018).

AI Solutions for Public Health Program Management

Public health professionals are focused on solutions for more efficient and effective administration of programs, policies, and services; disease outbreak detection and surveillance; and research. Relevant AI solutions are being experimented with in a number of areas.

Disease Surveillance

The range of AI solutions that can improve disease surveillance is considerable. For a number of years, researchers have tracked and refined the options for tracking disease outbreaks using search engine query data. Some of these approaches rely on the search terms that users type into Internet search engines (e.g., Google Flu Trends). At the same time, caution is warranted with these approaches. Relying on data not collected for scientific purposes (e.g., Internet search terms) to predict flu outbreaks has been fraught with error (Lazer et al., 2014). Nontransparent search algorithms that change constantly cannot be easily replicated and studied.

These changes may occur due to business needs (rather than the needs of a flu outbreak detection application) or due to changes in search behavior of consumers. Finally, relying on such methods exclusively misses the opportunity to combine them and co-develop them in conjunction with more traditional methods. As Lazer et al. (2014) detail, combining traditional and innovative methods (e.g., Google Flu Trends) performs better than either method alone.

Researchers and solution developers have experimented with the integration of case- and event-based surveillance (e.g., news and online media, sensors, digital traces, mobile devices, social media, microbiological labs, and clinical reporting) to arrive at dashboards and analysis approaches for threat verification. Such approaches have been referred to as digital epidemiological surveillance and can produce timelier data and reduce labor hours of investigation (Kostokova, 2013; Zhao et al., 2015). Such analyses rely on AI's capacities in spatial and spatiotemporal profiling, environmental monitoring, and signal detection (i.e., from wearable sensors). They have been successfully implemented to build early warning systems for adverse drug events, falls detection, and air pollution (Mooney and Pejaver, 2018). The ability to rely on unstructured data such as photos, physicians' notes, sensor data, and genomic information, when enabled by AI, may lead to additional, novel approaches in disease surveillance (Figge, 2018).

Moreover, participatory systems such as social media and listservs could be relied on to solicit information from individuals as well as groups in particular geographic locations. For example, such approaches may encourage a reduction in unsafe behaviors that put individuals at risk for human immunodeficiency virus (HIV) infection (Rubens et al., 2014; Young et al., 2017). For example, it has been demonstrated that psychiatric stressors can be detected from Twitter posts in select populations through keyword-based retrieval and filters and the use of neural networks (Du et al., 2018). However, how such AI solutions could improve the health of populations or communities is less clear, due to the lack of context for some tweets and because tweets may not reflect the true underlying mental health status of a person who tweeted. Studies that retroactively analyze the tweeting behavior of individuals with known suicide attempts or ideation, or other mental health conditions, may allow refinement in such approaches.

Finally, AI and machine learning have been used to develop a dashboard to provide live insight into opioid usage trends in Indiana (Bostic, 2018). This tool enabled prediction of drug positivity for small geographic areas (i.e., hot spots), allowing for interventions by public health officials, law enforcement, or program managers in targeted ways. A similar dashboarding approach supported by AI solutions has been used in Colorado to monitor HIV surveillance and outreach interventions and their impact after implementation (Snyder et al., 2016). This tool integrated data on regional resources with near-real-time visualization of complex information to support program planning, patient management, and resource allocation.

Environmental and Occupational Health

AI has already made inroads into environmental and occupational health by leveraging data generated by sensors, nanotechnology, and robots. For example, water-testing sensors with AI tools have been paired with microscopes to detect bacterial contamination in treatment plants through hourly water sampling and analysis. This significantly reduces the time traditionally spent sending water samples for laboratory testing and lowers the cost of certain automated systems (Leider, 2018).

In a similar fashion, remote sensing from meteorological sensors, combined with geographic information systems, has been used to measure and analyze air pollution patterns in space and over time. This evolving field of inquiry has been termed geospatial AI because it combines innovations in spatial science with the rapid growth of methods in AI, including machine learning and deep learning. In another approach to understanding environmental factors, images of Google StreetView have been analyzed using deep learning mechanisms to analyze urban greenness as a predictor and enabler of exercise (e.g., walking, cycling) (Lu, 2018).

Robots enabled by AI technology have been successfully deployed in a variety of hazardous occupational settings to improve worker safety and prevent injuries that can lead to costly medical treatments or short- and long-term disability. Robots can replace human labor in highly dangerous or tedious jobs that are fatiguing and could represent health risks to workers—reducing injuries and fatalities. Similarly, the construction industry has relied on AI-enabled robots for handling hazardous materials, handling heavy loads, working at elevation or in hard-to-reach places, and completing tasks that require difficult work postures, risking injury (Hsiao et al., 2017). Some of these robotic deployments are replacing human labor; in other instances, humans collaborate with robots to carry out such tasks. Hence, the deployment of robots requires workers to develop new skills in directing and managing robots and managing interactions between different types of robots or equipment, all operating in dynamic work environments.

AI SOLUTIONS FOR HEALTH CARE BUSINESS ADMINISTRATORS

Coordination and payment for care in the United States is highly complex. It involves the patient, providers, health care facilities, laboratories, hospitals, pharmacies, benefit administrators, payers, and others. Before, during, and after a patient encounter, administrative coordination occurs around scheduling, billing, and payment. Collectively, we call this the administration of care, or administrative workflow. AI might be used in this setting in the form of machine learning models that can work alongside administrative personnel to perform mundane, repetitive tasks in a more efficient, accurate, and unbiased fashion.

Newer methods in AI, known generally as deep learning, have advantages over traditional machine learning, especially in the analysis of text data. The use of deep learning is particularly powerful in a workflow where a trained professional reviews narrative data and makes a decision about a clear action plan. A vast number of prior authorizations exist, with decisions and underlying data; these data provide the ideal substrate to train an AI model. Textual information used for prior authorization can be used for training a deep learning model that reaches or even exceeds the ability of human reviewers, perhaps with even more consistency than human reviewers. AI for health care administration will likely be utilized extensively, even beyond those solutions deployed for direct clinical care. "While all AI solutions give some false positives and false negatives, in administration, these will mostly produce annoyances, but should be monitored closely to ensure that patient safety is never impacted."

As AI solutions become more sophisticated and automated, it may happen that a variety of AI methodologies will be deployed for a given solution. For example, a request by a patient to refill a prescription might involve speech recognition or AI chatbots, a rules-based system to determine if prior authorization is required, automated provider outreach, and a deep learning system for prior authorization when needed. It is worth noting that deep learning systems already drive many of today's speech recognition, translation, and chatbot programs.

We provide illustrative (non-exhaustive) examples in Table 3-2 for different types of applications of AI solutions to support routine health care administration processes.

Prior Authorization

Most health plans and pharmacy benefit managers require prior authorization of devices, durable equipment, labs, and procedures. The process includes the submission of patient information along with the proposed request, along with justification. Determinations require professional skill, analysis, and judgment. Automating this process can reduce biased decisions and improve speed, consistency, and quality of decisions.

There are a number of different ways that AI is applied today. For example, AI could simply be used to sort cases to the appropriate level of reviewer (e.g., nurse practitioner, physician advisor, medical director). Or, AI could identify and highlight the specific, relevant information in long documents or narratives to

TABLE 3-2 | Illustrative Examples of Artificial Intelligence Solutions to Aid in Health Care Administration Processes

Topic	Example Opportunity	Value	Output/ Intervention	Data
Prior authorization (Rowley, 2016; Wince, 2018; Zieger, 2018)	Automate decisions on drugs, labs, or procedures	Reduced cost, efficiency, improved quality, reduce bias	Authorization or rejection	Relevant patient electronic health record (EHR) data
Fraud, waste (Bauder and Khoshgoftaar, 2017; da Rosa, 2018; He et al., 1997)	Identify appropriate or fraudulent claims	Reduced cost, improved care	Identification of targets for investigation	Provider claims data
Provider directory management	Maintain accurate information on providers	Reduced patient frustration through accurate provider availability, avoid Medicare penalties	Accurate provider directory	Provider data from many sources
Adjudication	Determine if a hospital should be paid for an admission versus observation	Improved compliance, accurate payments	Adjudication decision	Relevant patient EHR record data
Automated coding (Huang et al., 2019; Li et al., 2018; Shi et al., 2017; Xiao et al., 2018)	Automate ICD-10[a] coding of patient encounters	Improved compliance, accurate payments	ICD-10 coding	Relevant patient EHR record data
Chart abstraction (Gehrmann et al., 2017)	Summarize redundant data into a coherent narrative or structured variables	Reduced cost, efficiency, improved quality	Accurate, clean narrative/ problem list	Relevant patient EHR record data
Patient scheduling (Jiang et al., 2018; Nelson et al., 2019; Sharma, 2016)	Identify no-shows and optimize scheduling	Improved patient satisfaction, faster appointments, provider efficiency	Optimized physician schedule	Scheduling history, EHR data

[a] The ICD-10-CM (*International Classification of Diseases, 10th Revision, Clinical Modification*) is a system used by physicians and other health care providers to classify and code all diagnoses, symptoms, and procedures recorded in conjunction with hospital care in the United States.

produce information regarding estimated costs or benefit/risk assessment to aid a consumer in a decision.

Automation of prior authorization could reduce administrative costs, frustration, and idle time for provider and payer alike. Ultimately, such a process could lead to fewer appeals as well, which is a costly outcome of any prior authorization decision. A prior authorization model would need to work in near real time, because the required decisions are typically time sensitive.

The use of prior authorization limits liability, but AI implementation could create some liability risk. Some AI models are or become biased, and examples of this have been featured in the news recently. There has been coverage of AI models discriminating on names associated with particular ethnic groups, mapping same-day delivery routes to avoid high-crime areas, discriminating in lending practices, etc. (Hamilton, 2019; Ingold and Soper, 2016; Ward-Foxton, 2019; Williamson-Lee, 2018).

Automated Coding

Coding is an exacting, expert-driven process that extracts information from EHRs for claims submissions and risk adjustment. These are called ICD-10 codes, from the *International Classification of Diseases, 10th Revision* (ICD-10). It is a human labor–intensive process that requires an understanding of language, expertise in clinical terminology, and a nuanced, expert understanding of administrative coding of medical care. Of note, codes are often deleted and added, and their assignment to particular medical descriptions often changes. Computer-assisted coding has existed for more than a decade; it typically has used more traditional, semantic-based NLP. Proximity and other methods are used to identify appropriate codes to assist or pre-populate manual coding.

The accuracy of coding is very important, and the process of assigning an unspecified number of multiple labels to an event is a complex one. It can lead to false negatives and false positives. False negatives in coding may result in a denial of reimbursement. False positives may lead to overcharges, compliance issues, and excess cost to payers.

There are opportunities for AI techniques to be applied to this administrative coding. Notes and patient records can be vectorized within this space, using tools such as Word2vec, so that they might be used in deep learning and other AI predictive models along with a wide variety of structured data, such as medication orders, laboratory tests, and vital signs.

Because of the complexity of multilabel prediction, humans will have to supervise and review the process for the foreseeable future. This also increases the need for transparency in the algorithmic outputs as part of facilitating human review. This is especially important in the review of coding in long EHR narratives. Transparency will also be helpful for monitoring automated processes because treatments and medical standards change over time and algorithms have to be retrained. This is a topic discussed in more detail in Chapter 6.

In the short term, AI coding solutions may help coders and create checks for payers. In the long term, increasing automation may be achieved for some or many types of encounters/hospitalizations. This automation will be reliant on data comprehensiveness, public acceptance, algorithm accuracy, and appropriate regulatory frameworks.

AI Solutions for Research and Development Professionals

The uses of AI technologies in research are broad; they frequently drive the development of new machine learning algorithms. To narrow this massive landscape, we focus our discussion on research institutions with medical training facilities. These medical school–affiliated health care providers often house massive and multiple large-scale data repositories (such as biobanks, Digital Imaging and Communications in Medicine or DICOM systems, and EHR systems).

Mining EHR Data

Research with EHR data offers promising opportunities to advance biomedical research and improve health care by interpreting structured, unstructured (e.g., free text), genomic, and imaging data.

Machine Learning

Extracting practical information from EHR data is challenging because such data are highly dimensional, heterogeneous, sparse, and often of low quality (Jensen et al., 2012; Zhao et al., 2017). Nevertheless, AI technologies are being applied to EHR data. AI techniques used on these data include a vast array of data mining approaches, from clustering and association rules to deep learning. We focus our discussion in the sections below on areas of present key importance.

Deep Learning

Deep learning algorithms rely on the large quantities of data and massive computer resources, both of which are newly possible in this era. Deep learning can identify underlying patterns in data well beyond the pattern-perceiving capacities of humans. Deep learning and its associated techniques have become popular in many data-driven fields of research. The principal difference between deep and traditional (i.e., shallow) machine learning paradigms lies in the ability of deep learning algorithms to construct latent data representations from a large number of raw features, often through deep architectures (i.e., many layers) of artificial neural networks. This "unsupervised feature extraction" sometimes permits highly accurate predictions. Recent research on EHR data has shown that deep learning predictive models can outperform traditional clinically used predictive models for predicting early detection of heart failure onset (Choi et al., 2017), various cancers (Miotto et al., 2016), and onset of and weaning from intensive care unit interventions (Suresh et al., 2017).

Nevertheless, the capacity of deep learning is a double-edged sword. The downside of deep learning comes from exactly where its superiority to other learning paradigms originates—that is, its ability to build and learn features. Model complexity means that human interpretability of deep learning models is almost nonexistent, because it is extremely hard to infer how the model makes its predictions so well. Deep learning models are "black box" models, where the internal workings of the algorithms remain unclear or mysterious to users of these models. As in other black box AI approaches, there is significant resistance to implementing deep learning models in the health care delivery process.

Applications to Imaging Data

Detecting abnormal brain structure is much more challenging for humans and machines than detecting a broken bone or a fracture. Exciting things are being done in this area with deep learning. One recent study predicted age from brain images (Cole et al., 2017). Multimodal image recognition analysis has discovered novel impairments not visible from a single view of the brain (e.g., structural MRI versus functional MRI) (Plis et al., 2018). Companies such as Avalon AI[1] are commercializing this type of work.

Effective AI use does not always require new modeling techniques. Some work at Massachusetts General Hospital in Boston uses a large selection of images and combines established machine learning techniques with mature brain-image analysis tools to explore what is normal for a child's developing brain (NITRC, 2019; Ou et al., 2017). Other recent applications of AI to radiology data include using machine learning on electrocardiogram data to characterize types of heart failure (Sanchez-Martinez et al., 2018). In addition, AI can aid in reducing noise in real images (e.g., endoscopy) via "adversarial training." It can smooth out erroneous signals in images to enhance prediction accuracy (Mahmood et al., 2018). AI is also being applied to moving images; gait analysis has long been done by human observation alone, but it now can be performed with greater accuracy by AI that uses video and sensor data. These techniques are being used to detect Parkinson's disease, to improve geriatric care, for sports rehabilitation, and in other areas (Prakash et al., 2018). AI can also improve video-assisted surgery, for example, by detecting colon polyps in real time (Urban et al., 2018)

---

[1] See http://avalonai.mystrikingly.com.

Learning from Practice Patterns

AI can assist in analyzing clinical practice patterns from EHR data to develop clinical practice models before such research can be distilled into literature or made widely available in clinical decision support tools. This notion of "learning from the crowd" stems from Condorcet's jury theorem, which states that the average decisions of a crowd of unbiased experts are more correct than any individual's decisions. (Think of the "jellybeans in a jar" challenge—the average of everyone's guesses is surprisingly close to the true number.)

The most straightforward approach uses association rule mining to find patterns, but this tends to find many false associations (Wright et al., 2010). Therefore, some researchers have attempted to use more AI approaches such as Bayesian network learning and probabilistic topic modeling (Chen et al., 2017; Klann et al., 2014).

Phenotyping

A phenotype refers to an observable trait of an organism, resulting from its genetic code and surrounding environment, and the interactions between them. It is becoming increasingly popular to identify patient cohorts by trait for clinical and genomic research. Although EHR data are often incomplete and inaccurate, they do convey enough information for constructing clinically relevant sets of observable characteristics that define a disease, or a phenotype.

EHR phenotyping uses the information in a patient's health records to infer the presence of a disease (or lack thereof). This is done by using algorithms that apply predetermined rules, machine learning, and statistical methods to derive phenotypes.

Rule-based phenotyping is time-consuming and expensive, and so applying machine learning methods to EHR data makes sense. The principal mechanism in this approach transforms raw EHR data (e.g., diagnostic codes, laboratory results, clinical notes) into meaningful features that can predict the presence of a disease. Machine learning–based solutions mine both structured and unstructured data stored in EHRs for phenotyping. NLP algorithms have been used in research to extract relevant features from EHRs. For example, Yu et al. (2015, 2017) used NLP to identify candidate clinical features from a pool of comprehensive medical concepts found in publicly available online knowledge sources.

When the set of features is extracted, different classification algorithms can be used to predict or classify the phenotype. Choice of the classification algorithm in supervised learning relies on the characteristics of the data on which the algorithm will be trained and tested. Feature selection and curation of gold-standard training sets includes two rate-limiting factors. Curating annotated datasets to train supervised algorithms requires involvement from domain experts, which hampers generalizability and scalability of phenotyping algorithms. As a result, the classification algorithms for phenotyping research has been limited so far to regularized algorithms that can address overfitting, which is what happens when an algorithm that uses many features is trained on small training sets.

Regularized classifiers penalize more features in favor of model parsimony. To overcome this limitation, new research is investigating the application of hybrid approaches (known as semi-supervised) to create semi-automatically annotated training sets and the use of unsupervised methods to scale up EHR phenotyping. The massive amounts of data in EHRs, if processed through deep neural networks, may soon permit the computation of phenotypes from a wider vector of features.

As mentioned previously, large national initiatives are now combining biobanks of genomic information with these phenotypes. For example, eMerge frequently uses genomic analyses such as genome-wide association studies in combination with phenotyping algorithms to define the gold-standard cohort or to study genetic risk factors in the phenotyped population (Gottesman et al., 2013; McCarty et al., 2011).

Drug Discovery

Machine learning has the capacity to make drug discovery faster, cheaper, and more effective. Drug designers frequently apply machine learning techniques to extract chemical information from large compound databases and to design drugs with important biological properties. Machine learning can also improve drug discovery by permitting a more comprehensive assessment of cellular systems and potential drug effects. With the emergence of large chemical datasets in recent years, machine and deep learning methods have been used in many areas (Baskin et al., 2016; Chen et al., 2018; Lima et al., 2016; Zitnik et al., 2018). These include

- predicting synthesis,
- biological activity of new ligands,
- drug selectivity,
- pharmacokinetic and toxicological profiles,
- modeling polypharmacy side effects (due to drug–drug interactions), and
- designing de novo molecular structures and structure-activity models.

Large chemical databases have made drug discovery faster and cheaper. EHR databases have brought millions of patients' lives into the universe of statistical learning. Research initiatives to link structured patient data with biobanks, radiology images, and notes are creating a rich and robust analytical playground for discovering new knowledge about human disease. Deep learning and other new techniques are creating solutions that can operate on the scale required to digest these multiterabyte datasets. The accelerating pace of discovery will probably challenge the research pipelines that translate new knowledge back into practice.

KEY CONSIDERATIONS

Although it is difficult to predict the future in a field that is changing so quickly, we offer the following ideas about how AI will be used and considerations for optimizing the success of AI for health.

Augmented Intelligence

AI will change health care delivery less by replacing clinicians than by supporting or augmenting clinicians in their work. AI will support clinicians with less training in performing tasks currently relegated to specialists. It filters out normal or noncomplex cases so that specialists can focus on a more challenging case load.

AI will support humans in tasks that suffer from inattention, cause fatigue, and are physically difficult to perform. AI will substitute for humans by facilitating screening and evaluation in areas with limited access to medical expertise. Some AI tools, like those for self-management or population health support, will be useful in spite of lower accuracy.

When an AI tool assists human cognition, it will initially need to explain the connections it has drawn, allowing for an understanding of a pathway to effects. With sufficient accuracy, humans will begin to trust the AI output and will require less transparency and explanation. In situations where AI substitutes for medical expertise, the workflow should include a human in the loop to identify misbehavior and provide accountability (Rahwan, 2018).

Partnerships

The central focus of health care will continue to expand from health care delivery systems to a dispersed model that aggregates information about behavior, traits, and environment in addition to medical symptoms and test results.

Market forces and privacy concerns or regulations may impede data sharing and analysis (Roski et al., 2014). Stakeholders will need to creatively balance competing demands. More national-level investments similar to the National Institutes of Health's All of Us program can facilitate and accelerate these partnerships. More ethical and legal guidelines are needed for successful data sharing and analysis (see Chapters 1 and 7).

Interoperability

AI tools will continue to be developed by industry, research, government, and individuals. With emerging standards such as SMART on FHIR (Substitutable Medical Apps, Reusable Technology on Fast Healthcare Interoperability Resource), these tools will increasingly be implemented across platforms regardless of the EHR vendor, brand of phone, etc. This will most likely speed the adoption of AI.

Clinical Practice Guidelines

AI will probably discover associations that have not yet been detected by humans and make predictions that differ from prevailing knowledge and expertise. As a result, some currently accepted practices may be abandoned, and best practice guidelines will be adjusted.

If the output of AI systems is going to influence international guidelines, developers of the applications will require fuller and more representative datasets for training and testing.

Clinical Evidence and Rate of Innovation

The dissemination of innovation will occur rapidly, which on the one hand may advance the adoption of new scientific knowledge but on the other may encourage the rushed adoption of innovation without sufficient evidence.

Bias and Trust

As AI increasingly infiltrates the field of health, biases inherent in clinical practice will appear in the datasets used in AI models. The discovery of existing bias will open the door to changing practices, but it may also produce public disillusionment and mistrust.

Important growth areas for AI include platforms designed for and accessible by the people most in need of additional support. This includes older adults, people living with multiple comorbid conditions, and people in low-resource settings.

REFERENCES

Accenture. 2018. *Consumer survey on digital health: US results.* https://www.accenture. com/t20180306T103559Z__w__/us-en/_acnmedia/PDF-71/accenture-health-2018-consumer-survey-digital-health.pdf (accessed November 12, 2019).

Alzheimers.net. 2017. *Alzheimer's statistics.* https://www.alzheimers.net/resources/alzheimers-statistics (accessed March 26, 2019).

Barrett, M., V. Combs, J. G. Su, K. Henderson, M. Tuffli, and AIR Louisville Collaborative. 2018. AIR Louisville: Addressing asthma with technology, crowdsourcing, cross-sector collaboration, and policy. *Health Affairs (Millwood)* 37(4):525–534.

Baskin, I. I., D. Winkler, and I. V. Tetko. 2016. A renaissance of neural networks in drug discovery. *Expert Opinion on Drug Discovery* 11(8):785–795.

Bauder, R. A., and T. M. Khoshgoftaar. 2017. Medicare fraud detection using machine learning methods. In *2017 16th IEEE International Conference on Machine Learning and Applications.* https://doi. org/10.1109/icmla.2017.00-48.

Best, J. 2017. AI that knows you're sick before you do: IBM's five-year plan to remake healthcare. *ZDNet.* https://www.zdnet.com/article/ai-that-knows-youre-sick-before-you-do-ibms-five-year-plan-to-remake-healthcare (accessed November 12, 2019).

Borzykowski, B. 2016. Truth be told, we're more honest with robots. *BBC WorkLife.* https://www.bbc.com/worklife/article/20160412-truth-be-told-were-more-honest-with-robots (accessed November 12, 2019).

Bostic, B. 2018. Using artificial intelligence to solve public health problems. *Beckers Hospital Review.* https://www.beckershospitalreview.com/healthcare-information-technology/using-artificial-intelligence-to-solve-public-health-problems.html (accessed November 12, 2019).

Brown, D. 2018. RSNA 2018: Researchers use AI to predict cancer survival, treatment response. *AI in Healthcare News.* https://www.aiin.healthcare/topics/research/research-ai-cancer-survival-treatment-response (accessed November 12, 2019).

Bryant, M. 2018. Hospitals turn to chatbots, AI for care. *Healthcare Dive.* https://www.healthcaredive.com/news/chatbots-ai-healthcare/516047 (accessed November 12, 2019).

Cabitza, F., R. Rasoini, and G. F. Gensini. 2017. Unintended consequences of machine learning in medicine. *JAMA* 318(6):517–518.

Cappella, J. N. 2017. Vectors into the future of mass and interpersonal communication research: Big data, social media, and computational social science. *Human Communication Research* 43(4):545–558.

CDC (Centers for Disease Control and Prevention). 2018. Prevalence of disabilities and health care access by disability status and type among adults—United States, 2016. *Morbidity and Mortality Weekly Report* 67(32):882–887.

CDC Foundation. 2019. *What is public health?* https://www.cdcfoundation.org/what-public-health (accessed November 12, 2019).

Chen, H., O. Engkvist, Y. Wang, M. Olivecrona, and T. Blaschke. 2018. The rise of deep learning in drug discovery. *Drug Discovery Today* 23(6):1241–1250.

Chen, J. H., M. K. Goldstein, S. M. Asch, L. Mackey, and R. B. Altman. 2017. Predicting inpatient clinical order patterns with probabilistic topic models vs conventional order sets. *Journal of the American Medical Informatics Association* 24(3):472–480.

Choi, E., S. Biswal, B. Malin, J. Duke, W. F. Stewart, and J. Sun. 2017. Generating multi-label discrete electronic health records using generative adversarial networks. *arXIV*. http://arxiv.org/abs/1703.06490 (accessed December 7, 2019).

Cole, J. H., R. P. K. Poudel, D. Tsagkrasoulis, M. W. A. Caan, C. Steves, T. D. Spector, and G. Montana. 2017. Predicting brain age with deep learning from raw imaging data results in a reliable and heritable biomarker. *NeuroImage* 163(December):115–124.

Contreras, I., and J. Vehi. 2018. Artificial intelligence for diabetes management and decision support: Literature review. *Journal of Medical Internet Research* 20(5):e10775.

da Rosa, R. C. 2018. *An Evaluation of Unsupervised Machine Learning Algorithms for Detecting Fraud and Abuse in the US Medicare Insurance Program.* Ph.D. dissertation, Florida Atlantic University, Boca Raton. https://pqdtopen.proquest.com/doc/2054014362.html?FMT=ABS (accessed November 12, 2019).

Dankwa-Mullan, I., M. Rivo, M. Sepulveda, Y. Park, J. Snowdon, and K. Rhee. 2019. Transforming diabetes care through artificial intelligence: The future is here. *Population Health Management* 22(3). http://doi.org/10.1089/pop.2018.0129.

Du, J., Y. Zhang, J. Luo, Y. Jia, Q. Wei, C. Tao, and H. Xu. 2018. Extracting psychiatric stressors for suicide from social media using deep learning. *BMC Medical Informatics and Decision Making* 18(Suppl 2):43.

Elliott, J. H., T. Turner, O. Clavisi, J. Thomas, J. P. Higgins, C. Mavergames, and R. L. Gruen. 2014. Living systematic reviews: An emerging opportunity to narrow the evidence-practice gap. *PLoS Medicine* 11(2):e1001603.

Family Caregiver Alliance. 2019. *Caregiver Statistics: Demographics. National Center on Caregiving.* https://www.caregiver.org/caregiver-statistics-demographics (accessed March 26, 2019).

Figge, H. 2018. Deploying artificial intelligence against infectious disease. *U.S. Pharmacist* 43(3):21–24.

Fiorini, N., K. Canese, G. Starchenko, E. Kireev, W. Kim, V. Miller, M. Osipov, M. Kholodov, R. Ismagilov, S. Mohan, J. Ostell, and Z. Lu. 2018. Best Match: New relevance search for PubMed. *PLoS Biology* 16(8):e2005343.

Fitzpatrick, K. K., A. Darcy, and M. Vierhile. 2017. Delivering cognitive behavior therapy to young adults with symptoms of depression and anxiety using a fully automated conversational agenda (Woebot): A randomized controlled trial. *JMIR Mental Health* 4(2):e19.

Gehrmann, S., F. Dernoncourt, Y. Li, E. T. Carlson, J. T. Wu, J. Welt, J. Foote, E. T. Moseley, D. W. Grant, P. D. Tyler, and L. A. Celi. 2017. Comparing rule-based and deep learning models for patient phenotyping. *arXiv preprint*. 1703.08705.

Gelichgerrcht, E., B. Munsell, S. Bhatia, W. Vandergrift, C. Rorden, C. McDonalid, J. Edwards, R. Kuzniecky, L. Bonilha. 2018. Deep learning applied to whole-brain connectome to determine seizure control after epilepsy surgery. *Epilepsia* 59(9):1643–1654.

Gottesman, O., H. Kuivaniemi, G. Tromp, W. A. Faucett, R. Li, T. A. Manolio, S. C. Sanderson, J. Kannry, R. Zinberg, M. A. Basford, M. Brilliant, D. J. Carey, R. L. Chisholm, C. G. Chute, J. J. Connolly, D. Crosslin, J. C. Denny, C. J. Gallego, J. L. Haines, H. Hakonarson, J. Harley, G. P. Jarvik, I. Kohane, I. J. Kullo, E. B. Larson, C. McCarty, M. D. Ritchie, D. M. Roden, M. E. Smith, E. P. Böttinger, M. S. Williams, and eMERGE Network. 2013. The electronic medical records and genomics (eMERGE) network: Past, present, and future. *Genetics in Medicine* 15(10):761–771.

Hamilton, E. 2019. *AI perpetuating human bias in the lending space.* https://www.techtimes.com/articles/240769/20190402/ai-perpetuating-human-bias-in-the-lending-space.htm (accessed November 12, 2019).

Hammana, I., L. Lepanto, T. Poder, C. Bellemare, and M. S. Ly. 2015. Speech recognition in the radiology department: A systematic review. *Health Informatics Management* 44(2):4–10.

He, H., J. Wang, W. Graco, and S. Hawkins. 1997. Application of neural networks to detection of medical fraud. *Expert Systems with Applications* 13(4):329–336.

Hindorff, L. A., V. L. Bonham, L. C. Brody, M. E. C. Ginoza, C. M. Hutter, T. A. Manolio, and E. D. Green. 2018. Prioritizing diversity in human genomics research. *Nature Reviews Genetics* 19:175–185.

Hixson, J., D. Barnes, K. Parko, T. Durgin, S. Van Bebber, A. Graham, and P. Wicks. 2015. Patients optimizing epilepsy management via an online community. *Neurology* 85(2):129–136. https://doi.org/10.1212/WNL.0000000000001728.

Hsiao, H., H. Choi, J. Sammarco, S. Earnest, D. Castillo, and G. Hill. 2017. *NIOSH presents: An occupational safety and health perspective on robotics applications in the workplace.* https://blogs.cdc.gov/niosh-science-blog/2017/12/05/robot_ safety_conf (accessed December 13, 2019).

Huang, J., C. Osorio, and L. W. Sy. 2019. An empirical evaluation of deep learning for ICD-9 code assignment using MIMIC-III clinical notes. *Computer Methods and Programs in Biomedicine* 177:141–153.

Imler, T. D., J. Morea, T. F. Imperiale. 2014. Clinical decisions support with natural language processing facilitates determination of colonscopy surveillance intervals. *Clinical Gastroenterology and Hepatology* 12(7):1130–1136.

Ingold, D., and S. Soper. 2016. Amazon doesn't consider the race of its customers. Should it? *Bloomberg.* https://www.bloomberg.com/graphics/2016-amazon-same-day (accessed November 12, 2019).

Jackson, G. L., B. J. Powers, R. Chatterjee, J. P. Bettger, A. R. Kemper, V. Hasselblad, R. J. Dolor, J. Irvine, B. L. Heidenfelder, A. S. Kendrick, R. Gray, and J. W. Williams. 2013. The patient-centered medical home: A systematic review. *Annals of Internal Medicine* 158:169–178.

Jensen, P. B., L. J. Jensen, and S. Brunak. 2012. Mining electronic health records: Towards better research applications and clinical care. *Nature Reviews Genetics* 13(6):395–405.

Jiang, S., K. S. Chin, and K. L. Tsui. 2018. A universal deep learning approach for modeling the flow of patients under different severities. *Computer Methods and Programs in Biomedicine* 154:191–203.

Joffe, E., O. Havakuk, J. R. Herskovic, V. L. Patel, and E. V. Bernstam. 2012. Collaborative knowledge acquisition for the design of context-aware alert systems. *Journal of the American Medical Informatics Association* 219(6):988–994.

Johnson, J. 2018. *Designing technology for an aging population.* Presentation at Stanford Center on Longevity meeting at Trcsidder Oak Lounge. http://longevity.stanford.edu/2018/10/17/designing-technology-for-an-aging-population (accessed December 7, 2019).

Kasthurirathne, S. N., J. R. Vest, N. Menachemi, P. K. Halverson, and S. J. Grannis. 2018. Assessing the capacity of social determinants of health data to augment predictive models identifying patients in need of wraparound social services. *Journal of the American Medical Informatics Association* 25(1):47–53.

Kindig, D., and G. Stoddart. 2003. What is population health? *American Journal of Public Health* 93(3):380–383.

Klann, J. G., P. Szolovits, S. M. Downs, and G. Schadow. 2014. Decision support from local data: Creating adaptive order menus from past clinician behavior. *Journal of Biomedical Informatics* 48:84–93.

Kostokova, P. 2013. A roadmap to integrated digital public health surveillance: The vision and the challenges. In *WWW '13 Companion Proceedings of the*

22nd International Conference on World Wide Web. New York: CMS. Pp. 687–694. https://www.researchgate.net/publication/250963354_A_roadmap_to_integrated_digital_public_health_surveillance_The_vision_and_the_challenges (accessed November 12, 2019).

Laranjo, L., A. G. Dunn, H. L. Tong, A. B. Kocaballi, J. Chen, R. Bashir, D. Surian, B. Gallego, F. Magrabi, and A. Coiera. 2018. Conversational agents in healthcare: A systematic review. *Journal of the American Medical Informatics Association* 25(9):1248–1258.

Lazer, D., R. Kennedy, G. King, and A. Vespignani. 2014. The parable of Google flu: Traps in big data analysis. *Science* 343(6176):1203–1205.

Leider, N. 2018. AI could protect public health by monitoring water treatment systems. *AI in Healthcare News.* https://www.aiin.healthcare/topics/artificial-intelligence/ai-public-health-monitoring-water-treatment (accessed November 12, 2019).

Li, M., Z. Fei, M. Zeng, F. Wu, Y. Li, Y. Pan, and J. Wang. 2018. Automated ICD-9 coding via a deep learning approach. *IEEE/ACM Transactions on Computational Biology and Bioinformatics* 16(4):1193–1202. https://doi.org/10.1109/TCBB.2018.2817488.

Lima, A. N., E. A. Philot, G. H. G. Trossini, L. P. B. Scott, V. G. Maltarollo, and K. M. Honorio. 2016. Use of machine learning approaches for novel drug discovery. *Expert Opinion on Drug Discovery* 11(3):225–239.

Liu, F., Z. Zhou, A. Samsonov, D. Blankenbaker, W. Larison, A. Kanarek, K. Lian, S. Kambhampati, and R. Kijowski. 2018. Deep learning approach for evaluating knee MR images: Achieving high diagnostic performance for cartilage lesion detection. *Radiology* 289(1):160–169.

Lu, Y. 2018. The association of urban greenness and walking behavior: Using Google StreetView and deep learning techniques to estimate residents' exposure to urban greenness. *International Journal of Environmental Health Research and Public Health* 15:1576.

Maharana, A., and E. O. Nsoesie. 2018. Use of deep learning to examine the association of the built environment with prevalence of neighborhood adult obesity. *JAMA Network Open* 1(4):e181535. https://doi.org/10.1001/jamanetworkopen.2018.1535.

Mahmood, F., R. Chen, and N. J. Durr. 2018. Unsupervised reverse domain adaptation for synthetic medical images via adversarial training. *IEEE Transactions on Medical Imaging* 37(12):2572–2581. https://doi.org/10.1109/TMI.2018.2842767.

Matheson, R. 2018. Machine-learning system determines the fewest, smallest doses that could still shrink brain tumors. *MIT News.* http://news.mit.edu/2018/artificial-intelligence-model-learns-patient-data-cancer-treatment-less-toxic-0810.

McCarty, C. A., R. L. Chisholm, C. G. Chute, I. J. Kullo, G. P. Jarvik, E. B. Larson, R. Li, D. R. Masys, M. D. Ritchie, D. M. Roden, J. P. Struewing, W. A. Wolf, and eMERGE Team. 2011. The eMERGE network: A consortium of biorepositories linked to electronic medical records data for conducting genomic studies. *BMC Medical Genomics* 4:13.

McCoy, A. B., E. J. Thomas, M. Krousel-Wood, and D. F. Sittig. 2014. Clinical decision support alert appropriateness: A review and proposal for improvement. *Ochsner Journal* 14(2):195–202.

Miotto, R., L. Li, B. A. Kidd, and J. I. T. Dudley. 2016. Deep patient: An unsupervised representation to predict the future of patients from the electronic health records. *Scientific Reports* 6:26094.

Mooney, S. J., and V. Pejaver. 2018. Big data in public health: Terminology, machine learning, and privacy. *Annual Review of Public Health* 39:95–112.

Moyle, W., C. J. Jones, J. E. Murfield, L. Thalib, E. R. A. Beattie, D. K. H. Shum, S. T. O'Dwyer, M. C. Mervin, and B. M. Draper. 2017. Use of a robotic seal as a therapeutic tool to improve dementia symptoms: A cluster-randomized controlled trial. *Journal of the American Medical Directors Association* 18(9):766–773.

Nahum-Shani, I., E. B. Hekler, and D. Spruijt-Metz. 2015. Building health behavior models to guide the development of just-in-time adaptive interventions: A pragmatic framework. *Health Psychology* 34S:1209–1219. https://doi.org/10.1037/hea0000306.

Nelson, A., D. Herron, G. Rees, and P. Nachev. 2019. Predicting scheduled hospital attendance with artificial intelligence. *NPJ Digital Medicine* 2(1):26.

Newmarker, C. 2018. Digital surgery touts artificial intelligence for the operating room. *Medical Design & Outsourcing.* https://www.medicaldesignandout sourcing.com/digital-surgery-touts-artificial-intelligence-for-the-operating-room (accessed November 12, 2019).

NITRC (Neuroimaging Tools & Resources Collaboratory). 2019. *MGH Neonatal/Pediatric ADC Atlases.* https://www.nitrc.org/projects/mgh_adcatlases (accessed October 18, 2019).

Ou, Y., L. Zöllei, K. Retzepi, V. Castro, S. V. Bates, S. Pieper, K. P. Andriole, S. N. Murphy, R. L. Gollub, and P. E. Grant. 2017. Using clinically acquired MRI to construct age-specific ADC atlases: Quantifying spatiotemporal ADC changes from birth to 6-year old. *Human Brain Mapping* 38(6):3052–3068.

Parakh, A., H. Lee, J. H. Lee, B. H. Eisiner, D. V. Sahani, and S. Do. 2019. Urinary stone detection on CT images using deep convolutional neural networks: Evaluation of model performance and generalization. *Radiology: Artificial Intelligence* 1(4). https://doi.org/10.1148/ryai.2019180066.

Payne, T. H., L. E. Hines, R. C. Chan, S. Hartman, J. Kapusnik-Uner, A. L. Russ, B. W. Chaffee, C. Hartman, V. Tamis, B. Galbreth, and P. A. Glassman. 2015. Recommendations to improve the usability of drug-drug interaction clinical decision support alerts. *Journal of the American Medical Informatics Association* 22(6):1243–1250.

Plis, S. M., F. Amin, A. Chekroud, D. Hjelm, E. Damaraju, H. J. Lee, J. R. Bustillo, K. Cho, G. D. Pearlson, and V. D. Calhoun. 2018. Reading the (functional) writing on the (structural) wall: Multimodal fusion of brain structure and function via a deep neural network based translation approach reveals novel impairments in schizophrenia. *NeuroImage* 181:734–747.

Poon, H., C. Quirk, K. Toutanova, and S. Wen-tau Yih. 2018. *AI for precision medicine*. Project Hanover. https://hanover.azurewebsites.net/#machineReading (accessed November 12, 2019).

Prakash, C., R. Kumar, and N. Mittal. 2018. Recent developments in human gait research: Parameters, approaches, applications, machine learning techniques, datasets and challenges. *Artificial Intelligence Review* 49(1):1–40.

Rabbitt, S. M., A. E. Kazdin, and B. Scassellati. 2015. Integrating socially assistive robotics into mental healthcare interventions: Applications and recommendations for expanded use. *Clinical Psychology Review* 35:35–46.

Rahwan, I. 2018. Society-in-the-loop: Programming the algorithmic social contract. *Ethics and Information Technology* 20(1):5–14. https://doi.org/10.1007/s10676-017-9430-8.

Reps, J. M., M. J. Schuemie, M. A. Suchard, P. B. Ryan, and P. R. Rijnbeek. 2018. Design and implementation of a standardized framework to generate and evaluate patient-level prediction models using observational healthcare data. *Journal of the American Medical Informatics Association* 25(8):969–975.

Roski, J., G. Bo-Linn, and T. Andrews. 2014. Creating value in healthcare through big data: Opportunities and policy implications. *Health Affairs* 33(7):1115–1122.

Roski, J., B. Gillingham, E. Juse, S. Barr, E. Sohn, and K. Sakarcan. 2018. Implementing and scaling artificial intelligence solutions: Considerations for policy makers and decision makers. *Health Affairs (Blog)*. https://www.healthaffairs.org/do/10.1377/hblog20180917.283077/full (accessed November 12, 2019).

Rowley, R. 2016. Can AI reduce the prior authorization burden in healthcare? *Health IT*. https://hitconsultant.net/2016/07/11/34693/#.Xd6pD25Fw2w (accessed November 12, 2019).

Rubens, M., A. Ramaamoorthy, A. Saxena, and N. Shehadeh. 2014. Public health in the 21st century: The role of advanced technologies. *Frontiers in Public Health* 2:1–4.

Sanchez-Martinez, S., N. Duchateau, T. Erdei, G. Kunszt, S. Aakhus, A. Degiovanni, P. Marino, E. Carluccio, G. Piella, A. G. Fraser, and B. H. Bijnens. 2018. Machine learning analysis of left ventricular function to characterize heart failure with preserved ejection fraction. *Circulation: Cardiovascular Imaging* 11(4):e007138.

Schuler, A., A. Callahan, K. Jung, and N. Shah. 2018. Performing an informatics consult: Methods and challenges. *Journal of the American College of Radiology* 15:563–568.

Schulman-Marcus, J., S. Mookherjee, L. Rice, and R. Lyubarova. 2019. New approaches for the treatment of delirium: A case for robotic pets. *American Journal of Medicine* 132(7):781–782. https://doi.org/10.1016/j.amjmed.2018.12.039.

Sennaar, K. 2018. Machine learning medical diagnostics—4 current applications. *Emerj Artificial Intelligence Research.* https://emerj.com/ai-sector-overviews/machine-learning-medical-diagnostics-4-current-applications (accessed November 12, 2019).

Shademan, A., R. S. Decker, J. D. Opfermann, S. Leonard, A. Krieger, and P. C. W. Kim. 2016. Supervised autonomous robotic soft tissue surgery. *Science Translational Medicine* 8(337):337ra64.

Shanafelt, T. D., L. N. Dyrbye, C. Sinsky, O. Hasan, D. Satele, J. Sloan, and C. P. West. 2016. Relationship between clerical burden and characteristics of the electronic environment with physician burnout and professional satisfaction. *Mayo Clinic Proceedings* 91(7):836–848.

Sharma, M. 2016. Benefits of an AI-based patient appointments service for hospitals. *Medium.* https://medium.com/@HCITExpert/benefits-of-an-ai-based-patient-appointments-service-for-hospitals-by-msharmas-617fdb2498e0 (accessed November 12, 2019).

Shen, H., C. Wang, L. Xie, S. Zhou, L. Gu, and H. Xie. 2018. A novel remote-controlled robotic system for cerebrovascular intervention. *International Journal of Medical Robotics and Computer Assisted Surgery* 14(6):e1943.

Shi, H., P. Xie, Z. Hu, M. Zhang, and E. P. Xing. 2017. Towards automated ICD coding using deep learning. *arXiv preprint.* 1711.04075.

Shin, E. K., R, Mahajan, O. Akbilgic, and A. Shaban-Nejad. 2018. Sociomarkers and biomarkers: Predictive modeling in identifying pediatric asthma patients at risk of hospital revisits. *Nature Medicine* 50(1). doi: 10.1038/s41746-018-0056-y.

Snyder, L., D. McEwen, M. Thrun, and A. Davidson. 2016. Visualizing the local experience: HIV Data to Care Tool. *Online Journal of Public Health Informatics* 8(1):e39.

Spruijt-Metz, D., and W. Nilsen. 2014. Dynamic models of behavior for just-in-time adaptive interventions. *IEEE Pervasive Computing* 13(3):13–17.

Stahl, B. C., and M. Coeckelbergh. 2016. Ethics of healthcare robotics: Towards responsible research and innovation. *Robotics and Autonomous Systems* 86:152–161.

Suresh, H., N. Hunt, A. Johnson, L. A. Celi, P. Szolovits, and M. Ghassemi. 2017. Clinical intervention prediction and understanding with deep neural networks. In *Proceedings of Machine Learning for Healthcare 2017*, JMLR W&C Track Vol. 68, edited by F. Doshi-Velez, J. Fackler, D. Kale, R. Ranganath, B. Wallace, and J. Wiens. Pp. 322–337. http://mucmd.org/CameraReadySubmissions/65%5CCameraReadySubmission%5Cclinical-intervention-prediction%20(4).pdf (accessed May 13, 2020).

Urban, G., P. Tripathi, T. Alkayali, M. Mittal, F. Jalali, W. Karnes, and P. Baldi. 2018. Deep learning localizes and identifies polyps in real time with 96% accuracy in screening colonoscopy. *Gastroenterology* 155(4):1069–1078

Waljee, A. K., P. D. R. Higgins, and A. G. Singal. 2014. A primer on predictive models. *Clinical and Translational Gastroenterology* 5:e44.

Wang, D., A. Khosla, R. Gargeya, H. Irshad, and A. H. Beck. 2016. Deep learning for identifying metastatic breast cancer. *arXIV.* https://arxiv.org/abs/1606.05718 (accessed November 12, 2019).

Ward-Foxton, S. 2019. Reducing bias in AI models for credit and loan decisions. *EE Times.* https://www.eetimes.com/document.asp?doc_id=1334632# (accessed November 12, 2019).

Wetzel, R. C. 2018. Is it ethical to let patients develop relationships with robots? *AI Medicine.* http://ai-med.io/ethical-patients-relationships-robots (accessed November 12, 2019).

Wicks, P., D. Keininger, M. Massagli, C. de la Loge, C. Brownstein, J. Isojärvi, and J. Heywood. 2012. Perceived benefits of sharing health data between people with epilepsy on an online platform. *Epilepsy & Behavior* 23(1):16–23. https://doi.org/10.1016/j.yebeh.2011.09.026.

Wiggers, K. 2018. CB Insights: AI health care startups have raised $4.3 billion since 2013. *VentureBeat.* https://venturebeat.com/2018/09/13/cb-insights-ai-health-care-startups-have-raised-4-3-billion-since-2013 (accessed November 12, 2019).

Williamson-Lee, J. 2018. How machines inherit their creators' biases: A.I. doesn't have to be conscious to be harmful. *Medium.* https://medium.com/coinmonks/ai-doesnt-have-to-be-conscious-to-be-harmful-385d143bd311 (accessed November 12, 2019).

Wince, R. 2018. Why AI is the future of prior auths. *insideBIGDATA.* https://insidebigdata.com/2018/12/21/ai-future-prior-auths (accessed November 12, 2019).

Wright, A., E. S. Chen, and F. L. Maloney. 2010. An automated technique for identifying associations between medications, laboratory results and problems. *Journal of Biomedical Informatics* 43(6):891–901.

Xiao, C., E. Choi, and J. Sun. 2018. Opportunities and challenges in developing deep learning models using electronic health records data: A systematic review. *Journal of the American Medical Informatics Association* 25(10):1419–1428.

YellRobot. 2018. *Robot pets for elderly and dementia patients.* https://yellrobot.com/robot-pets-for-elderly (accessed December 7, 2019).

Young, S. D., W. Yu, and W. Wang. 2017. Toward automating HIV identification: Machine learning for rapid identification of HIV-related social media data. *Journal of Acquired Immune Deficiency Syndrome* 74(Suppl 2):128–131.

Yu, S., P. K. Liao, S. Y. Shaw, V. S. Gainer, S. E. Churchill, P. Szolovits, S. N. Murphy, I. S. Kohane, and T. Cai. 2015. Toward high-throughput phenotyping: Unbiased automated feature extraction and selection from knowledge sources. *Journal of the American Medical Informatics Association* 22(5):993–1000.

Yu, S., A. Chakrabortty, K. P. Liao, T. Cai, A. N. Ananthakrishnan, V. S. Gainer, S. E. Churchill, P. Szolovits, S. N. Murphy, I. S. Kohane, and T. Cai. 2017. Surrogate-assisted feature extraction for high-throughput phenotyping. *Journal of the American Medical Informatics Association* 24(e1):e143–e149.

Zauderer, M. G., A. Gucalp, A. S. Epstein, A. D. Seidman, A. Caroline, S. Granovsky, J. Fu, J. Keesing, S. Lewis, H. Co, J. Petri, M. Megerian, T. Eggebraaten, P. Bach, and M. G. Kris. 2014. Piloting IBM Watson Oncology within Memorial Sloan Kettering's regional network. *Journal of Clinical Oncology* 32(15 Suppl):e17653.

Zellweger, M. J., A. Tsirkin, V. Vasilchenko, M. Failer, A. Dressel, M. E. Kleber, P. Ruff, and W. März. 2018. A new non-invasive diagnostic tool in coronary artery disease: Artificial intelligence as an essential element of predictive, preventive, and personalized medicine. *EPMA Journal* 9(3):235–247.

Zhao, J., P. Papapetrou, L. Asker, and H. Boström. 2017. Learning from heterogeneous temporal data in electronic health records. *Journal of Biomedical Informatics* 65(January):105–119.

Zhao, J., G. Wang, Z. Jiang, C. Jiang, J. Liu, J. Zhou, and J. Li. 2018. Robotic gastrotomy with intracorporeal suture for patients with gastric gastrointestinal stromal tumors located at cardia and subcardiac region. *Surgical Laparoscopy Endoscopy Percutaneous Technology* 28(1):e1–e7.

Zhao, L., J. Chen, F. Chen, W. Wang, C. T. Lu, and N. Ramakrishnan. 2015. SimNest: Social media nested epidemic simulation via online semi-supervised learning. In *Proceedings of the IEEE International Conference on Data Mining.* Pp. 639–648. doi:10.1109/ICDM.2015.39.

Zick, R. G., and J. Olsen. 2001. Voice recognition software versus a traditional transcription service for physician charting in the ED. *American Journal of Emergency Medicine* 19(4):295–298.

Zieger, A. 2018. Will payers use AI to do prior authorization? And will these AIs make things better? *Healthcare IT Today.* https://www.healthcareittoday.com/2018/12/27/will-payers-use-ai-to-do-prior-authorization-and-will-these-ais-make-things-better (accessed November 12, 2019).

Zitnik, M., M. Agrawal, and J. Leskovec. 2018. Modeling polypharmacy side effects with graph convolutional networks. *Bioinformatics* 34(13):i457–i466.

Suggested citation for Chapter 3: Roski, J., W. Chapman, J. Heffner, R. Trivedi, G. Del Fiol, R. Kukafka, P. Bleicher, H. Estiri, J. Klann, and J. Pierce. 2020. How artificial intelligence is changing health and health care. In *Artificial intelligence in health care: The hope, the hype, the promise, the peril.* Washington, DC: National Academy of Medicine.

4

POTENTIAL TRADE-OFFS AND UNINTENDED CONSEQUENCES OF ARTIFICIAL INTELLIGENCE

Jonathan Chen, Stanford University; Andrew Beam, Harvard University; Suchi Saria, Johns Hopkins University; and Eneida A. Mendonça, Regenstrief Institute

INTRODUCTION

Chapter 3 highlights the vast potential for artificial intelligence (AI)-driven solutions to systematically improve the efficiency, efficacy, and equity of health and medicine. Although we optimistically look forward to this future, we address fears over potentially unintended (but predictable) consequences of an AI future in human health, with key considerations about how to recognize and mitigate credible risks.

This chapter reviews how hype cycles can promote interest in the short term but inadvertently impede progress when disillusionment sets in from unmet expectations as in the AI Winters discussed in Chapter 2. We further explore the potential harms of poorly implemented AI systems, including misleading models, bias, and vulnerability to adversarial actors, all of which warrant an intentional process for validation and monitoring. We round out this chapter with a discussion of the implications of technological automation to improve health care efficiency and access to care, even as we expect AI to redefine job roles and potentially exacerbate existing inequities without dedicated investments into human workforce development.

HYPE VERSUS HOPE

One of the greatest near-term risks in the current development of AI tools in medicine is not that it will cause serious unintended harm, but that it simply cannot meet the incredible expectations stoked by excessive hype. Indeed, so-called AI

expectations

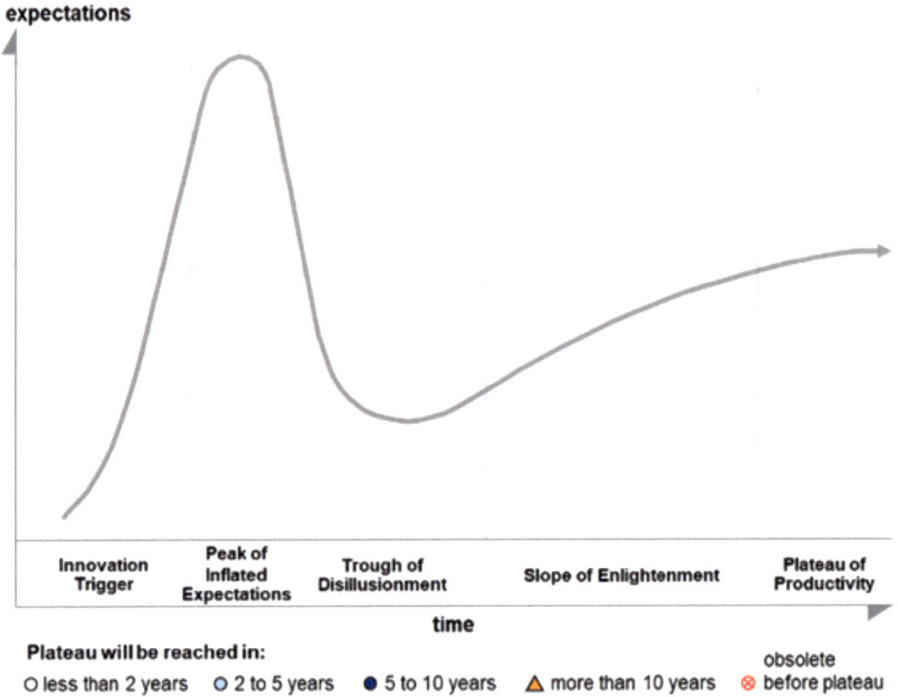

| Innovation Trigger | Peak of Inflated Expectations | Trough of Disillusionment | Slope of Enlightenment | Plateau of Productivity |

time

Plateau will be reached in:

O less than 2 years   ⊙ 2 to 5 years   ● 5 to 10 years   ▲ more than 10 years   ⊗ obsolete before plateau

FIGURE 4-1 | Gartner Hype Cycle.
SOURCE: Gartner Hype Cycle HD, Gartner, Inc. 2017.

technologies such as deep learning and machine learning are riding atop the utmost peak of inflated expectations for emerging technologies, as noted by the Gartner Hype Cycle, which tracks relative maturity stages for emerging technologies (Chen and Asch, 2017; Panetta, 2017) (see Figure 4-1). Without an appreciation for both the capabilities and limitations of AI technology in medicine, we will predictably crash into a "trough of disillusionment." The greatest risk of all may be a backlash that impedes real progress toward using AI tools to improve human lives.

Over the past decade, several factors have led to increasing interest in and escalating hype of AI. There have been legitimate discontinuous leaps in computational capacity, electronic data availability (e.g., ImageNet [Russakovsky et al., 2015] and digitization of medical records), and perception capability (e.g., image recognition [Krizhevsky et al., 2017]). Just as algorithms can now automatically name the breed of a dog in a photo and generate a caption of a "dog catching a frisbee" (Vinyals et al., 2017), we are seeing automated recognition of malignant skin lesions (Esteva et al., 2017) and pathology specimens (Ehteshami et al., 2017). Such functionality is incredible but can easily lead one to mistakenly assume that the computer "knows" what skin cancer is and that a surgical excision is being considered. It is expected that an intelligent human who can recognize an object in a photo can also naturally understand and explain the context of what they are seeing, but the narrow, applied AI algorithms atop the current hype cycle have no such general comprehension. Instead, these algorithms are each designed to complete specific tasks, such as answering well-formed multiple-choice questions.

With Moore's law of exponential growth in computing power, the question arises whether it is reasonable to expect that machines will soon possess greater computational power than human brains (Saracco, 2018). This comparison may not even make sense with the fundamentally different architectures of computer processors and biological brains, because computers already can exceed human brains by measures of pure storage and speed (Fischetti, 2011). Does this mean that humans are headed toward a technological singularity (Shanahan, 2015; Vinge, 1993) that will spawn fully autonomous AI systems that continually self-improve beyond the confines of human control? Roy Amara, co-founder of Institute for the Future, reminds us that "we tend to overestimate the effect of a technology in the short run and underestimate the effect in the long run" (Ridley, 2017). Among other reasons however, intelligence is not simply a function of computing power. Increasing computing speed and storage makes a better *calculator*, but not a better *thinker*. For the near future at least, this leaves us with fundamental design and concept issues in (general) AI research that have remained unresolved for decades (e.g., common sense, framing, abstract reasoning, creativity; Brooks, 2017).

Explicit advertising hyperbole may be one of the most direct triggers for unintended consequences of hype. While such promotion is important to drive interest and motivate progress, it can become counterproductive in excess. Hyperbolic marketing of AI systems that will "outthink cancer" (Brown, 2017) can ultimately set the field back when confronted by the hard realities in attempting to deliver changes in actual patient lives (Ross and Swetlitz, 2017). Modern advances do reflect important progress in AI software and data, but can shortsightedly discount the "hardware" of a health care delivery system (people, policies, and processes) needed to actually execute care. Limited AI systems can fail to provide insights to clinicians beyond what they already knew, undercutting many hopes for early warning systems and screening asymptomatic patients for rare diseases (Butterfield, 2018). Ongoing research has a tendency to promote the latest technology as a cure-all (Marcus, 2018), even if there is a "regression to regression" where well-worn methods backed by a good data source can be as, or more, useful than "advanced" AI methods in many applications (Razavian et al., 2015).

A combination of technical and subject domain expertise is needed to recognize the credible potential of AI systems and avoid the backlash that will come from overselling them. Yet, there is no need for pessimism if our benchmark is improving on the current state of human health. Algorithms and AI systems cannot provide "guarantees of fairness, equitability, or even veracity" (Beam and Kohane, 2018), but no humans can either. The "Superhuman Human Fallacy" (Kohane, 2017) is to dismiss computerized systems (or humans) that do not achieve an unrealizable standard of perfection or improve on the best performing human. For example, accidents attributed to self-driving cars receive outsized media attention even though they occur far less frequently than accidents attributed to human–driven cars (Felton, 2018). Yet, the potential outsized impact of automated technologies reasonably makes us demand a higher standard of reliability (Stewart, 2019) even if the necessary degree is unclear and may even cost more lives in opportunity cost while awaiting perfection (Kalra and Groves, 2017). In health care, it is possible to determine where even imperfect AI clinical augmentation can improve care and reduce practice variation. For example, gaps exist now where humans commonly misjudge the accuracy of screening tests for rare diagnoses (Manrai et al., 2014), grossly overestimate patient life expectancy (Christakis and Lamont, 2000; Glare et al., 2003), and deliver care of widely varied intensity in the last 6 months of life (Barnato et al., 2007; Dartmouth Atlas Project, 2018). There is no need to overhype the potential of AI in medicine when there is ample opportunity (as reviewed in Chapter 3) to address existing issues with undesirable variability, crippling costs, and impaired access to quality care (DOJ and FTC, 2015).

To find opportunities for automated predictive systems, stakeholders should consider where important decisions hinge upon humans making predictions with a clear outcome (Bates et al., 2014; Kleinberg et al., 2016). Though human intuition is powerful, it is inevitably variable without a support system. One could identify scarce interventions that are known to be valuable and use AI tools to assist in identifying patients most likely to benefit. For example, an intensive outpatient care team need not attend to everyone, but can be targeted to only those patients that AI systems predict are at high risk of morbidity (Zulman et al., 2017). In addition, there are numerous opportunities to deploy AI workflow support to assist humans to rapidly answer or complete repetitive information tasks (e.g., documentation, scheduling, and other back-office administration).

HOW COULD IMPROPER AI HURT PATIENTS AND THE HEALTH SYSTEM?

The evolution of AI techniques applied to medical-use cases parallels better processing power and cheaper storage capabilities (Deo, 2015) and the exponential increase in health data generated from scientific and clinical systems (e.g., electronic health records [EHRs], picture archiving and communication systems, and -omics) if not directly from patients (e.g., mobile sensors and social media interactions). Most of the conceptual foundations for AI are not new, but the combined advances can finally now translate theoretical models into usable technologies.

This will mark a fundamental change in the expectations for the next generation of physicians (Silver et al., 2018). Though there is much upside in the potential for the use of AI systems to improve health and health care, like all technologies, implementation does not come without certain risks. This section outlines some ways in which AI in health care may cause harm in unintended ways.

Correlation or Causation? Prediction Versus Action?

Poorly constructed or interpreted models from observational data can harm patients. Incredible advances in learning algorithms are now toppling world-class professional humans in games such as chess, go (Silver et al., 2018), poker (Brown and Sandholm, 2018), and even complex real-time strategy games (AlphaStar Team, 2019). The key distinction is that these can be reliably simulated with clear outcomes of success and failure. Such simulations allow algorithms to generate a virtually unlimited amount of data and experiments. In contrast, accurate simulations of novel medical care with predictable outcomes may well be impossible, meaning medical data collection requires high-cost, high-stakes experiments on real people. In addition, high-fidelity, reliably measured outcomes are not always achievable, because AI systems are constrained to learning from available observational health data.

The implementation of EHRs and other health information systems has provided scientists with rich longitudinal, multidimensional, and detailed records about an individual's health data. However, these data are noisy and biased because they are produced for different purposes in the process of documenting care. Health care data scientists must be careful to apply the right types of modeling approaches based on the characteristics and limitations of the underlying data.

Correlation can be sufficient for diagnosing problems and *predicting* outcomes in certain cases. In most scenarios, however, patients and clinicians are not interested in just *predicting* outcomes given "usual care" or following a "natural history." Often, the whole point of paying attention to health data is to *intervene* to *change* the expected outcomes.

Predictive models already help decision makers assess patient risk. However, methods that primarily learn associations between inputs and outputs can be unreliable, if not overtly dangerous when used for driving medical decisions (Schulam and Saria, 2017). There are three common reasons why this is the case. First, performance of association-based models tends to be susceptible to even minor deviations between the development and the implementation datasets. The learned associations may memorize dataset-specific patterns that do not generalize as the tool is moved to new environments where these patterns no longer hold (Subbaswamy et al., 2019). A common example of this phenomenon is shifts in provider practice with the introduction of new medical evidence, technology, and epidemiology. If a tool heavily relies on a practice pattern to be predictive, as practice changes, the tool is no longer valid (Schulam and Saria, 2017). Second, such algorithms cannot correct for biases due to feedback loops that are introduced when learning continuously over time (Schulam and Saria, 2017). In particular, if the implementation of an AI system changes patient exposures, interventions, and outcomes (often as intended), it can cause data shifts or changes in the distribution of the data that degrade performance. Finally, it may be tempting to treat the proposed predictors as factors one can manipulate to change outcomes, but these are often misleading.

Consider, for instance, the finding discussed by Caruana et al. (2015) regarding risk of death among those who develop pneumonia. Their goal was to build a model that predicts risk of death for a hospitalized individual with pneumonia so that those at high risk could be treated and those at low risk could be safely sent home. The model applying supervised learning counterintuitively learned that patients who have asthma and pneumonia are less likely to die than patients who only have asthma. They traced the result back to an existing policy that patients who have asthma and pneumonia should be directly admitted to the intensive care unit, therefore receiving more aggressive treatment that in turn improved their prognosis (Cabitza et al., 2017). The health care system and research team noted this confounded finding, but had such a model been deployed to assess risk, then sicker patients might have been triaged to a lower level of care, putting them at greater risk. In this example, the association–based algorithm learned risk conditioned on the triage policy in the development dataset that persisted in the implementation environment. However, as providers begin to rely on these types of tools, practice patterns deviate (a phenomenon called practice policy shift) from those observed in the development data. This shift hurts the validity and reliability of the tool (Brown and Sandholm, 2018).

In another example, researchers observed that the time a lab value is measured can often be more predictive than the value itself (Agniel et al., 2018). For instance, the fact that a hospital test was done at 2:00 a.m. was more predictive of patient outcomes than the actual results of the test, because the implied emergency that prompted the test was at an unusual time. Similarly, a mortality prediction model may learn that patients visited by the chaplain have an increased risk of death (Chen and Altman, 2014; Choi et al., 2015).

Finally, a prostate screening test can be determined to be "protective" of near-term mortality, not because the actual test does anything, but because patients who receive that screening test are those who are already fairly healthy and have a longer life expectancy (Agniel et al., 2018). A model based on associations may very well be learning about the way local clinical operations run but not generalize well when moving across hospitals or units with different practice patterns (Schulam and Saria, 2017). More broadly, both humans and predictive models can fail to generalize from training to implementation environments because of many different types of *dataset shift*—shift in dataset characteristics over time, in practice pattern, or across populations—posing a threat to model reliability and the safety of downstream decisions made in practice (Subbaswamy and Saria, 2018). Recent works have proposed that *proactive learning* techniques are less susceptible to dataset shifts (Schulam and Saria, 2017; Subbaswamy et al., 2019). These algorithms proactively correct for likely shifts in data.

In addition to learning a model once, an alternative approach is to update models over time so that they continuously adapt to local and recent data. Such adaptive algorithms offer constant vigilance and monitoring for changing behavior. However, this may exacerbate disparities when only well-resourced institutions can deploy the expertise to do so in an environment. In addition, regulation and law, as reviewed in Chapter 7, faces significant challenges in addressing approval and certification for continuously evolving systems.

Rule-based systems are explicitly authored by human knowledge engineers, encoding their understanding of an application domain into a computing inference engine. These are generally more explicit and interpretable in their intent, making these easier to audit for safety and reliability. On the other hand, they take less advantage of relationships that can be automatically inferred through data-driven models and therefore are often less accurate. Integrating domain-knowledge within learning-based frameworks, and combining these with methods for measuring and proactively eliminating bias, provides a promising path forward (Subbaswamy and Saria, 2018). Much of the literature on predictive modeling is based on black box models that memorize associations. Increases in model complexity can reduce both the interpretability and ability of the user to respond to predictions in practical ways (Obermeyer and Emanuel, 2016). As a result, these models are susceptible to unreliability, leading to harmful suggestions. Evaluating for reliability and actionability are key in developing models that have the potential to affect health outcomes. These issues are at the core of the tension between "black box" and "interpretable" model algorithms that afford end users some explanation for why certain predictions are favored.

Training reliable models depends on training datasets to be representative of the population where the model will be applied. Learning from real-world data— where insights can be drawn from patients similar to a given index patient—has the benefit of leading to inferences that are more relevant, but it is important to characterize populations where there are inadequate data to support robust conclusions. For example, a tool may show acceptable performance on average across individuals captured within a dataset but may perform poorly for specific subpopulations because the algorithm has not had enough data to learn from.

In genetic testing, minority groups can be disproportionately adversely affected when recommendations are made based on data that do not adequately represent them (Manrai et al., 2016). Test-time auditing tools that can identify individuals for whom the model predictions are likely to be unreliable can reduce the likelihood of incorrect decision making due to model bias (Schulam and Saria, 2017).

Amplification or Exacerbation?

AI systems will generally make people more efficient at what they are already doing, whether that is good or bad. Bias is not inherently undesirable, because the whole point of learning from (clinical) practices is that there is an underlying assumption that human experts are making nonrandom decisions biased toward achieving desirable effects. Machine learning relying on observational data will generally have an amplifying effect on our existing behavior, regardless of whether that behavior is beneficial or only exacerbates existing societal biases. For instance, Google Photos, an app that uses machine learning technology to organize images, incorrectly identified people with darker skin tones as "gorillas," an animal that has historically been used as a racial slur (Lee, 2018). Another study found that machine translation systems were biased against women due to the way in which women were described in the data used to train the system (Prates et al., 2018). In another example, Amazon developed a hiring algorithm based on its prior hiring practices, which recapitulated existing biases against women (Dastin, 2018). Although some of these algorithms were revised or discontinued, the underlying issues will continue to be significant problems, requiring constant vigilance, as well as algorithm surveillance and maintenance to detect and address them (see Chapter 6). The need for continuous assessment about the ongoing safety of systems is discussed in Chapter 7, including a call for significant changes in regulatory compliance. Societal biases reflected in health care data may be amplified as automated systems drive more decisions, as further addressed in Chapters 5 and 6.

AI Systems Transparency

Transparency is a key theme underlying deeper issues related to privacy and consent or notification for patient data use, and to potential concerns on the part of patients and clinicians around being subject to algorithmically driven decisions. Consistent progress will only be feasible if health care consumers and health care systems are mutually recognized as trusted data partners.

As discussed in detail in Chapter 7, there are tensions that exist between the desire for robust data aggregation to facilitate the development and validation of novel AI models and the need to protect consumer privacy as well as demonstrate respect for consumer preferences through informed consent or notification procedures. However, lack of transparency about data use and privacy practices runs the risk of fostering a situation that lacks clear consent when patient data are used in ways that patients do not understand, realize, or accept. Current consent practices for the use of EHRs and claims data are generally based on models focused on the Health Insurance Portability and Accountability Act (HIPAA) privacy rules, and some argue that HIPAA needs updating (Cohen and Mello, 2018). The progressive integration of other sources of patient-related data (e.g., genetic information, social determinants of health) and the facilitated access to highly granular and multidimensional data are changing the protections provided by the traditional mechanisms. For instance, with more data available, reidentification becomes easier to perform (Cohen and Mello, 2019). As discussed further in Chapter 7, regulations need to be updated and consent processes will need to be more informative of those added risks. Educating patients about the value of having their data used to help advance science and care, but also being explicit about the potential risks of data misuse or unintended negative effects is crucial.

In addition to issues related to data use transparency, peer and community review of publications that describe AI tools, with dissemination of code and source data, is necessary to support scientific reproducibility and validation. The risks of "stealth research" (Ioannidis, 2015), where claims regarding important, high-stakes medical advancements are made outside of the peer-reviewed scientific literature, are too great. While there will be claims of commercial concerns for proprietary intellectual property and even controversial concerns over "research parasites" (Longo and Drazen, 2016), some minimal level of transparency must be expected. Before clinical acceptance of systems can be expected, peer-reviewed publication of model performance and sources of training data should be expected just as much as population descriptions in randomized controlled trials. This is necessary to clarify the representativeness of any models and what populations to which they can reasonably be expected to apply.

For review of AI model development and validation, different models of accountability can be considered, such as the development of review agencies for automated AI and other systems in medicine. If not through existing structures such as the U.S. Food and Drug Administration (FDA) or Clinical Laboratory Improvement Amendments (CLIA), these can be modeled after the National Transportation Safety Board. In the latter case, such an agency has no direct enforcement authority, but in the event of any adverse event that could harm people, full disclosure of all data and information to the review board is required to ensure that the community can learn from mistakes. Refer to Chapter 7 for additional reading related to current and necessary policies and regulations in the use of AI systems in health care.

Cybersecurity Vulnerabilities Due to AI Automation

Vulnerabilities

Most of this chapter focuses on the side effects of nonmalicious actors using ethically neutral AI technology. Chapter 1 discusses some of the challenges in the ethical uses of health care AI tools. However, it is also important to consider how increasing automation opens new risks for bad actors to directly induce harm, such as through overt fraud. E-mail gave us new ways to communicate and increased productivity, but it also enabled new forms of fraud through spam and phishing. Likewise, new health care technology may open up new streams for fraud and abuse. After the widespread adoption of digital health records, data breaches resulting in the release of millions of individuals' private medical information have become commonplace (Patil and Seshadri, 2014). These breaches will likely increase in an era when our demand for health data exceeds its supply in the public sector (Jiang and Bai, 2019; Perakslis, 2014). Health care systems are increasingly vigilant, but ongoing attacks demonstrate that safeguarding against a quickly evolving threat landscape remains exceedingly difficult (Ehrenfeld, 2017). The risk to personal data safety will continue to increase as AI becomes mainstream and commercialized. Engaging the public on how and when their secondary data are being used will be crucial to preventing public backlash as we have seen with the Facebook–Cambridge Analytica data scandal (Cadwalladr and Graham-Harrison, 2018). A recent study also indicates that hospital size and academic environment could be associated with increased risk for breaches, calling for better data breach statistics (Fabbri et al., 2017).

Health care data will not be the only target for attackers; the AI systems themselves will become the subject of assault and manipulation. FDA has already approved several AI systems for clinical use, some of which can operate without the oversight of a physician. In parallel, the health care economy in the United States is projected to represent 20 percent of the gross domestic product by 2025 (Papanicolas et al., 2018), making automated medical AI systems a natural target for manipulation as they drive decisions that move billions of dollars through the health care system.

Though recent advances in AI have made impressive progress on clinical tasks, the fact remains that these systems as currently conceived are exceptionally brittle, making them easy to mislead and manipulate with seemingly slight variations in input. Medical images that have small but intentionally crafted modifications (imperceptible to the human eye) can be used to create error in the diagnoses that an AI system provides (Finlayson et al., 2018, 2019). Such attacks allow the attacker to exert arbitrary control over the AI model by modifying the input provided to the system. Figure 4-2 demonstrates how such an attack may be carried out.

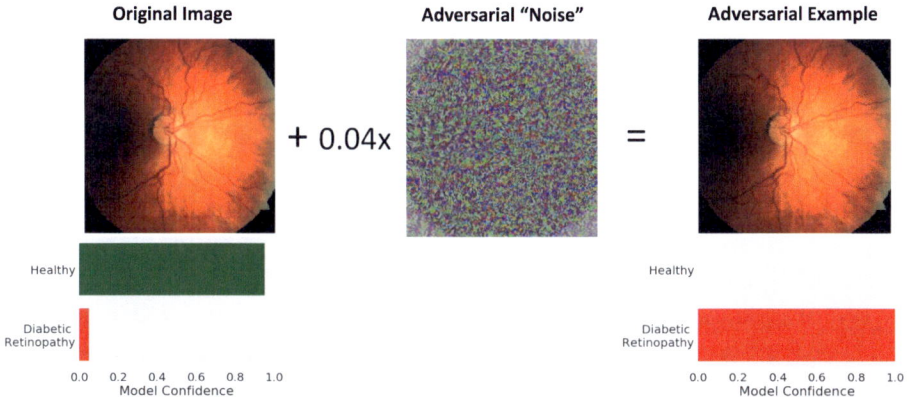

FIGURE 4-2 | Construction of an "adversarial example." Left: An unaltered fundus image of a healthy retina. The AI system (bottom left) correctly identifies it as a healthy eye. Middle: Adversarial "noise" that is constructed with knowledge of the AI system is added to the original image. Right: Resulting adversarial image that superimposes the original image and the adversarial noise. Though the original image is indistinguishable from the adversarial example to human eyes, the AI system has now changed the diagnosis to diabetic retinopathy with essentially 100 percent confidence.

SOURCE: Image was provided by Samuel Finlayson.

These kinds of attacks can give potential adversaries an opportunity to manipulate the health care system. For instance, suppose that AI has become ubiquitous in the health care system and payers require that an AI system evaluate and confirm an imaging-based diagnosis before a reimbursement is granted. Under such a system, a motivated provider could be incentivized to modify "borderline" cases to allow them to perform a procedure in pursuit of reimbursement. These kinds of attacks could be conducted on a larger scale where similar large financial gains are at stake. Consider that clinical trials that are based on imaging endpoints (e.g., tumor burden in X-rays) will likely be evaluated by AI systems in the future to ensure "objectivity." Any entity could intentionally ensure a positive result by making small and untraceable adversarial changes to the image, which would cause the AI system to think that tumor burden had been reduced. It is unlikely that the hypothetical scenarios discussed above will happen in the near term, but they are presented as cautionary examples to encourage a proactive dialogue and to highlight limitations of current AI technology.

Adversarial Defenses

There are roughly two broad classes of possible defenses: infrastructural and algorithmic (Qiu et al., 2019; Yuan et al., 2018). Infrastructural defenses prevent image tampering or detect if it has occurred. For instance, an image hash, also known as a "digital fingerprint," could be generated and stored by the device as soon as an image is created. The hash would then be used to determine if the image had been altered in any way, because any modification would result in a new hash. This would require an update to hospital information technology (IT) infrastructure, which has historically been very difficult. However, a set of standards similar to ones for laboratories such as CLIA could be established to ensure that the medical imaging pipeline is secure.

Algorithmic defenses against adversarial attacks are a very active area of research within the broader machine learning community (Qiu et al., 2019; Yuan et al., 2018). As of yet, there are no defenses that have proven to be 100 percent effective, and new defenses are often broken almost as quickly as they are proposed. However, there have been successful defenses in specific domains or on specific datasets. On the handwritten digit dataset known as MNIST, several approaches have proven to be robust to adversarial attacks while retaining high levels of predictive accuracy (Kannan et al., 2018; Madry et al., 2017). It remains to be seen if some specific property of medical imaging (such as low levels of pose variance or restricted color spectrum) could be leveraged to improve robustness to adversarial attacks, but this is likely a fruitful direction for research in this area.

Both types of defenses, infrastructural and algorithmic, highlight the need for interdisciplinary teams of computer scientists, health care workers, and consumer representatives at every stage of design and implementation of these systems. Because these AI systems represent a new type of IT infrastructure, they must be treated as such and continually probed for possible security vulnerabilities. This will necessarily require deep collaborations between health care IT experts, computer scientists, the traditional health care workforce, and those the algorithm is designed to affect.

HOW COULD AI RESHAPE MEDICINE AND HEALTH IN UNINTENDED WAYS?

The examples in this chapter largely revolve around clinical cases and risks, but the implications reach far beyond to all of the application domains explored in Chapter 3. Public health, consumer health, and population health and/or risk management applications and risks are all foreseeable. Operational and administrative cases may be more viable early target areas with much more forgiving risk profiles for unintended harm, without high-stakes medical decisions depending on them. Even then, automated AI systems will have far-reaching implications for patient populations, health systems, and the workforce in terms of the efficiency and equity of delivering against the unmet and unlimited demands for health care.

Future of Employment and Displacement

"It's just completely obvious that in five years deep learning is going to do better than radiologists. It might be 10 years," according to Geoffrey Hinton, a pioneer in artificial neural network research (Mukherjee, 2017). How should health care systems respond to the statement by Sun Microsystems co-founder Vinod Khosla that "Machines will replace 80 percent of doctors in a health care future that will be driven by entrepreneurs, not medical professionals" (Clark, 2012)? With the advancing capabilities of AI, and a history of prior large-scale workforce disruptions through technology advances, it seems reasonable to posit that entire job categories may be replaced by automation (see Figure 4-3), including some of the most common (e.g., retail clerks and drivers) (Desjardins, 2017; Frey and Osborne, 2013).

Are job losses in medicine a credible consequence of advancing AI? In 1968, Warner Slack commented that "any doctor that can be replaced by a machine should be replaced by a machine" (deBronkart and Sands, 2018). This sentiment is often misinterpreted as an argument for replacing people with computer systems, when it is meant to emphasize the value a good human adds that a computer system does not. If one's job is restricted to relaying information and answering well-structured, verifiable multiple-choice questions, then it is likely those tasks should be automated and the job eliminated. Most clinical jobs and patient needs require much more cognitive adaptability, problem solving, and communication skills than a computer can muster. Anxiety over job losses due to AI and automation are likely exaggerated, but advancing technology will almost certainly change roles as certain tasks are automated. A conceivable future could eliminate manual tasks such as checking patient vital signs (especially with self-monitoring devices), collecting laboratory specimens, preparing medications for pickup, transcribing clinical documentation, completing prior authorization forms, scheduling appointments, collecting standard history elements, and making routine diagnoses. Rather than eliminate jobs, however, industrialization and technology typically yield net productivity gains to society, with increased labor demands elsewhere such as in software, technical, support, and related services work. Even within the same job category, many assumed automated teller machines would eliminate the need for bank tellers. Instead, the efficiencies gained enabled expansion of branches and even greater demand for tellers that could focus on higher cognitive tasks (e.g., interacting with customers, rather than simply counting money) (Pethokoukis, 2016). Health care is already the fastest growing and now largest employment sector in the nation (outstripping retail), but most of that growth is not in clinical professionals such as doctors and nurses, but rather in home care support and administrative staff (Thompson, 2018).

The future of employment

About half of today's jobs will likely be done by computers in a decade or two. Automation has so far taken over mostly well-defined routine tasks, shifting jobs from middle-income manufacturing to lower-income service jobs. As computers get better at for example perception – think self-driving cars – those services jobs are likely next up to be replaced by machines. Frey and Osborne (2013) estimate the probability of each job becoming automated. Here are how their predictions apply to 2016 US employment statistics. Black fields are jobs likely to be automated and white fields are jobs that are likely to remain.

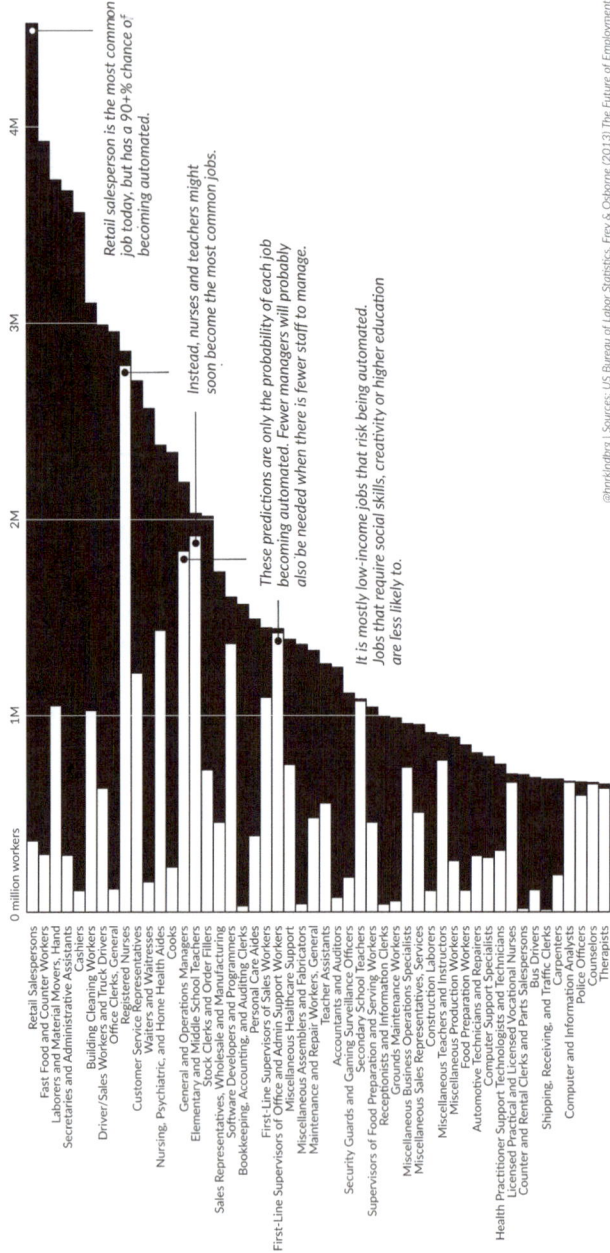

Retail salesperson is the most common job today, but has a 90+% chance of becoming automated.

Instead, nurses and teachers might soon become the most common jobs.

These predictions are only the probability of each job becoming automated. Fewer managers will probably also be needed when there is fewer staff to manage.

It is mostly low-income jobs that risk being automated. Jobs that require social skills, creativity or higher education are less likely to.

@mrkndbrg | Sources: US Bureau of Labor Statistics, Frey & Osborne (2013) The Future of Employment

FIGURE 4-3 | The future of employment.
SOURCE: Desjardins, 2017.

Filling the Gap for Human Expertise, the Scarcest Health Care Resource

Besides using AI automation to tackle obvious targets such as repetitive administrative tasks (clinical documentation, scheduling, etc.), more important is to consider the most valuable and limited resource in medicine, which is access to and time with a competent professional clinician. More than 25 million people in the United States alone have deficient access to medical specialty care (Woolhandler and Himmelstein, 2017). For everyone to receive levels of medical care that the insured metropolitan populations do, we already lack >30,000 doctors in the United States to meet that demand. With growing and aging populations, the demand for physicians continually outpaces supply, with shortfalls projected to be as much as 100,000 physicians in the United States alone by 2030 (Markit, 2017) (see Figure 4-4). The scarcity of available expertise runs even deeper in international and rural settings, where populations may not be able to reach even basic health care without prolonged travel. This pent-up and escalating demand for health care services should direct advances in telemedicine and AI automation to ultimately increase access and fill these shortfalls. At the same time, we should not feel satisfied with broad dissemination of lower quality services that may only widen inequity between affluent urban centers with ready access to multiple tiers of service and remote rural populations with more limited choices.

Instead of trying to replace medical workers, the coming era of AI automation can instead be directed toward enabling a broader reach of the workforce to do more good for more people, given a constrained set of scarce resources.

Net Gains, Unequal Pains

Even with the optimistic perspective that increasing automation through AI technology will be net beneficial in the end, the intervening processes of displacement can be painful, disruptive, and can widen existing inequality (Acemoglu and Restrepo, 2018). Automation reflects a movement of production from labor to capital. This tends to mean unequal distribution of benefits, as productivity starts coming from those holding the capital while the labor force (wage workers) is progressively constrained into a narrower set of tasks, not sharing as much in the control or growth in overall income (Acemoglu and Restrepo, 2018).

Everyone is enriched when something needed (e.g., food or medical care) becomes less expensive to produce through automation (Herrendorf et al., 2009). The response to such technological shocks can be slow and painful, however, with costly reallocation and retraining of workers. This can be particularly challenging when there is a mismatch between new technology and workforce skills. Such disruptive

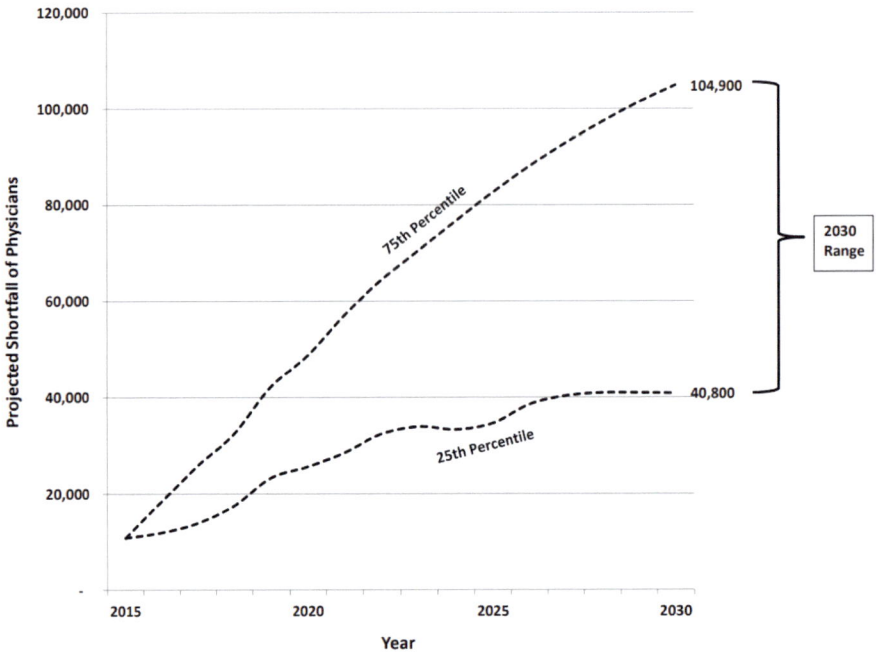

FIGURE 4-4 | Projected total physician shortfall range, 2015–2030.
SOURCE: LaPointe, 2017.

changes tend to be harder on small (usually under-represented) groups who are already on the margins, amplifying existing inequity. Those who can adapt well to different economies and structures are likely those who already have better resources, education, and socioeconomic stability. Advances in health care AI technologies may well create more jobs (e.g., software development, health care system analysts) than are eliminated (e.g., data entry, scribing, scheduling), but those in the jobs that are easy to automate are unlikely to be the ones able to easily adopt the skills needed for the new jobs created. The fallout from a growing mismatch between employer skill set demand and employee training are reflected with only one in four employees feeling that they are getting training to adapt to an AI tech world (Giacomelli and Shukla, 2018).

Although the above example is on the individual worker level, even at the system level, we are likely to see increasing disparities. Well-resourced academic medical centers may be in a position to build and deploy adaptive learning AI systems, whereas smaller health care systems that care for the majority of the population are unlikely to have the resources to assemble the on-site expertise and data infrastructure needed for more than out-of-the-box systems that are subject to all of the modeling risks previously discussed.

While it is important to measure total and average improvement in human outcomes, it is equally important to also measure equitable distribution of such benefits (e.g., Gini index [Gastwirth, 1972]). By analogy to a "food apartheid," if we only optimize for production of total calories per acre (Haspel, 2015), all can get fatter with more empty calories, but the poor are less likely to access actual nutrition (Brones, 2018). If high-tech health care is only available and used by those already plugged in socioeconomically, such advances may inadvertently reinforce a "health care apartheid" (Thadaney and Verghese, 2019).

New Roles in an AI Future

Prior advances in technology and automation have resulted in transitions of jobs from agricultural to manufacturing to service. Where will medical workers go when even service jobs are automated? Most of the near-term changes discussed are largely applied AI in terms of data analytics for prediction, decision making, logistics, and pattern recognition. These remain unlikely to displace many human skills such as complex reasoning, judgment, analogy-based learning, abstract problem solving, physical interactions, empathy, communication, counseling, and implicit observation. There will thus likely be a shift in health care toward jobs that require direct physical (human) interaction, which are not so easily automated. The advent of the AI era will even require the creation of new job roles (Wilson et al., 2017), including

- **Trainers:** Teaching AI systems how to perform will require deliberate effort to evaluate and stress test them. AI systems can automate tasks and find patterns in data, but still require humans to provide meaning, purpose, and direction.
- **Explainers:** Advancing AI algorithms often have a "black box" nature, making suggestions without clear explanations, requiring humans versed in both the technical and application domains to explain how such algorithms can be trusted to drive practical decisions.
- **Sustainers:** The intelligence needs of human endeavors will continually evolve, preventing the advent of "completed" AI systems. Humans must continue to maintain, interpret, and monitor the behavior and unintended consequences of AI systems.

Deskilling of the Health Care Workforce

Even if health-related jobs are not replaced by AI, deskilling ("skill rot") is a risk of over-reliance on computer-based systems (Cabitza et al., 2017). While clinicians may not be totally displaced, the fear is that they may lose "core competencies" considered vital to medical practice. In light of the rapid advancements of AI capabilities in reading X-rays (Beam and Kohane, 2016; Gulshan et al., 2016), will radiologists of the future be able to perform this task without the aid of a computer? The very notion of a core competency is an evolving one that professionals will need to adapt as technology changes roles (Jha and Topol, 2016).

As the skills needed in imaging-based specialties change rapidly, radiologists and pathologists "must be willing to be displaced to avoid being replaced" (Jha and Topol, 2016). Jha and Topol (2016) articulate a future in which physicians in these specialties no longer operate as image readers as they currently do, but have evolved to be "information specialists" that manage complex AI systems and integrate the various pieces of information they might provide. Indeed, they argue that radiology and pathology will be affected by AI in such a similar manner that these specialties might be merged under the unified banner of information specialists, to more accurately reflect the skills needed by these physicians in the AI-enabled future. While this may be extreme due to the significantly different clinical information required in the two disciplines, it highlights that this era of health care is likely to be substantially disrupted and transformed.

Need for Education and Workforce Development

Advancing technologies in health care can bring substantial societal benefits, but will require significant training or retraining of the workforce for roles that emphasize where humans and machines have different strengths. The Industrial Revolution illustrated the paradox of overall technological advance and productivity growth, which first passed through a period of stagnated wages, reduced share to laborers, expanding poverty, and harsh living conditions (Mokyr, 1990). An overall beneficial shift only occurred after mass schooling and other investments in human capital to expand skills of the workforce. Such adjustments are impeded if the educational system is not able to provide the newly relevant skills.

A graceful transition into the AI era of health care that minimizes the unintended consequences of displacement will require deliberate redesign of training programs. This ranges from support for a core basis of primary education in science, technology, engineering, and math literacy in the broader population to continuing professional education in the face of a changing environment. Any professional's job changes over time as technology and systems evolve. While complete replacement of health-related jobs by AI computer systems is unlikely, a lack of adaptation will result in a growing skill set mismatch, decreases in efficiency, and increasing cost of care delivery. In the face of the escalating complexity in medicine and computerization of data, medical training institutions already acknowledge that emphasizing rote memorization and repetition of information is suboptimal in an information age, requiring large-scale transformation. Health care workers in the AI future will need to learn how to use and interact with information systems, with foundational education in information retrieval and synthesis, statistics and evidence-based medicine appraisal, and interpretation of predictive models in terms of diagnostic performance measures. Institutional organizations (e.g., the National Institutes of Health, health care systems, professional organizations, universities, and medical schools) should shift focus from skills that are easily replaced by AI automation to specific education and workforce development programs for work in the AI future with emphasis in science, technology, engineering, and medicine and data science skills and human skills that are hard to replace with a computer. Along with the retraining required to effectively integrate AI with existing roles, new roles will be created as well (e.g., trainers, explainers, sustainers), creating the need to develop and implement training programs to address these roles.

Moravec's paradox notes that "it is comparatively easy to make computers exhibit adult level performance on intelligence tests or playing checkers, and difficult or impossible to give them the skills of a one-year-old when it comes to perception and mobility" (Moravec, 2018). Respectively, clinicians will need to be selected for, and emphasize training in, more distinctly "human" skills of counseling, physical examination, communication, management, and coordination.

AI System Augmentation of Human Tasks

Anxieties over the potential for automated AI systems to replace jobs rests in a false dichotomy. Humans and machines can excel in distinct ways that the other cannot, meaning that the two combined can accomplish what neither could do alone. In one example of a deep learning algorithm versus an expert pathologist identifying metastatic breast cancer, the high accuracy of the algorithm was impressive enough, but more compelling was that combining the algorithm with the human expert outperformed both (Wang et al., 2016).

HOW WILL AI TRANSFORM PATIENT, PROVIDER, AND COMPUTER INTERACTIONS?

The progressive digitization of U.S. medicine underwent a massive shift in just the last decade with the rapid adoption of EHRs spurred by the Health Information Technology for Economic and Clinical Health (HITECH) Act of 2009 (HHS, 2017). This transformation creates much of the digital infrastructure that will make AI in medicine possible, but the pace of change was so rapid that we may not have yet achieved the maturity to effectively benefit from new technology without compromising core values of the profession. Advancing AI systems will depend on massive data streams for their power, but even relatively basic billing processes, quality reporting, and business analytics that current EHRs support is burning out a generation of clinical professionals because of increased electronic workflow requirements (Downing et al., 2018; Hill et al., 2013; Verghese, 2018).

As AI medical guidance systems driven by automated sensors increasingly direct medical care, there is concern that a result will be greater separation of patients from clinicians by digital intermediaries (Gawande, 2018). The future may see patients asking for advice and receiving direction from automated chatbots (Miner et al., 2016, 2017) while doctors and patients attentively analyze and recommend treatments for "iPatient" avatars that represent the data of their patients but are not the physical human beings (Verghese, 2008).

WHAT WILL HAPPEN TO ACCEPTANCE, TRUST, AND LIABILITY IN A HUMAN AND MACHINE AI FUTURE?

Information retrieval systems will increase democratization of medical knowledge, likely to the point where fully automated systems, chatbots, or intelligent agents are able to triage and dispense information and give health advice to patients (Olson, 2018). Less clear is how this disrupts conventions of who and what to trust. Widespread distribution of information comes with a respective risk of circulating misinformation in digital filter bubbles and echo chambers (Cashin-Garbutt, 2017).

Who is sued when something goes wrong, but all there is to point at is a faceless automation backed by a nebulous bureaucracy? Regulatory and guidance frameworks (see Chapter 7) must adapt, or leave us in an ethically ambiguous space (Victory, 2018).

HOW WILL HEALTH CARE PROVIDER ROLES BE CONCEPTUALIZED?

The classical ideal of a clinician evokes an image of a professional laying his or her stethoscope on patients for skillful examination, fulfilling a bonding and healing role. The gap between this image and reality may only widen further with advancing AI technology in medicine. The patient's ability to tell his or her story to a live person could change in a world with voice-recognition software and AI chatbots. This may actually allow patients to be more honest in their medical interactions (Borzykowski, 2016), but could diminish one of the most effective therapeutic interventions, that of simply feeling that you are being listened to by an attentive and empathetic human being. In an AI-enabled world, the role of clinician will likely move progressively toward manager, coordinator, and counselor, challenging the classical perception of what their role is and what should be counted among one's core competencies. Digitization of medicine is intended to improve care delivery, particularly at the population level, but these benefits may not be felt on the frontlines of care. Instead, it can turn clinical professionals into data entry clerks, feeding data-hungry machines (optimized for billing incentives rather than clinical care). This may escalate as AI tools need even more data, amid a policy climate imposing ever more documentation requirements to evaluate and monitor metrics of health care quality.

The transition to more IT solutions, computerized data collection, and algorithmic feedback should ultimately improve the consistency of patient care quality and efficiency. However, will the measurable gains necessarily outweigh the loss of harder-to-quantify human qualities of medicine? Will it lead to different types of medical errors when health care relies on technology-driven test interpretations and care recommendations instead of human clinical assessment, interpretation, and management? These are provocative questions, but acknowledging that these are public concerns and addressing them are important from a societal perspective.

More optimistically, perhaps such advancing AI technologies can instead enhance human relationships. Multiple companies are exploring remote and automating approaches to "auto-scribe" for clinical encounters (Cashin-Garbutt, 2017), allowing patient interactions to focus on direct care instead of note-taking and data entry. Though such promise is tantalizing, it is also important to be aware of the unintended consequences or overt actions of bad actors who could exploit such passive monitoring, intruding on confidential physician–patient conversations that could make either party unwilling to discuss important issues. Health care AI developments may be better suited in the near term to back-office administrative tasks (e.g., coding, prior authorization, supply chain management, and scheduling). Rather than developing patches like scribes for mundane administrative tasks, a holistic system redesign may be needed to reorient incentives and eliminate the need for low-value tasks altogether. Otherwise, AI systems may just efficiently automate low-value tasks, further entrenching those tasks in the culture, rather than facilitating their elimination.

WHY SHOULD THIS TIME BE ANY DIFFERENT?

A special article in the *New England Journal of Medicine* proclaimed that

> Rapid advances in the information sciences, coupled with the political commitment to broad extensions of health care, promise to bring about basic changes in the structure of medical practice. Computing science will probably exert its major effects by augmenting and, in some cases, largely replacing the intellectual functions of the physician. (Schwartz, 1970)

This was published in 1970. Will excitement over the current wave of AI technology only trigger the next AI Winter? Why should this time be any different? General AI systems will remain elusive for the foreseeable future, but there are credible reasons to expect that narrow, applied AI systems will still transform many areas of medicine and health in the next decade. Although many foundational concepts for AI systems were developed decades ago, only now is there availability of the key ingredient: data. Digitization of medical records, aggregated Internet crowdsourcing, and patient-generated data streams provide the critical fuel to power modern AI systems. Even in the unlikely event that no further major technological breakthroughs follow, the coming decades will be busy translating existing technological advances (e.g., image recognition, machine translation, voice recognition, predictive modeling) into practical solutions for increasingly complex problems in health.

KEY CONSIDERATIONS

Though this chapter is meant to highlight potential risks and unintended consequences of the developing AI future of medicine, it should not be read as pessimism or discouragement of progress. Complexity and challenges in health care are only escalating (IOM, 2013) as is global competition in AI technology (Metz, 2019). "If we don't change direction soon, we'll end up where we're going" (Horne, 2016). Doing nothing has its own risks and costs in terms of missed opportunities. Leaders can integrate the key considerations outlined below to develop strategies and thinking around effective use of AI.

Viewed through a medical ethics framework (Gillon, 1994), these considerations are guided by four principles:

- **Beneficence:** Use AI systems to do good and consider that it would even be a harmful missed opportunity to neglect their use.
- **Non-maleficence:** Avoid unintentional harm from misinterpreting poorly constructed models or the overt actions of bad actors.
- **Autonomy:** Respect individual decisions and participation, including as they pertain to transparency in personal data collection and the applicability of AI-driven decisions.
- **Justice:** Act on the basis of fair adjudication between competing claims, so that AI systems can help reduce rather than exacerbate existing disparities in access to quality health resources.

The review in this chapter seeks to soften any crash into a trough of disillusionment over the unintended consequences of health care AI, so that we may quickly move on to the slope of enlightenment that follows the hype cycle (Chen and Asch,

2017; see Figure 4-1) where we effectively use all information and data sources to improve our collective health. To that end are the following considerations:

1. **Beware of marketing hype, but recognize real opportunities.** There is no need to *over*-hype the potential of AI in health care when there is ample opportunity (as reviewed in Chapter 3) to address existing issues from undesirable variability, to crippling costs, to impaired access to quality care.

2. **Seek out robust evaluations of model performance, utility, vulnerabilities, and bias.** Developers must carefully probe models for unreliable behavior due to shifts in population, practice patterns, or other characteristics that do not generalize from the development to the deployment environment. Even within a contained deployment environment, it is important to measure robustness of machine learning approaches relative to shifts in the real-world, data-generating processes and sustain efforts to address the underlying human practices and culture from which the algorithms are learning.

3. **Respective effort should be deliberately allocated to identify, mitigate, and correct biases in decision-making tools.** Computers/algorithms are effective at learning statistical structure, patterns, organization, and rules in complex data sources, but they do not offer meaning, purpose, or a sense of justice or fairness. Recognize that algorithms trained on biased datasets will likely just amplify those biases (Rajkomar et al., 2018; Zou and Schiebinger, 2018).

4. **Demand transparency in data collection and algorithm evaluation processes.** The trade-offs between innovation and safety and between progress and regulation are complex, but transparency should be demanded along the way, as more thoroughly explored in Chapter 7.

5. **Develop AI systems with adversaries (bad actors) in mind.** Take inspiration from the cybersecurity industry with arms races between "white hats" versus "black hats." Deep collaborations between "white hat" health care IT experts, computer scientists, and the traditional health care workforce are needed to sniff out system vulnerabilities and fortify them before the "black hat" bad actors identify and exploit vulnerabilities in live systems (Symantec, 2019).

6. **Prioritize education reform and workforce development.** A graceful transition into the AI era of medicine that minimizes displacement will require deliberate redesign of training programs and workforce development toward roles that emphasize where humans have different strengths than computers.

7. **Identify synergy rather than replacement.** Humans and machines can excel in distinct ways that the other cannot, meaning that the two combined can accomplish what neither could do alone. Rather than replacement, consider applications where there is limited access to a scarce resource (e.g., clinical expertise) that AI systems can relieve.

8. **Use AI systems to engage, rather than stifle, uniquely human abilities.** AI-based automation of mundane administrative tasks and efficient health-related operations can improve system efficiency to give more time for human patients and clinicians to do what they are better at (e.g., relationship building, information elicitation, counseling, and management). As explored in Chapter 6, avoid systems that disrupt human workflows.

9. **Use automated systems to reach patients where existing health systems do not.** Even as there is unique value in an in-person clinician–patient interaction, more than 90 percent of a patient's life will not be in a hospital or doctor's office. Automated systems and remote care frameworks (e.g., telemedicine and self-monitoring) can attend to, guide, and build patient relationships to monitor chronic health issues, meeting many who were previously not engaged at all.

REFERENCES

Acemoglu, D., and P. Restrepo. 2018. *Artificial intelligence, automation and work.* Working Paper 24196. National Bureau of Economic Research. https://doi.org/10.3386/w24196.

Agniel, D., I. S. Kohane, and G. M. Weber. 2018. Biases in electronic health record data due to processes within the healthcare system: Retrospective observational study. *BMJ* 361:k1479.

AlphaStar Team. 2019. AlphaStar: Mastering the real-time strategy game StarCraft II. *DeepMind.* https://deepmind.com/blog/alphastar-mastering-real-time-strategy-game-starcraft-ii (accessed November 12, 2019).

Barnato, A. E., M. B. Herndon, D. L. Anthony, P. M. Gallagher, J. S. Skinner, J. P. W. Bynum, and E. S. Fisher. 2007. Are regional variations in end-of-life care intensity explained by patient preferences? A study of the US Medicare population. *Medical Care* 45(5):386–393.

Bates, D. W., S. Saria, L. Ohno-Machado, A. Shah, and G. Escobar. 2014. Big data in health care: Using analytics to identify and manage high-risk and high-cost patients. *Health Affairs* 33:1123–1131.

Beam, A. L., and I. S. Kohane. 2016. Translating artificial intelligence into clinical care. *JAMA* 316:2368–2369.

Beam, A. L., and I. S. Kohane. 2018. Big data and machine learning in health care. *JAMA* 319:1317–1318.

Borzykowski, B. 2016. Truth be told, we're more honest with robots. *BBC WorkLife.* https://www.bbc.com/worklife/article/20160412-truth-be-told-were-more-honest-with-robots (accessed November 12, 2019).

Brones, A. 2018. Food apartheid: The root of the problem with America's groceries. *The Guardian.* https://www.theguardian.com/society/2018/may/15/food-apartheid-food-deserts-racism-inequality-america-karen-washington-interview (accessed November 12, 2019).

Brooks, R. 2017. The seven deadly sins of AI predictions. *MIT Technology Review.* https://www.technologyreview.com/s/609048/the-seven-deadly-sins-of-ai-predictions (accessed November 12, 2019).

Brown, J. 2017. Why everyone is hating on IBM Watson—including the people who helped make it. *Gizmodo.* https://gizmodo.com/why-everyone-is-hating-on-watson-including-the-people-w-1797510888 (accessed November 12, 2019).

Brown, N., and T. Sandholm. 2018. Superhuman AI for heads-up no-limit poker: Libratus beats top professionals. *Science* 359:418–424.

Butterfield, S. 2018. Let the computer figure it out. *ACP Hospitalist.* https://acphospitalist.org/archives/2018/01/machine-learning-computer-figure-out.htm (accessed November 12, 2019).

Cabitza, F., R. Rasoini, and G. F. Gensini. 2017. Unintended consequences of machine learning in medicine. *JAMA* 318(6):517–518.

Cadwalladr, C., and E. Graham-Harrison. 2018. *Revealed: 50 million Facebook profiles harvested for Cambridge Analytica in major data breach.* https://www.theguardian.com/news/2018/mar/17/cambridge-analytica-facebook-influence-us-election (accessed December 7, 2019).

Caruana, R., P. Koch, Y. Lou, M. Sturm, J. Gehrke, and N. Elhadad. 2015. Intelligible models for healthcare: Predicting pneumonia risk and hospital 30-day readmission. In *Proceedings of the 21th ACM SIGKDD International Conference on Knowledge Discovery and Data Mining.* New York: ACM. Pp. 1721–1730. https://doi.org/10.1145/2783258.2788613.

Cashin-Garbutt, A. 2017. Could smartglass rehumanize the physician patient relationship? *News-Medical.net.* https://www.news-medical.net/news/20170307/Could-smartglass-rehumanize-the-physician-patient-relationship.aspx (accessed November 12, 2019).

Chen, J. H., and R. B. Altman. 2014. Automated physician order recommendations and outcome predictions by data-mining electronic medical records. In *AMIA Summits on Translational Science Proceedings.* Pp. 206–210.

Chen, J., and S. Asch. 2017. Machine learning and prediction in medicine—Beyond the peak of inflated expectations. *New England Journal of Medicine* 376:2507–2509.

Choi, P. J., F. A. Curlin, and C. E. Cox. 2015. "The patient is dying, please call the chaplain": The activities of chaplains in one medical center's intensive care units. *Journal of Pain and Symptom Management* 50:501–506.

Christakis, N. A., and E. B. Lamont. 2000. Extent and determinants of error in physicians' prognoses in terminally ill patients: Prospective cohort study. *Western Journal of Medicine* 172:310–313.

Clark, L. 2012. Machines will replace 80 percent of doctors. *Wired.* https://www.wired.co.uk/article/doctors-replaced-with-machines (accessed December 13, 2019).

Cohen, G., and M. Mello. 2018. HIPAA and protecting health information in the 21st century. *JAMA* 320(3):231–232.

Cohen, G., and M. Mello. 2019. Big data, big tech, and protecting patient privacy. *JAMA* 322(12):1141–1142.

Dartmouth Atlas Project. 2018. *Dartmouth Atlas of Health Care.* http://www.dartmouthatlas.org (accessed November 12, 2019).

Dastin, J. 2018. Amazon scraps secret AI recruiting tool that showed bias against women. *Reuters.* https://www.reuters.com/article/us-amazon-com-jobs-automation-insight/amazon-scraps-secret-ai-recruiting-tool-that-showed-bias-against-women-idUSKCN1MK08G (accessed on November 12, 2019).

deBronkart, D., and D. Sands. 2018. Warner Slack: "Patients are the most underused resource." *BMJ* 362:k3194.

Deo, R. C. 2015. Machine learning in medicine. *Circulation* 132:1920–1930.

Desjardins, J. 2017. Visualizing the jobs lost to automation. *Visual Capitalist.* http://www.visualcapitalist.com/visualizing-jobs-lost-automation/?link=mktw (accessed November 12, 2019).

DOJ and FTC (U.S. Department of Justice and Federal Trade Commission). 2015. Executive summary [updated]. *Improving health care: A dose of competition.* https://www.justice.gov/atr/executive-summary (accessed February 11, 2019).

Downing, N. L., D. W. Bates, and C. A. Longhurst. 2018. Physician burnout in the electronic health record era: Are we ignoring the real cause? *Annals of Internal Medicine* 169:50–51.

Ehrenfeld, J. M. 2017. WannaCry, cybersecurity and health information technology: A time to act. *Journal of Medical Systems* 41:104.

Ehteshami, B. B., M. Veta, P. J. van Diest, B. van Finneken, N. Karssemeijer, G. Litjens, J. A. W. M. van der Laak, the CAMELYON16 Consortium, M. Hermsen, Q. F. Manson, M. Balkenhol, O. Geessink, N. Stathonikos, M. C. Van Dijk, P. Bult, F. Beca, A. H. Beck, D. Wang, A. Khosla, R. Gargeya, H. Irshad, A. Zhong, Q. Dou, Q. Li, H. Chen, H. J. Lin, P. A. Heng, C. Hab, E. Bruni, Q. Wong, U. Halici, M. U. Oner, R. Cetin-Atalay, M. Berseth, V. Khvatkov, A. Vylegzhanin, O. Kraus, M. Shaban, N. Rajpoot, R. Awan, K. Sirinukunwattana, T. Qaiser, Y. W. Tsang, D. Tellez, J. Annuscheit, P. Hufnagl, M. Valkonen, K. Kartasalo, L. Latonen, P. Ruusuvuoiri, K. Kiimatainen, S. Albargouni, B. Mungal, A. George,

S. Demirci, N. Navab, S. Watanabe, S. Seno, Y. Takenaka, H. Matsuda, H. Ahmady Phoulady, V. Kovalev, A. Kalinovsky, V. Liauchuk, G. Bueno, M. M. Fernandez-Carrobles, I. Serrano, O. Deniz, D. Racoceanu, and R. Venancio. 2017. Diagnostic assessment of deep learning algorithms for detection of lymph node metastases in women with breast cancer. *JAMA* 318:2199–2210.

Esteva, A., B. Kuprel, R. A. Novoa, J. Ko, S. M. Sweter, H. M. Blau, and S. Thrun. 2017. Dermatologist-level classification of skin cancer with deep neural networks. *Nature* 542:115–118.

Fabbri, D., M. E. Frisse, and B. Malin. 2017. The need for better data breach statistics. *JAMA Internal Medicine* 177(11):1696.

Felton, R. 2018. The problem isn't media coverage of semi-autonomous car crashes. *Jalopnik.* https://jalopnik.com/the-problem-isn-t-media-coverage-of-semi-autonomous-car-1826048294 (accessed November 12, 2019).

Finlayson, S. G., H. W. Chung, I. S. Kohane, and A. L. Beam. 2018. Adversarial attacks against medical deep learning systems. *arXiv.org.* https://arxiv.org/abs/1804.05296 (accessed November 12, 2019).

Finlayson, S. G., J. D. Bowers, J. Ito, J. L. Zittrain, A. L. Beam, and I. S. Kohane. 2019. Adversarial attacks on medical machine learning. *Science* 363:1287–1289.

Fischetti, M. 2011. Computers versus brains. *Scientific American.* https://www.scientificamerican.com/article/computers-vs-brains (accessed November 12, 2019).

Frey, C., and M. Osborne. 2013. *The future of employment: How susceptible are jobs to computerisation?* Working Paper. Oxford Martin Programme on Technology and Employment.

Gastwirth, J. L. 1972. The estimation of the Lorenz curve and Gini index. *Review of Economics and Statistics* 54:306–316.

Gawande, A. 2018. Why doctors hate their computers. *The New Yorker.* https://www.newyorker.com/magazine/2018/11/12/why-doctors-hate-their-computers (accessed November 12, 2019).

Giacomelli, G., and P. Shukla. 2018. How AI can combat labor displacement. *Information Week.* https://www.informationweek.com/big-data/how-ai-can-combat-labor-displacement-/a/d-id/1331997 (accessed November 12, 2019).

Gillon, R. 1994. Medical ethics: Four principles plus attention to scope. *BMJ* 309:184–188.

Glare, P., K. Virik, M. Jones, M. Hudson, S. Eychmuller, J. Simes, and N. Christakis. 2003. A systematic review of physicians' survival predictions in terminally ill cancer patients. *BMJ* 327:195–198.

Gulshan, V., L. Peng, M. Coram, M. C. Stumpe, D. Wu, A. Narayanaswamy, S. Venugopalan, K. Widner, T. Madams, J. Cuadros, R. Kim, R. Raman, P. C. Nelson, J. L. Mega, and D. R. Webster. 2016. Development and validation of a deep learning algorithm for detection of diabetic retinopathy in retinal fundus photographs. *JAMA* 316:2402–2410.

Haspel, T. 2015. In defense of corn, the world's most important food crop. *The Washington Post.* https://www.washingtonpost.com/lifestyle/food/in-defense-of-corn-the-worlds-most-important-food-crop/2015/07/12/78d86530-25a8-11e5-b77f-eb13a215f593_story.html (accessed November 12, 2019).

Herrendorf, B., R. Rogerson, and A. Valentinyi. 2009. *Two perspectives on preferences and structural transformation.* Working Paper 15416, National Bureau of Economic Research. https://doi. org/10.3386/w15416.

HHS (U.S. Department of Health and Human Services). 2017. *HITECH Act enforcement interim final rule.* https://www.hhs.gov/hipaa/for-professionals/special-topics/hitech-act-enforcement-interim-final-rule/index.html (accessed December 26, 2018).

Hill, R. G., Jr., L. M. Sears, and S. W. Melanson. 2013. 4000 Clicks: A productivity analysis of electronic medical records in a community hospital ED. *American Journal of Emergency Medicine* 31:1591–1594.

Horne, F. 2016. If we don't change direction soon, we'll end up where we're going. *Healthcare Management Forum* 29:59–62.

Ioannidis, J. P. A. 2015. Stealth research. *JAMA* 313:663.

IOM (Institute of Medicine). 2013. *Best care at lower cost: The path to continuously learning health care in America.* Washington, DC: The National Academies Press. https://doi.org/10.17226/13444.

Jha, S., and E. J. Topol. 2016. Adapting to artificial intelligence: Radiologists and pathologists as information specialists. *JAMA* 316:2353–2354.

Jiang, J. X., and G. Bai. 2019. Types of information comprised in breaches of protected health information. *Annals of Internal Medicine.* https://doi. org/10.7326/M19-1759 (accessed November 12, 2019).

Kalra, N., and D. G. Groves. 2017. *The enemy of good: Estimating the cost of waiting for nearly perfect autonomous vehicles.* Santa Monica, CA: RAND Corporation. https://www.rand.org/pubs/research_reports/RR2150.html (accessed November 12, 2019).

Kannan, H., A. Kurakin, and I. Goodfellow. 2018. Adversarial logit pairing. *arXiv.org.* https://arxiv.org/ abs/1803.06373 (accessed November 12, 2019).

Kleinberg, J., J. Ludwig, and S. Mullainathan. 2016. A guide to solving social problems with machine learning. *Harvard Business Review.* https://hbr. org/2016/12/a-guide-to-solving-social-problems-with-machine-learning (accessed November 12, 2019).

Kohane, I. 2017. What my 90-year-old mom taught me about the future of AI in health care. *CommonHealth.* https://www.wbur.org/commonhealth/2017/06/16/managing-mom-weight-algorithm.

Krizhevsky, A., I. Sutskever, and G. E. Hinton. 2017. ImageNet classification with deep convolutional neural networks. *Communications of the ACM* 60:84–90.

LaPointe, J. 2017. Physician shortage projected to grow to 104k providers by 2030. *RevCycle Intelligence.* https://revcycleintelligence.com/news/physician-shortage-projected-to-grow-to-104k-providers-by-2030 (accessed December 13, 2019).

Lee, N. T. 2018. Detecting racial bias in algorithms and machine learning. *Journal of Information, Communication and Ethics in Society* 16:252–260.

Longo, D. L., and J. M. Drazen. 2016. Data sharing. *New England Journal of Medicine* 374:276–277.

Madry, A., A. Makelov, L. Schmidt, D. Tsipras, and A. Vladu. 2017. Towards deep learning models resistant to adversarial attacks. *arXiv.org.* https://arxiv.org/abs/1706.06083 (accessed November 12, 2019).

Manrai, A. K., G. Bhatia, J. Strymish, I. S. Kohane, and S. H. Jain. 2014. Medicine's uncomfortable relationship with math: Calculating positive predictive value. *JAMA Internal Medicine* 174:991–993.

Manrai, A. K., B. H. Funke, H. L. Rehm, M. S. Olesen, B. A. Maron, P. Szolovits, D. M. Margulies, J. Loscalzo, and I. S. Kohane. 2016. Genetic misdiagnoses and the potential for health disparities. *New England Journal of Medicine* 375:655–665.

Marcus, G. 2018. Deep learning: A critical appraisal. *arXiv.org.* https://arxiv.org/abs/1801.00631 (accessed November 13, 2019).

Markit, I. 2017. *The complexities of physician supply and demand: Projections from 2015 to 2030. Final report.* Washington, DC: Association of American Medical Colleges. https://aamc-black.global.ssl.fastly.net/production/media/filer_public/a5/c3/a5c3d565-14ec-48fb-974b-99fafaeecb00/aamc_projections_update_2017.pdf (accessed November 12, 2019).

Metz, C. 2019. A.I. shows promise assisting physicians. *The New York Times.* https://www.nytimes.com/2019/02/11/health/artificial-intelligence-medical-diagnosis.html (accessed November 12, 2019).

Miner, A. S., A. Milstein, S. Schueller, R. Hegde, C. Mangurian, and E. Linos. 2016. Smartphone-based conversational agents and responses to questions about mental health, interpersonal violence, and physical health. *JAMA Internal Medicine* 176:619–625.

Miner, A. S., A. Milstein, and J. T. Hancock. 2017. Talking to machines about personal mental health problems. *JAMA* 318:1217–1218.

Mokyr, J. 1990. *The lever of riches: Technological creativity and economic progress.* New York: Oxford University Press.

Moravec, H. 1990. *Mind children: The future of robot and human intelligence.* Cambridge, MA: Harvard University Press. http://www.hup.harvard.edu/catalog.php?isbn=9780674576186 (accessed November 12, 2019).

Mukherjee, S. 2017. A.I. versus M.D. *The New Yorker.* https://www.newyorker.com/magazine/2017/04/03/ai-versus-md (accessed November 12, 2019).

Obermeyer, Z., and E. J. Emanuel. 2016. Predicting the future—Big data, machine learning, and clinical medicine. *New England Journal of Medicine* 375:1216–1219.

Olson, P. 2018. This health startup won big government deals—but inside, doctors flagged problems. *Forbes Magazine.* https://www.forbes.com/sites/parmyolson/2018/12/17/this-health-startup-won-big-government-dealsbut-inside-doctors-flagged-problems/#5d4ddbeeabba (accessed November 12, 2019).

Panetta, K. 2017. Top trends in the Gartner Hype Cycle for emerging technologies, 2017. *Gartner.* https://www.gartner.com/smarterwithgartner/top-trends-in-the-gartner-hype-cycle-for-emerging-technologies-2017 (accessed December 13, 2019).

Papanicolas, I., L. R. Woskie, and A. K. Jha. 2018. Health care spending in the United States and other high-income countries. *JAMA* 319:1024–1039.

Patil, H. K., and R. Seshadri. 2014. Big data security and privacy issues in healthcare. In *2014 IEEE International Congress on Big Data.* Pp. 762–765. https://doi.org/10.1109/BigData.Congress.2014.112.

Perakslis, E. D. 2014. Cybersecurity in health care. *New England Journal of Medicine* 371:395–397.

Pethokoukis, J. 2016. What the story of ATMs and bank tellers reveals about the "rise of the robots" and jobs. *AEIdeas Blog.* https://www.aei.org/publication/what-atms-bank-tellers-rise-robots-and-jobs (accessed November 12, 2019).

Prates, M. O. R., P. H. C. Avelar, and L. Lamb. 2018. Assessing gender bias in machine translation—A case study with Google Translate. *arXiv.org.* https://arxiv.org/abs/1809.02208 (accessed November 12, 2019).

Qiu, S., L. Qihe, Z. Shijie, and W. Chunjiang. 2019. Review of artificial intelligence adversarial attack and defense technologies. *Applied Sciences* 9(5):909.

Rajkomar, A., M. Hardt, M. D. Howell, G. Corrado, and M. H. Chin. 2018. Ensuring fairness in machine learning to advance health equity. *Annals of Internal Medicine* 169:866–872.

Razavian, N., S. Blecker, A. M. Schmidt, A. Smith-McLallen, S. Nigam, and D. Sontag. 2015. Population-level prediction of type 2 diabetes from claims data and analysis of risk factors. *Big Data* 3:277–287.

Ridley, M. 2017. Amara's Law. *MattRidleyOnline.* http://www.rationaloptimist.com/blog/amaras-law (accessed December 13, 2019).

Ross, C., and I. Swetlitz. 2017. IBM pitched its Watson supercomputer as a revolution in cancer care. It's nowhere close. *STAT.* https://www.statnews.com/2017/09/05/watson-ibm-cancer (accessed November 12, 2019).

Russakovsky, O., J. Deng, H. Su, J. Krause, S. Satheesh, S. Ma, Z. Huang, A. Karpathy, A. Khosla, M. Bernstein, A. C. Berg, and L. Fei-Fei. 2015. ImageNet large scale visual recognition challenge. *arXiv.org*. https://arxiv.org/abs/1409.0575 (accessed November 12, 2019).

Saracco, R. 2018. What is the computational power of our brain? *EIT Digital*. https://www.eitdigital.eu/newsroom/blog/article/what-is-the-computational-power-of-our-brain (accessed November 12, 2019).

Schulam, P., and S. Saria. 2017. Reliable decision support using counterfactual models. *Advances in Neural Information Processing Systems* 30:1697–1708.

Schwartz, W. B. 1970. Medicine and the computer. The promise and problems of change. *New England Journal of Medicine* 283:1257–1264.

Shanahan, M. 2015. *The technological singularity*. Cambridge, MA: MIT Press. https://mitpress.mit.edu/books/technological-singularity (accessed November 12, 2019).

Silver, D., T. Hubert, J. Schrittwieser, I. Antonoglou, M. Lai, A. Guez, M. Lanctot, L. Sifre, D. Kumaran, T. Graepel, T. Lillicrap, K. Simonyan, and D. Hassabis. 2018. A general reinforcement learning algorithm that masters chess, Shogi, and Go through self-play. *Science* 362:1140–1144.

Stewart, E. 2019. Self-driving cars have to be safer than regular cars. The question is how much. *Vox*. https://www.vox.com/recode/2019/5/17/18564501/self-driving-car-morals-safety-tesla-waymo (accessed November 12, 2019).

Subbaswamy, A., and S. Saria. 2018. Counterfactual normalization: Proactively addressing dataset shift and improving reliability using causal mechanisms. *arXiv.org*. https://arxiv.org/abs/1808.03253 (accessed November 13, 2019).

Subbaswamy, A., P. Schulam, and S. Saria. 2019. Preventing failures due to dataset shift: Learning predictive models that transport. *Proceedings of Machine Learning Research* 89:3118–3127.

Symantec. 2019. What is the difference between black, white and grey hat hackers? *Norton Security Center*. https://us.norton.com/internetsecurity-emerging-threats-what-is-the-difference-between-black-white-and-grey-hat-hackers.html (accessed November 12, 2019).

Thadaney, S., and A. Verghese. 2019. Humans and AI, not humans versus AI. *Stanford Medicine*. http://medicine.stanford.edu/2019-report/humans-and-ai.html (accessed November 12, 2019).

Thompson, D. 2018. Health care just became the U.S.'s largest employer. *The Atlantic*. https://www.theatlantic.com/business/archive/2018/01/health-care-america-jobs/550079 (accessed on November 12, 2019).

Verghese, A. 2008. Culture shock—Patient as icon, icon as patient. *New England Journal of Medicine* 359:2748–2751.

Verghese, A. 2018. How tech can turn doctors into clerical workers. *The New York Times.* https://www.nytimes.com/interactive/2018/05/16/magazine/health-issue-what-we-lose-with-data-driven-medicine.html (accessed November 12, 2019).

Victory, J. 2018. What did journalists overlook about the Apple Watch "'heart monitor'" feature? *HealthNewsReview.org.* https://www.healthnewsreview.org/2018/09/what-did-journalists-overlook-about-the-apple-watch-heart-monitor-feature (accessed November 13, 2019).

Vinge, V. 1993. The coming technological singularity: How to survive in the post-human era. *National Aeronautics and Space Administration.* https://ntrs.nasa.gov/archive/nasa/casi.ntrs.nasa.gov/19940022856.pdf (accessed November 12, 2019).

Vinyals, O., A. Toshev, S. Bengio, and D. Erhan. 2017. Show and tell: Lessons learned from the 2015 MSCOCO image captioning challenge. *IEEE Transactions on Pattern Analysis and Machine Intelligence* 39:652–663.

Wang, D., A. Khosla, R. Gargeya, H. Irshad, and A. H. Beck. 2016. Deep learning for identifying metastatic breast cancer. *arXiv.org.* https://arxiv.org/abs/1606.05718 (accessed November 13, 2019).

Wilson, H. J., P. R. Daugherty, and N. Morini-Bianzino. 2017. The jobs that artificial intelligence will create. *MIT Sloan Management Review.* https://sloanreview.mit.edu/article/will-ai-create-as-many-jobs-as-it-eliminates (accessed November 12, 2019).

Woolhandler, S., and D. U. Himmelstein. 2017. The relationship of health insurance and mortality: Is lack of insurance deadly? *Annals of Internal Medicine* 167:424–431.

Yuan, X., H. Pan, Q. Zhu, and X. Li. 2018. Adversarial examples: Attacks and defenses for deep learning. *arXiv.org.* https://arxiv.org/pdf/1712.07107.pdf (accessed November 12, 2019).

Zou, J., and L. Schiebinger. 2018. Design AI so that it's fair. *Nature* 559:324–326. https://www.nature.com/magazine-assets/d41586-018-05707-8/d41586-018-05707-8.pdf (accessed November 12, 2019).

Zulman, D. M., C. P. Chee, S. C. Ezeji-Okoye, J. G. Shaw, T. H. Holmes, J. S. Kahn, and S. M. Asch. 2017. Effect of an intensive outpatient program to augment primary care for high-need veterans affairs patients: A randomized clinical trial. *JAMA Internal Medicine* 177:166–175.

Suggested citation for Chapter 4: Chen, J., A. Beam, S. Saria, and E. A. Mendonça. 2020. Potential trade-offs and unintended consequences of artificial intelligence. In *Artificial intelligence in health care: The hope, the hype, the promise, the peril.* Washington, DC: National Academy of Medicine.

5

ARTIFICIAL INTELLIGENCE MODEL DEVELOPMENT AND VALIDATION

Hongfang Liu, Mayo Clinic; Hossein Estiri, Harvard University; Jenna Wiens, University of Michigan; Anna Goldenberg, University of Toronto; Suchi Saria, Johns Hopkins University; and Nigam Shah, Stanford University

INTRODUCTION

This chapter provides an overview of current best practices in model development and validation. It gives readers a high-level perspective of the key components of development and validation of artificial intelligence (AI) solutions in the health care domain but should not be considered exhaustive. The concepts discussed here apply to the development and validation of an algorithmic agent (or, plainly, an algorithm) that is used to diagnose, prognose, or recommend actions for preventive care as well as patient care in outpatient and inpatient settings.

Overall, Chapters 5, 6, and 7 represent the process of use case and needs assessment, conceptualization, design, development, validation, implementation, and maintenance within the framework of regulatory and legislative requirements. Each of these chapters engages readers from a different perspective within the ecosystem of AI tool development, with specific considerations from each lens (see Figure 1-6 in Chapter 1).

A complete evaluation of an AI solution in health care requires an assessment of utility, feasibility given available data, implementation costs, deployment challenges, clinical uptake, and maintenance over time. This chapter focuses on the process necessary to develop and validate a model, and Chapter 6 covers the issues of implementation, clinical use, and maintenance.

This chapter focuses on how to identify tasks that can be completed or augmented by AI, on challenges in developing and validating AI models for health care, and on how to develop AI models that can be deployed. First, all stakeholders must understand the needs coming from clinical practice, so that proposed AI systems address the needs of health care delivery. Second, it is necessary that such models be developed and validated through a team effort involving AI experts and health care providers. Throughout the process, it is important to be mindful of the fact that the datasets used to train AI are heterogeneous, complex, and nuanced in ways that are often subtle and institution specific. This affects how AI tools are monitored for safety and reliability, and how they are adapted for different locations and over time. Third, before deployment at the point of care, AI systems should be rigorously evaluated to ensure their competency and safety, in a process similar to that done for drugs, medical devices, and other interventions.

Illustrative Use Case

Consider the case of Vera, a 60-year-old woman of Asian descent with a history of hypertension, osteoporosis, diabetes, and chronic obstructive pulmonary disease, entering the doctor's office with symptoms of shortness of breath and palpitations. Her primary care physician must diagnose and treat the acute illness, but also manage the risks associated with her chronic diseases. Ideally, decisions regarding *if to treat* are guided by risk stratification tools, and decisions of *how to treat* are guided by evidence-based guidelines. However, such recommendations are frequently applied to patients not represented in the data used in those recommendations' development. For example, best practices to manage blood pressure come from randomized controlled trials enrolling highly homogeneous populations (Cushman et al., 2016), and methods for risk stratification (e.g., assessment via the atherosclerotic cardiovascular disease risk equation) frequently do not generalize well to diverse populations (Yadlowsky et al., 2018). Moreover, there are care delivery gaps from clinical inertia, provider familiarity with treatments, and patient preferences that result in the lack of management or under-treatment of many conditions.

Vera's experience would improve if an automated algorithm could support health care teams to accurately (1) classify and precisely recognize existing conditions (accounting for her age, race, and genetic makeup more broadly), (2) predict risks of specific events (e.g., 1-year risk of stroke) given the broad context (e.g., comorbidities such as osteoporosis) and not just the current symptoms, and (3) recommend specific interventions.

Even for well-understood clinical situations, such as the monitoring of surgical site infections, current care delivery falls woefully short. For example, the use of automated text-processing and subsequent reasoning on both the text-derived content as well as other structured data in the electronic health record (EHR) resulted in better tools for monitoring surgical site infections in real time (Ke et al., 2017; Sohn et al., 2017). Such automation can significantly increase the capacity

TABLE 5-1 | Example of Artificial Intelligence Applications by the Primary Task and Main Stakeholder

	Classify (Diagnose)	Predict (Prognose)	Treat
Payers	Identify which patients will not adhere to a treatment plan	Estimate risk of a "no-show" for a magnetic resonance imaging appointment	Select the best second line agent for managing diabetes after Metformin given a specific clinical history
Patients and caregivers	Estimate risk of having an undiagnosed genetic condition (e.g., familial hypercholesterolemia)	Estimate risk of a postsurgical complication	Identify a combination of anticancer drugs that will work for a specific tumor type
Providers	Identify patients with unrecognized mental health needs	Determine risk of acute deterioration needing heightened care	Establish how to manage an incidentally found atrial septal defect

of a care team to provide quality care or, at the very least, free up their time from the busy work of reporting outcomes. Below, additional examples are discussed regarding applications driving the use of algorithms to classify, predict, and treat, which can guide users in figuring out for whom to take action and when. These applications may be driven by needs of providers, payers, or patients and their caregivers (see Table 5-1).

MODEL DEVELOPMENT

Establishing Utility

One of the most critical components of developing AI for health care is to define and characterize the problem to be addressed and then evaluate whether it can be solved (or is worth solving) using AI and machine learning. Doing so requires an assessment of utility, feasibility given available data, implementation costs, deployment challenges, clinical uptake, and maintenance over time. This chapter focuses on the process necessary to develop and validate a model, and Chapter 6 covers the issues of implementation, clinical use, and maintenance.

It is useful to think in terms of how one would act given a model's output when considering the utility of AI in health care. Factors affecting the clinical utility of a predictive model may include lead time offered by the prediction, the existence of a mitigating action, the cost and ease of intervening, the logistics of the intervention, and incentives (Amarasingham et al., 2014; Meskó et al., 2018; Yu et al., 2018). While model evaluation typically focuses on metrics such as positive predictive value, sensitivity (or recall), specificity, and calibration, constraints on the action triggered by the model's output (e.g., continuous rhythm monitoring might be constrained by availability of Holter monitors) often can have a much larger influence in determining model utility (Moons et al., 2012).

For example, if Vera was suspected of having atrial fibrillation based on a personalized risk estimate (Kwong et al., 2017), the execution of follow-up action (such as rhythm monitoring for 24 hours) depends on availability of the right equipment. In the absence of the ability to follow up, having a personalized estimate of having undiagnosed atrial fibrillation does not improve Vera's care.

Therefore, a framework for assessing the utility of a prediction-action pair resulting from an AI solution is necessary. During this assessment process, there are several key conceptual questions that must be answered (see Box 5-1). Quantitative answers to these questions can drive analyses for optimizing the desired outcomes, adjusting components of the expected utility formulation and fixing variables that are difficult to modify (e.g., the cost of an action) to derive the bounds of optimal utility.

For effective development and validation of AI/machine learning applications in health care, one needs to carefully formulate the problem to be solved, taking into consideration the properties of the algorithm (e.g., positive predictive value) and the properties of the resulting action (e.g., effectiveness), as well as the constraints on the action (e.g., costs, capacity), given the clinical and psychosocial environment.

If Vera's diagnosis was confirmed and subsequently the CHADS2 risk score indicated a high 1-year risk of ischemic stroke, the utility of treating using anticoagulants has to be determined in the light of the positive predictive value of the CHADS2 score and the known (or estimated) effectiveness of anticoagulation in preventing the stroke as well as the increased risk of bleeding incurred from anticoagulant use in the presence of hypertension.

BOX 5-1

Key Considerations in Model Development

- What will the downstream interventions be?
- Who is the target user of the model's output?
- What are the mechanics of executing the intervention?
- What is the risk of failure and adverse events?
- What is the capacity to intervene given existing resources?
- What accuracy is needed, and are false positives or negatives less desirable?
- What is the desired outcome change following intervention?

Choices Before Beginning Model Development

After the potential utility has been established, there are some key choices that must be made prior to actual model development. Both model developers and model users are needed at this stage in order to maximize the chances of succeeding in model development because many modeling choices are dependent on the context of use of the model. Although clinical validity is discussed in Chapter 6, we note here that the need for external validity depends on what one wishes to do with the model, the degree of agency ascribed to the model, and the nature of the action triggered by the model.

The Two Cultures of Data Modeling and Algorithmic Modeling

Expert-driven systems attempt to capture knowledge and derive decisions through explicit representation of expert knowledge. These types of systems make use of established biomedical knowledge, conventions, and relationships. The earliest AI systems in health care were all expert-driven systems, given the paucity of datasets to learn from (e.g., MYCIN) (Shortliffe, 1974).

Modern AI systems often do not attempt to encode prior medical knowledge directly into the algorithms but attempt to uncover these relationships during model learning. Inexpensive data storage, fast processors, and advancements in machine learning techniques have made it feasible to use large datasets, which can uncover previously unknown relationships. They have also been shown to outperform expert-driven approaches in many cases, as illustrated through the latest digital medicine focus in *Nature Medicine* (Esteva et al., 2019; Gottesman et al., 2019; He et al., 2019). However, learning directly from the data carries the risk of obtaining models with decreased interpretability, getting potentially counterintuitive (to a clinical audience) models and models that are overfitted and fail to generalize, and propagating biased decision making by codifying the existing biases in the medical system (Char et al., 2018; Chen et al., 2019; Vellido, 2019; Wang et al., 2018).

In addition, when a model is learning from (or being fitted to) the available data, there are often conflicting views that lie at two ends of a spectrum (Breiman, 2001). At one end are approaches that posit a causal diagram of which variables influence other variables, in such a way that this "model" is able to faithfully represent the underlying process that led to the observed data—that is, we attempt to model the process that produced the data (Breiman, 2001). At the other end of the spectrum are approaches that treat the true mechanisms that produced the observed data as unknown and focus on learning a mathematical function that maps the given set of input variables to the observed outcomes. Such models merely capture associations and make no claim regarding causality (Cleophas et al., 2013).

As an example, consider the situation of taking a dataset of observed characteristics on 1 million individuals and building a model to assess the risk of a heart attack in 1 year. The causal approach would require that the variables we collect—such as age, race, gender, lipid levels, and blood pressure—have some underlying biological role in the mechanisms that lead to heart attacks. Once a model learns from the data, the variables that are most associated with the outcome "have a role" in causing the outcome; modifying those variables (e.g., lowering lipid levels) reduces the risk of the outcome (the heart attack). Typically, such models also have external validity in the sense that the risk equation learned once (e.g., from the Framingham Heart Study in New Hampshire) works in a different geography (e.g., California) decades later (Fox, 2010; Mason et al., 2012). If one is interested purely in associations, one might include every variable available, such as hair color, and also tolerate the fact that some key items such as lipid levels are missing. In this case the model—the mathematical function mapping inputs to outcomes—learns to weigh "hair color" as an important factor for heart attack risk and learns that people with white or gray hair have a higher risk of heart attacks. Clearly, this is a cartoon example, as coloring people's hair black does nothing to reduce their heart attack risk. However, if one needs to estimate financial risk in insuring our hypothetical population of 1 million individuals, and a large fraction of that population has white or gray hair, a model need not be "causal." As Judea Pearl writes, "Good predictions need not have good explanations. The owl can be a good hunter without understanding why the rat always goes from point A to point B" (Pearl and Mackenzie, 2018).

Ideally, one can combine prior medical knowledge of causal relationships with learning from data in order to develop an accurate model (Schulam and Saria, 2017; Subbaswamy et al., 2018). Such combination of prior data can take multiple forms. For example, one can encode the structure fully and learn the parameters from data (Sachs et al., 2005). Alternatively, one could develop models that faithfully represent what is known about the disease and learn the remaining structure and parameters (Schulam and Saria, 2017; Subbaswamy et al., 2018).

Model learning that incorporates prior knowledge automatically satisfies construct validity and is less likely to generate counterintuitive predictions. Many view the use of prior knowledge or causal relationships as impractical for any sufficiently complex problem, in part because the full set of causal relationships is rarely known. However, recent works show that even when we have established only partial understanding of causal relationships, we can improve generalizability across environments by removing spurious relationships that are less likely to be generalizable, thereby reducing the risk of catastrophic prediction failures (Schulam and Saria, 2017; Subbaswamy et al., 2018).

The topic of interpretability deserves special discussion because of ongoing debates around interpretability, or the lack of it (Licitra et al., 2017; Lipton, 2016; Voosen, 2017). Interpretability can mean different things to the individuals who build the models and the individuals who consume the model's output. To the model builder, interpretability often means the ability to explain which variables and their combinations, in what manner, led to the output produced by the model (Friedler et al., 2019). To the clinical user, interpretability could mean one of two things: a sufficient enough understanding of what is going on, so that they can trust the output and/or be able to get liability insurance for its recommendations; or enough causality in the model structure to provide hints as to what mitigating action to take. The Framingham risk equation satisfies all three meanings of interpretability (Greenland et al., 2001). Interpretability is not always necessary, nor is it sufficient for utility. Given two models of equal performance, one a black box model and one an interpretable model, most users prefer the interpretable model (Lipton, 2016). However, in many practical scenarios, models that may not be as easily interpreted can lead to better performance. Gaining users' trust has often been cited as a reason for interpretability (Abdul, 2018). The level of users' trust highly depends on the users' understanding of the target problems. For example, one does not need to have an interpretable model for a rain forecast in order to rely on it when deciding whether to carry an umbrella, as long as the model is correct enough, often enough, because a rain forecast is a complex problem beyond the understanding of individuals. For non-expert users, as long as the model is well validated, the degree of interpretability often does not affect user trust in the model, whereas expert users tend to demand a higher degree of model interpretability (Poursabzi-Sangdeh, 2018).

To avoid wasted effort, it is important to understand what kind of interpretability is needed in a particular application. For example, consider the prediction of 24-hour mortality using a deep neural network (Rajkomar et al., 2018). It can take considerably more effort to train and interpret deep neural networks, while linear models, which are arguably more interpretable, may yield sufficient performance. If interpretability is deemed necessary, it is important to understand why interpretability is needed. In Rajkomar et al. (2018), the neural networks for predicting high 24-hour mortality risk were interrogated to interpret their predictions and highlight the reasons for the high mortality risk. For a patient with high 24-hour mortality risk, in one case, the reasons provided were the presence of metastatic breast cancer with malignant pleural effusions and empyema. Such engineering interpretability, while certainly valid, does not provide suggestions for what to do in response to the high-mortality prediction.

A black box model may suffice if the output was *trusted*, and the recommended intervention was known to affect the outcome. Trust in the output can be obtained by rigorous testing and prospective assessment of how often the model's predictions are correct and calibrated, and for assessing the impact of the interventions on the outcome. At the same time, prospective assessment can be costly. Thus, doing all one can to vet the model in advance (e.g., by inspecting learned relationships) is imperative.

Augmentation Versus Automation

In health care, physicians are accustomed to augmentations. For example, a doctor is supported by a team of intelligent agents, including specialists, nurses, physician assistants, pharmacists, social workers, case managers, and other health care professionals (Meskó et al., 2018). While much of the popular discussion of AI focuses on how AI tools will replace human workers, in the foreseeable future, AI will function in an augmenting role, adding to the capabilities of the technology's human partners. As the volume of data and information available for patient care grows exponentially, AI tools will naturally become part of such a care team. They will provide task-specific expertise in the data and information space, augmenting the capabilities of the physician and the entire team, making their jobs easier and more effective, and ultimately improving patient care (Herasevich et al., 2018; Wu, 2019).

There has been considerable ongoing discussion about the level of autonomy that AI can or should have within the health care environment (Verghese et al., 2018). The required performance characteristics and latitude of use of AI models is substantially different when the model is operating autonomously versus when a human is using it as an advisor and making the final decision. This axis also has significant policy, regulatory, and legislative considerations, which are discussed in Chapter 7. It is likely that progress in health care AI will proceed more rapidly when these AI systems are designed with the human in the loop, with attention to the prediction-action pairing, and with considerations of the societal, clinical, and personal contexts of use. The utility of those systems highly depends on the ability to augment human decision-making capabilities in disease prevention, diagnosis, treatment, and prognosis.

Selection of a Learning Approach

The subfield of AI focused on learning from data is known as machine learning. Machine learning can be grouped into three main approaches: (1) supervised, (2) unsupervised, and (3) reinforcement learning. Each approach can address different needs within health care.

Supervised learning focuses on learning from a collection of labeled examples. Each example (i.e., patient) is represented by input data (e.g., demographics, vital signs, laboratory results) and a label (such as being diabetic or not). The learning algorithm then seeks to learn a mapping from the inputs to the labels that can generalize to new examples. There have been many successful applications of supervised learning to health care. For example, Rajpurkar et al. (2018) developed an AI system that classified 14 conditions in chest radiographs at a performance level comparable to that of practicing radiologists. Based on the training data, their system learned which image features were most closely associated with the different diagnoses. Such systems can also be used to train models that predict future events. For example, Rajkomar et al. (2018) used supervised learning to learn a mapping from the structured as well as textual contents of the EHR to a patient's risk for mortality, readmission, and diagnosis with specific *International Classification of Diseases, Ninth Revision*, codes by discharge (Rajkomar et al., 2018). This method of training a model is popular in settings with a clear outcome and large amounts of labeled data. However, obtaining labeled data is not always straightforward. Unambiguous labels may be difficult to obtain for a number of reasons: the outcome or classification may be ambiguous, with little interclinician agreement; the labeling process may be labor intensive and costly; or labels may simply be unavailable. In many settings, there may not be a large enough dataset to confidently train a model. In such settings, weakly supervised learning can be leveraged when noisy, weak signals are available. For example, to mitigate the burden of expensive annotations, one study used weak supervision to learn a severity score for acute deterioration (Dyagilev and Saria, 2016). In another study where it was not possible to acquire gold-standard labels, weak supervision was used to learn a disease progression score for Parkinson's disease (Zhan et al., 2018). Various other strategies, including semi-supervised learning and active learning, can be deployed to reduce the amount of labeled data needed (Zhou, 2017).

Unsupervised learning seeks to examine a collection of unlabeled examples and group them by some notion of shared commonality. Clustering is one of the common unsupervised learning tasks. Clustering algorithms are largely used for exploratory purposes and can help identify structure and substructure in the data. For example, Williams et al. (2018) clustered data pertaining to more than 10,000 pediatric intensive care unit admissions, identifying clinically relevant clusters. Unsupervised learning can also be used to stage or subtype heterogeneous disease (Doshi-Velez et al., 2014; Goyal et al., 2018; Saria and Goldenberg, 2015). Here, the difficulty lies not in obtaining the grouping—although such techniques similarly suffer from small datasets—but in evaluating it. When given a dataset and a clustering algorithm, we always get a grouping. The challenge, then, is whether the presence of the groups (i.e., clusters) or learning that a new patient is deemed a member of a certain group is actionable in the form of offering different treatment options. Most often, the ability to reproduce the same groups in another dataset is considered a sign that the groups are medically meaningful and perhaps they should be managed differently. If the fact that a new record belongs to a certain group allows an assignment of higher (or lower) risk of specific outcomes, that is considered a sign that the learned groups have meaning. For example, Shah et al. (2015) analyzed a group of roughly 450 patients who had heart failure with preserved ejection fraction in order to find three subgroups (Shah et al., 2015). In data that were not used to learn the groups, application of the grouping scheme sorted patients into high, medium, and low risk of subsequent mortality.

Reinforcement learning differs from supervised and unsupervised learning, because the algorithm learns through interacting with its environments rather than through observational data alone. Such techniques have had recent successes in game settings (Hutson, 2017). In games, an agent begins in some initial stage and then takes actions affecting the environment (i.e., transitioning to a new state) and receiving a reward. This framework mimics how clinicians may interact with their environment, adjusting medication or therapy based on observed effects. Reinforcement learning is most applicable in settings involving sequential decision making where the reward may be delayed (i.e., not received for several time steps). Although most applications consider online settings, recent work in health care has applied reinforcement learning in an offline setting using observational data (Komorowski et al., 2018). Reinforcement learning holds promise, although its current applications suffer from issues of confounding and lack of actionability (Saria, 2018).

LEARNING A MODEL

To illustrate the process of learning a model, we focus on a supervised learning task for risk stratification in health care. Assume we have n patients. Each patient is represented by a d-dimensional feature vector that lies in some feature space X (see rows in Figure 5-1). In addition, each patient has some label, y, representing that patient's outcome or condition (such as being diabetic or not). In some settings, we may have only a single label for each patient; in others we may have multiple labels that vary over time. We begin with the simple case of only a single binary label per patient. The task is to learn a mapping from the vector X to y. This mapping is called the model and is performed by a learning algorithm such as stochastic gradient descent.

As discussed earlier, the degree to which the resulting model is causal is the degree to which it is an accurate representation of the true underlying process, denoted by $f(x)$ in Figure 5-1. Depending on the data available, the degree of prior knowledge used in constraining the model's structure, and the specific learning algorithm employed, we learn models that support differing degrees of causal interpretation.

Once the model is learned, given a new patient represented by a feature vector, we can then estimate the probability of the outcome. The data used to learn the model are called training data, and the new data used to assess how well a model

BOX 5-2

Key Definitions in Model Development

- **Training dataset:** A dataset of instances used for learning parameters of a model.
- **Validation dataset:** A dataset of instances used to tune the hyperparameters of a model.
- **Test dataset:** A dataset that is independent of the training dataset but follows the same distribution as the training dataset. If part of the original dataset is set aside and used as a test set, it is also called **holdout dataset**.
- **K-fold cross validation:** A dataset is randomly partitioned into K parts and one part is set for testing, and the model is trained on the remaining K-1 parts, and the model is evaluated on the holdout part.
- **External cross validation:** Perform cross validation across various settings of model parameters and report the best result.
- **Internal cross validation:** Perform cross validation on the training data and train a model on the best set of parameters.
- **Sensitivity:** Proportion of actual positives that are correctly identified in a binary classification. It is also called the **true positive rate (TPR)**, the **recall**, or **probability of detection**.
- **Specificity:** Proportion of actual negatives that are correctly identified in a binary classification. It is also called the **true negative rate**.
- **Precision:** Proportion of predicted positives that are true positives. It is also called the **positive predictive value**.
- **Accuracy:** Proportion of correctly identified instances among all instances examined.
- **Receiver operating characteristic (ROC) curve:** Graphical plot created by plotting the TPR against a false positive rate. The **area under the ROC curve** is a measure of how well a parameter setting can distinguish between two groups.
- **Precision-recall (PR) curve:** Graphical plot created by plotting the precision against the recall to show the trade-off between precision and recall for different parameter settings. The **area under the PR curve** is a better measure for highly imbalanced classification tasks.

SOURCE: Bottou et al., 2018.

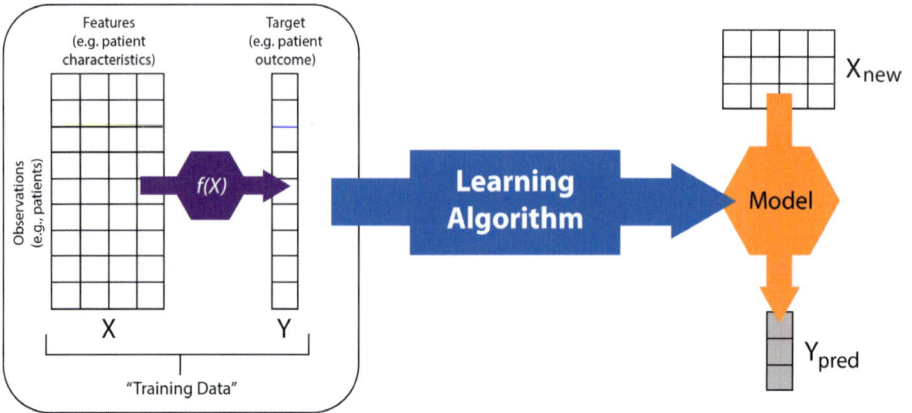

FIGURE 5-1 | What is a model?

NOTE: A model is a map from inputs *(X)* to an output *(y)*—mathematically, a function. We implicitly assume that there is a real data-generating function, *f(x)*, which is unknown and is what we are trying to represent at varying degrees of fidelity.

SOURCE: Developed by Alejandro Schuler and Nigam Shah for BIOMEDIN 215 at Stanford University.

performs are the test data (Wikipedia, 2019). Training data are often further split into training and validation subsets. Model selection, which is the selection of one specific model from among the many that are possible given the training data, is performed using the validation data.

Choosing the Data to Learn From

Bad data will result in bad models, recalling the age-old adage "garbage in, garbage out" (Kilkenny and Robinson, 2018). There is a tendency to hype AI as something magical that can learn no matter what the inputs are. In practice, the choice of data always trumps the choice of the specific mathematical formulation of the model.

In choosing the data for any model learning exercise, the outcome of interest (e.g., inpatient mortality) and the process for extracting it (e.g., identified using chart review of the discharge summary note) should be described in a reproducible manner. If the problem involves time-series data, the time at which an outcome is observed and recorded versus the time at which it needs to be predicted have to be defined upfront (see Figure 5-2). The window of data used to learn the model (i.e., observation window) and the amount of lead time needed from the prediction should be included.

It is necessary to provide a detailed description of the process of data acquisition, the criteria for subselecting the training data, and the description and prevalence of attributes that are likely to affect how the model will perform on a new dataset. For example, when building a predictive model, subjects in the training data may

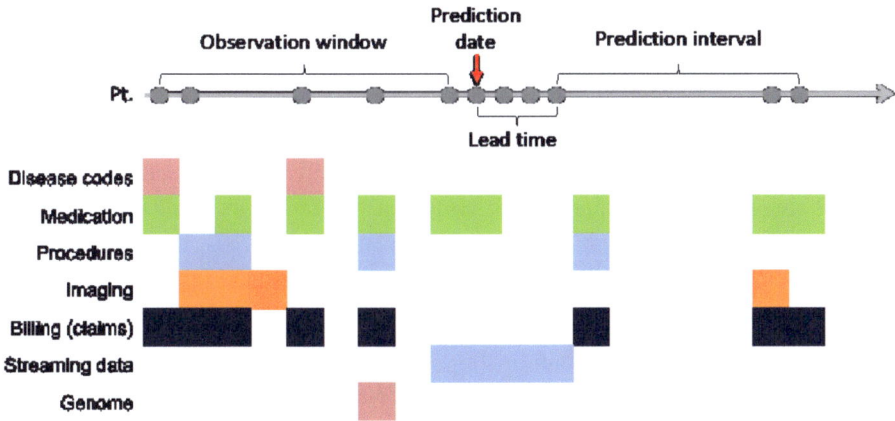

FIGURE 5-2 | Patient timeline and associated data–gathering opportunities.

NOTES: Specific events in the timeline are denoted by gray circles. The colored portions of the timeline below the gray line show the different types of data that may be collected at different encounters and the fact that not everything is collected at the same time. Almost no data source provides a continuous measurement of the patient's health except data streams of intensive care unit monitors used in short stretches. (Wearables increasingly promise such continuous data but their use in health care is just beginning.) The red arrow shows a chosen point in the timeline where a prediction attempt is made. Only data prior to that are available for model learning for that prediction. Each prediction offers the chance of taking some action before the predicted event happens. The time interval between the prediction data and the soonest possible occurrence of the predicted event indicates the lead time available to complete the necessary mitigating action.

SOURCE: Developed by Alejandro Schuler and Nigam Shah for BIOMEDIN 215 at Stanford University.

not be representative of the target population (i.e., selection bias). Meanwhile, errors in measuring exposure or disease occurrences can be an important source of bias (i.e., measurement bias), especially when using EHR data as a source of measurements (Gianfrancesco et al., 2018). Both selection bias and measurement bias can affect the accuracy as well as generalizability of a predictive model learned from the data (Suresh and Guttag, 2019).

The degree to which the chosen data affect generalization of a model learned from it depends on the method used for modeling and the biases inherent in the data during their acquisition. For example, models can be susceptible to provider practice patterns; most models trained using supervised learning assume that practice patterns in the new environment are similar to those in the development environment (Schulam and Saria, 2017). The degree of left censoring, right censoring, or missingness can also affect generalization (Dyagilev and Saria, 2016; Molenberghs and Kenward, 2007; Schulam and Saria, 2018). Finally, the processes by which the data are generated and collected also change over time. This change, known as nonstationarity in the data, can have a significant effect on model performance (Jung and Shah, 2015). Using stale data can lead to suboptimal learning by models, which then get labeled as biased or unfair.

The decisions made during the creation and acquisition of datasets will be reflected in downstream models. In addition to knowing the final features representing patient data (see Figure 5-1), any preprocessing steps should be clearly documented and made available with the model. Such data-wrangling steps (e.g., how one dealt with missing values or irregularly sampled data) are often overlooked or not reported. The choices made around data preparation and transformation into the analytical data representation can contribute significantly to bias that then gets incorporated into the AI algorithm (Suresh and Guttag, 2019).

Often, the users of the model's output hold the model itself responsible for such biases, rather than the underlying data and the model developer's design decisions surrounding the data (Char et al., 2018). In nonmedical fields, there are numerous examples in which model use has reflected biases inherent in the data used to train them (Angwin et al., 2016; Char et al., 2018; O'Neil, 2017). For example, programs designed to aid judges in sentencing by predicting an offender's risk of recidivism have shown racial discrimination (Angwin et al., 2016). In health care, attempts to use data from the Framingham Heart Study to predict the risk of cardiovascular events in minority populations have led to biased risk estimates (Gijsberts et al., 2015). Subtle discrimination inherent in health care delivery may be harder to anticipate; as a result, it may be more difficult to prevent an algorithm from learning and incorporating this type of bias (Shah et al., 2018). Such biases may lead to self-fulfilling prophesies: If clinicians always withdraw care from patients with certain findings (e.g., extreme prematurity or a brain injury), machine learning systems may conclude that such findings are always fatal. (Note that the degree to which such biases may affect actual patient care depends on the degree of causality ascribed to the model and to the process of choosing the downstream action.)

Learning Setup

In the machine learning literature, the dataset from which a model is learned is also called the training dataset. Sometimes a portion of this dataset may be set aside for tuning hyperparameters—the weights assigned to different variables and their combinations. This portion of the training data is referred to as the hyperparameter-validation dataset, or often just the validation dataset. The validation dataset confirms whether the choices of the values of the parameters in the model are correct or not. Note that the nomenclature is unfortunate, because these validation data have nothing to do with the notion of clinical validation or external validity.

Given that the model was developed from the training/validation data, it is necessary to evaluate its performance in classifying or making predictions on a "holdout" test set (see Figure 5-1). This test set is held out in the sense that it was not used to select model parameters or hyperparameters. The test set should be as close as possible to the data that the model would be applied to in routine use. The choice of metrics used to assess a model's performance is guided by the end goal of the modeling as well as the type of learning being conducted (e.g., unsupervised versus supervised). Here, we focus on metrics for supervised binary classifiers (e.g., patient risk stratification tools). The estimation of metrics can be obtained through cross validation where the whole dataset is split randomly into multiple parts with one part set as the test set and the remaining parts used for training a model.

Choosing Metrics of Model Performance

Recall and precision are two of the most debated performance metrics because they exhibit varying importance based on the use case. Sensitivity quantifies a classifier's ability to identify the true positive cases. Typically, a highly sensitive classifier can reliably rule out a disease when its result is negative (Davidson, 2002). Precision quantifies a classifier's ability to correctly identify a true positive case—that is, it estimates the number of times the classifier falsely categorizes a noncase as a case. Specificity quantifies the portion of actual negatives that are correctly identified as such. There is a trade-off between the recall, precision, and specificity measures, which needs to be resolved based on the clinical question of interest. For situations where we cannot afford to miss a case, high sensitivity is desired. Often, a highly sensitive classifier is followed up with a highly specific test to identify the false positives among those flagged by the sensitive classifier. The trade-off between specificity and sensitivity can be visually explored in the receiver operating characteristic (ROC) curve. The area under the ROC (AUROC) curve is the most popular index for summarizing the information in the ROC curves. When reporting results on the holdout test set, we recommend going beyond the AUROC curve and instead reporting the entire ROC curve as well as the sensitivity, specificity, positive predictive value, and negative predictive value at a variety of points on the curve that represent reasonable decision-making cutoffs (Bradley, 1997; Hanley and McNeil, 1982).

However, the limitations of the ROC curves are well known even though they continue to be widely used (Cook, 2007). Despite the popularity of AUROC curve and ROC curve for evaluating classifier performance, there are other important considerations. First, the utility offered by two ROC curves can be wildly different, and it is possible that classifiers with a lower overall AUROC curve have higher utility based on the shape of the ROC curve. Second, in highly imbalanced datasets, where negative and positive labels are not distributed equally, a precision-recall (PR) curve provides a better basis for comparing classifiers (McClish, 1989). Therefore, in order to enable meaningful comparisons, researchers should report both the AUROC curve and area under the PR curve, along with the actual curves, and error bars around the average classifier performance.

For decision making in the clinic, additional metrics such as calibration, net reclassification, and a utility assessment are necessary (Lorent et al., 2019; Shah et al., 2019; Steyerberg et al., 2010). While the ROC curves provide information about a classifier's ability to discriminate a true case from a noncase, calibration metrics quantify how well the predicted probabilities of a true case being a case agree with observed proportions of cases and noncases. For a well-calibrated classifier, 90 of 100 samples with a predicted probability of 0.9 will be correctly identified true cases (Cook, 2008).

When evaluating the use of machine learning models, it is also important to develop parallel baselines, such as a penalized regression model applied on the same data that are supplied to more sophisticated models such as deep learning or random forests. Given the non-obvious relationship between a model's positive predictive value, recall, and specificity to its utility, having these parallel models provides another axis of evaluation in terms of cost of implementation, interpretability, and relative performance.

Aside from issues related to quantifying the incremental value of using a model to improve care delivery, there are methodological issues in continuously evaluating or testing a model as the underlying data change. For example, a model for predicting 24-hour mortality could be retrained every week or every day as new data become available. It is unclear which metrics of the underlying data as well as of the model performance we should monitor to manage such continuously evolving models. It is also unclear how to set the retraining schedule, and what information should guide that decision. The issues of model surveillance and implementation are more deeply addressed in Chapter 6. Finally, there are unique regulatory issues that arise if a model might get retrained after it is approved and then behave differently, and some of the current guidance for these issues is discussed in Chapter 7.

DATA QUALITY

A variety of issues affect data integrity in health care. For example, the software for data retrieval, preprocessing, and cleaning is often lost or not maintained, making it impossible to re-create the same dataset. In addition, the data from the source system(s) may have been discarded or may have changed. The problem is further compounded by fast-changing data sources or changes over time in institutional data stores or governance procedures. Finally, silos of expertise and access around data sources create dependence on individual people or teams. When the collection and provenance of the data that a model is trained on is a black box, researchers must compensate with reliance on trusted individuals or teams, which is suboptimal and not sustainable in the long run. Developing AI based on bad data further amplifies the potential negative impacts of poor-quality data. Consider, for example, that race and ethnicity information is simply not recorded, is missing, or is wrong in more than 30 to 40 percent of the records at most medical centers (Huser et al., 2016, 2018; Khare et al., 2017). Given the poor quality of these data, arguments about unfairness of predictive models for ethnic groups remain an academic discussion (Kroll, 2018). As a community, we need to address the quality of data that the vast majority of the enterprise is collecting. The quality is highly variable and acknowledging this variability as well as managing it during model building is essential. To effectively use AI, it is essential to follow good data practices in both the creation and curation of retrospective datasets for model training and in the prospective collection of the data. The quality of these data practices affects the development of models and the successful implementation at the point of care.

It is widely accepted that the successful development of an AI system requires high-quality data. However, the assessment of the quality of data that are available and the methodology to create a high-quality dataset are not standardized or often are nonexistent. Methods to assess data validity and reproducibility are often ad hoc. Efforts made by large research networks such as the Observational Health Data Science and Informatics collaborative as well as the Sentinel project have begun to outline quality assurance practices for data used to train AI models. Ideally, data should be cross-validated from multiple sources to best determine trustworthiness. Also, multiple subject matter experts should be involved in data validation (for both outcome and explanatory variables). In manually abstracted and annotated datasets, having multiple trained annotators can provide an accurate assessment of the ambiguity and variability inherent in data. For example, when tasked with identifying surgical site infection, there was little ambiguity whether infection was present or not; however, there was little agreement about the severity of the infection (Nuttall et al., 2016). Insufficiently capturing the provenance and semantics of such outcomes in datasets is at best inefficient. At worst, it can be outright dangerous, because datasets may have unspecified biases or assumptions, leading to models that produce inappropriate results in certain contexts. Ultimately, for the predictions (or classifications) from models to be trusted for clinical use, the semantics and provenance of the data used to derive them must be fully transparent, unambiguously communicated, and available for validation.

An often-missed issue around data is that the data used for training the model must be such that they are actually *available* in the real-world environment where the AI trained on the data will be used. For example, an AI analyzing electrocardiogram (ECG) waveforms must have a way to access the waveforms at the point of care. For instance, waveforms captured on a Holter monitor may not be available for clinical interpretation for hours, if not days, due to the difficulty of processing the large amount of data, whereas an irregular heart rhythm presenting on a 12-lead ECG may be interpreted and acted upon within minutes. Therefore, AI development teams should have information technology (IT) engineers who are knowledgeable about the details of when and where certain data become available and whether the mechanics of data availability and access are compatible with the model being constructed.

Another critical point is that the acquisition of the data elements present in the training data must be possible without major effort. Models derived using datasets where data elements are manually abstracted (e.g., Surgical Risk Calculator from the American College of Surgeons) cannot be deployed without significant investment by the deploying site to acquire the necessary data elements for the patient for whom the model needs to be used. While this issue can be overcome with computational phenotyping methods, such methods struggle with portability due to EHR system variations resulting in different reporting schemes, as well as clinical practice and workflow differences. With the rise of interoperability standards such as the Fast Healthcare Interoperability Resource, the magnitude of this problem is likely to decrease in the near future. When computationally defined phenotypes serve as the basis for downstream analytics, it is important that computational phenotypes themselves be well managed and clearly defined and adequately reflect the target domain.

As a reasonable starting point for minimizing the data quality issues, data should adhere to the FAIR (findability, accessibility, interoperability, and reusability) principles in order to maximize the value of the data (Wilkinson et al., 2016). Researchers in molecular biology and bioinformatics put forth these principles, and, admittedly, their applicability in health care is not easy or straightforward.

One of the unique challenges (and opportunities) facing impactful design and implementation of AI in health care is the disparate data types that comprise today's health care data. Today's EHRs and wearable devices have greatly increased the volume, variety, and velocity of clinical data. The soon-to-be in-clinic promise of genomic data further complicates the problems of maintaining data provenance, timely availability of data, and knowing what data will be available for which patient at what time.

Always keeping a timeline view of the patient's medical record is essential (see Figure 5-2), as is explicitly knowing the times at which the different data types across different sources come into existence. It stands to reason that any predictive or classification model operating at a given point in the patient timeline can only expect to use data that have come into being prior to the time at which the model is used (Jung et al., 2016; Panesar, 2019). Such a real-life view of data availability is crucial when building models, because using clean data gives an overly optimistic view of models' performance and an unrealistic impression of their potential value. Finally, we note that the use of synthetic data, if created to mirror real-life data in its missingness and acquisition delay by data type, can serve as a useful strategy for a model builder to create realistic training and testing environments for novel methods (Carnegie Mellon University, 2018; Franklin et al., 2017; Schuler, 2018).

EDUCATION

It is critical that we educate the community regarding data science, AI, medicine, and health care. Progress is contingent on creating a critical mass of experts in data science and AI who understand the mission, culture, workflow, strategic plan, and infrastructure of health care institutions.

As decision makers in health care institutions invest in data, tools, and personnel related to data science and AI, there is enormous pressure for rapid results. Such pressures raise two extremes of issues. On the one hand, the relative ease of implementing newly developed AI solutions rapidly can lead to the implementation of solutions in routine clinical care without an adequate understanding of their validity and potential influence on care, raising the potential for wasted resources and even patient harm (Herper, 2017). On the other hand, holding the AI models to superhuman standards and constantly requiring that evaluations outcompete doctors is also a flawed attitude that could lead to valuable solutions never getting implemented. Vendors of health care IT have an incentive to overstate the value of data science and AI generally. Limited attention has been given to the significant risk of harm, from wasting resources as well as from relying on evaluation strategies decoupled from the action they influence (Abrams, 2019) or relying on evaluation regimes that avoid simple and obvious baseline comparisons (Christodoulou et al., 2019).

KEY CONSIDERATIONS

The rapid increase in the volume and variety of data in health care has driven the current interest in the use of AI (Roski et al., 2014). There is active discussion and interest in addressing the potential ethical issues in using AI (Char et al., 2018), the need for humanizing AI (Israni and Verghese, 2019), the potential unintended consequences (Cabitza et al., 2017), and the need to tamper the hype (Beam and Kohane, 2018). However, more discovery and work in these areas is essential. The way that AI is developed, evaluated, and utilized in health care must change. At present, most of the existing discussion focuses on evaluating the model from a technical standpoint. A critically underassessed area is the net benefit of the integration of AI into clinical practice workflow (see Chapter 6).

Establishing Utility

When considering the use of AI in health care, it is necessary to know how one would act given a model's output. While model evaluation typically focuses on metrics such as positive predictive value, sensitivity (or recall), specificity, and calibration, constraints on the action triggered by the model's output (e.g., continuous rhythm monitoring constraint based on availability of Holter monitors) often can have a much larger influence in determining model utility (Moons et al., 2012). Completing model selection, then doing a net-benefit analysis, and later factoring work constraints are suboptimal (Shah et al., 2019). Realizing the benefit of using AI requires defining potential utility upfront. Only by including the characteristics of actions taken on the basis of the model's predictions, and factoring in their implications, can a model's potential usefulness in improving care be properly assessed.

Model Learning

After the potential utility has been established, model developers and model users need to interact closely during model learning because many modeling choices are dependent on the context of use of the model (Wiens et al., 2019). For example, the need for external validity depends on what one wishes to do with the model, the degree of agency ascribed to the model, and the nature of the action triggered by the model.

It is well known that biased data will result in biased models, thus, the data that are selected to learn from matter far more than the choice of the specific mathematical formulation of the model. Model builders need to pay closer attention to the data they train on and need to think beyond the technical evaluation of models. Even in technical evaluation, it is necessary to look beyond the ROC curves and examine multiple dimensions of performance (see Box 5-2). For decision making in the clinic, additional metrics such as calibration, net reclassification, and a utility assessment are necessary. Given the non-obvious relationship between a model's positive predictive value, recall, and specificity to its utility, it is important to examine simple and obvious parallel baselines, such as a penalized regression model applied on the same data that are supplied to more sophisticated models such as deep learning.

The topic of interpretability deserves special discussion because of ongoing debates around interpretability, or the lack of it (Licitra et al., 2017; Lipton, 2016; Voosen, 2017). To the model builder, interpretability often means the ability to explain which variables and their combinations, in what manner, led to the output produced by the model (Friedler et al., 2019). To the clinical user, interpretability could mean one of two things: a sufficient enough understanding of what is going on, so that they can trust the output and/or be able to get liability insurance for its recommendations; or enough causality in the model structure to provide hints as to what mitigating action to take. To avoid wasted effort, it is important to understand what kind of interpretability is needed in a particular application. A black box model may suffice if the output was trusted, and trust can be obtained by prospective assessment of how often the model's predictions are correct and calibrated.

Data Quality

Bad data quality adversely affects patient care and outcomes (Jamal et al., 2009). A recent systematic review shows that the AI models could dramatically improve if four particular adjustments were made: use of multicenter datasets, incorporation of time-varying data, assessment of missing data as well as informative censoring, and development of metrics of clinical utility (Goldstein et al., 2017). As a reasonable starting point for minimizing the data quality issues, data should adhere to the FAIR principles in order to maximize the value of the data (Wilkinson et al., 2016). An often overlooked detail is when and where certain data become available and whether the mechanics of data availability and access are compatible with the model being constructed. In parallel, we need to educate the different stakeholders, and the model builders need to understand the datasets they learn from.

Stakeholder Education and Managing Expectations

The use of AI solutions presents a wide range of legal and ethical challenges, which are still being worked out (see Chapter 7). For example, when a physician makes decisions assisted by AI, it is not always clear where to place blame in the case of failure. This subtlety is not new to recent technological advancements, and in fact was brought up decades ago (Berg, 2010). However, most of the legal and ethical issues were never fully addressed in the history of computer-assisted decision support, and a new wave of more powerful AI-driven methods only adds to the complexity of ethical questions (e.g., the frequently condemned black box model) (Char et al., 2018).

The model builders need to better understand the datasets they choose to learn from. The decision makers need to look beyond technical evaluations and ask for utility assessments. The media needs to do a better job in articulating both immense potential and the risks of adopting the use of AI in health care. Therefore, it is important to promote a measured approach to adopting AI technology, which would further AI's role as augmenting rather than replacing human actors. This framework could allow the AI community to make progress while managing evaluation challenges (e.g., when and how to employ interpretable models versus black box models) as well as ethical challenges that are bound to arise as the technology is widely adopted.

REFERENCES

Abdul, A., J. Vermeulen, D. Wang, B. Y. Lim, and M. Kankanhalli. 2018. Trends and trajectories for explainable, accountable and intelligible systems: An HCI research agenda. In *Proceedings of the 2018 CHI Conference on Human Factors in Computing Systems.* New York: ACM. https://dl.acm.org/citation.cfm?id=3174156 (accessed November 13, 2019).

Abrams, C. 2019. Google's effort to prevent blindness shows AI challenges. *The Wall Street Journal.* https://www.wsj.com/articles/googles-effort-to-prevent-blindness-hits-roadblock-11548504004 (accessed November 13, 2019).

Amarasingham, R., R. E. Patzer, M. Huesch, N. Q. Nguyen, and B. Xie. 2014. Implementing electronic health care predictive analytics: Considerations and challenges. *Health Affairs* 33(7):1148–1154.

Angwin, J., J. Larson, S. Mattu, and L. Kirchner. 2016. Machine bias: There's software used across the country to predict future criminals. And it's biased against blacks. *ProPublica.* https://www.propublica.org/article/machine-bias-risk-assessments-in-criminal-sentencing (accessed November 13, 2019).

Beam, A. L., and I. S. Kohane. 2018. Big data and machine learning in health care. *JAMA* 319(13):1317–1318.

Berg, J. 2010. Review of "The Ethics of Consent, eds. Franklin G. Miller and Alan Wertheimer." *American Journal of Bioethics* 10(7):71–72.

Bottou, L., F. E. Curtis, and J. Nocedal. 2018. Optimization methods for large-scale machine learning. *SIAM Review* 60(2):223–311.

Bradley, A. P. 1997. The use of the area under the ROC curve in the evaluation of machine learning algorithms. *Pattern Recognition* 30(7):1145–1159.

Breiman, L. 2001. Statistical modeling: The two cultures (with comments and a rejoinder by the author). *Statistical Science* 16(3):199–231.

Cabitza, F., R. Rasoini, and G. F. Gensini. 2017. Unintended consequences of machine learning in medicine. *JAMA* 318(6):517–518.

Carnegie Mellon University. 2018. *Atlantic Causal Inference Conference—2018: Data Challenge.* https://www.cmu.edu/acic2018/data-challenge/index.html (accessed November 13, 2019).

Char, D. S., N. H. Shah, and D. Magnus. 2018. Implementing machine learning in health care—Addressing ethical challenges. *New England Journal of Medicine* 378(11):981–983.

Chen, I.Y., P. Szolovits, and M. Ghassemi. 2019. Can AI help reduce disparities in general medical and mental health care? *AMA Journal of Ethics* 21(2):167–179.

Christodoulou, E., J. Ma, G. S. Collins, E. W. Steyerberg, J. Y. Verbakel, and B. Van Calster. 2019. A systematic review shows no performance benefit of machine learning over logistic regression for clinical prediction models. *Journal of Clinical Epidemiology* 110:12–22.

Cleophas, T. J., A. H. Zwinderman, and H. I. Cleophas-Allers. 2013. *Machine learning in medicine.* New York: Springer. https://www.springer.com/gp/book/9789400758230 (accessed November 13, 2019).

Cook, N. R. 2007. Use and misuse of the receiver operating characteristic curve in risk prediction. *Circulation* 115(7):928–935.

Cook, N. R. 2008. Statistical evaluation of prognostic versus diagnostic models: Beyond the ROC curve. *Clinical Chemistry* 54(1):17–23.

Cushman, W. C., P. K. Whelton, L. J. Fine, J. T. Wright, Jr., D. M. Reboussin, K. C. Johnson, and S. Oparil. 2016. SPRINT trial results: Latest news in hypertension management. *Hypertension* 67(2):263–265.

Davidson, M. 2002. The interpretation of diagnostic tests: A primer for physiotherapists. *Australian Journal of Physiotherapy* 48(3):227–232.

Doshi-Velez, F., Y. Ge, and I. Kohane. 2014. Comorbidity clusters in autism spectrum disorders: An electronic health record time-series analysis. *Pediatrics* 133(1):54–63.

Dyagilev, K., and S. Saria. 2016. Learning (predictive) risk scores in the presence of censoring due to interventions. *Machine Learning* 102(3):323–348.

Esteva, A., A. Robicquet, B. Ramsundar, V. Kuleshov, M. DePristo, K. Chou, C. Cui, G. Corrado, S. Thrun, and J. Dean. 2019. A guide to deep learning in healthcare. *Nature Medicine* 25(1):24.

Fox, C. S. 2010. Cardiovascular disease risk factors, type 2 diabetes mellitus, and the Framingham Heart Study. *Trends in Cardiovascular Medicine* 20(3):90–95.

Franklin, J. M., W. Eddings, P. C. Austin, E. A. Stuart, and S. Schneeweiss. 2017. Comparing the performance of propensity score methods in healthcare database studies with rare outcomes. *Statistics in Medicine* 36(12):1946–1963.

Friedler, S. A., C. D. Roy, C. Scheidegger, and D. Slack. 2019. Assessing the local interpretability of machine learning models. *arXiv.org.* https://ui.adsabs.harvard.edu/abs/2019arXiv190203501S/abstract (accessed November 13, 2019).

Gianfrancesco, M., S. Tamang, and J. Yazdanzy. 2018. Potential biases in machine learning algorithms using electronic health record data. *JAMA Internal Medicine* 178(11):1544–1547.

Gijsberts, C. M., K. A. Groenewegen, I. E. Hoefer, M. J. Eijkemans, F. W. Asselbergs, T. J. Anderson, A. R. Britton, J. M. Dekker, G. Engström, G. W. Evans, and J. De Graaf. 2015. Race/ethnic differences in the associations of the Framingham risk factors with carotid IMT and cardiovascular events. *PLoS One* 10(7):e0132321.

Goldstein, B. A., A. M. Navar, M. J. Pencina, and J. Ioannidis. 2017. Opportunities and challenges in developing risk prediction models with electronic health records data: A systematic review. *Journal of the American Medical Informatics Association* 24(1):198–208.

Gottesman, O., F. Johansson, M. Komorowski, A. Faisal, D. Sontag, F. Doshi-Velez, and L. A. Celi. 2019. Guidelines for reinforcement learning in healthcare. *Nature Medicine* 25(1): 16–18.

Goyal, D., D. Tjandra, R. Q. Migrino, B. Giordani, Z. Syed, J. Wiens, and Alzheimer's Disease Neuroimaging Initiative. 2018. Characterizing heterogeneity in the progression of Alzheimer's disease using longitudinal clinical and neuroimaging biomarkers. *Alzheimer's & Dementia: Diagnosis, Assessment & Disease Monitoring* 10:629–637.

Greenland, P., S. C. Smith, Jr., and S. M. Grundy. 2001. Improving coronary heart disease risk assessment in asymptomatic people: Role of traditional risk factors and noninvasive cardiovascular tests. *Circulation* 104(15):1863–1867.

Hanley, J. A., and B. J. McNeil. 1982. The meaning and use of the area under a receiver operating characteristic (ROC) curve. *Radiology* 143(1):29–36.

He, J., S. L. Baxter, J. Xu, J. Xu, X. Zhou, and K. Zhang. 2019. The practical implementation of artificial intelligence technologies in medicine. *Nature Medicine* 25(1):30–36.

Herasevich, V., B. Pickering, and O. Gajic. 2018. How Mayo Clinic is combating information overload in critical care units. *Harvard Business Review.* https://www.bizjournals.com/albany/news/2018/04/23/hbr-how-mayo-clinic-is-combating-information.html (accessed November 13, 2019).

Herper, M. 2017. MD Anderson benches IBM Watson in setback for artificial intelligence in medicine. *Forbes.* https://www.forbes.com/sites/matthewherper/2017/02/19/md-anderson-benches-ibm-watson-in-setback-for-artificial-intelligence-in-medicine/#7a051f7f3774 (accessed November 13, 2019).

Huser, V., F. J. DeFalco, M. Schuemie, P. B. Ryan, N. Shang, M. Velez, R. W. Park, R. D. Boyce, J. Duke, R. Khare, and L. Utidjian. 2016. Multisite evaluation of a data quality tool for patient-level clinical data sets. *EGEMS (Washington, DC)* 4(1):1239.

Huser, V., M. G. Kahn, J. S. Brown, and R. Gouripeddi. 2018. Methods for examining data quality in healthcare integrated data repositories. *Pacific Symposium on Biocomputing.* 23:628–633.

Hutson, M. 2017. This computer program can beat humans at Go—with no human instruction. *Science Magazine.* https://www.sciencemag.org/news/2017/10/computer-program-can-beat-humans-go-no-human-instruction (accessed November 13, 2019).

Israni, S. T., and A. Verghese. 2019. Humanizing artificial intelligence. *JAMA* 321(1):29–30.

Jamal, A., K. McKenzie, and M. Clark. 2009. The impact of health information technology on the quality of medical and health care: A systematic review. *Health Information Management Journal* 38(3):26–37.

Jung, K., and N. H. Shah. 2015. Implications of non-stationarity on predictive modeling using EHRs. *Journal of Biomedical Informatics* 58:168–174.

Jung, K., S. Covington, C. K. Sen, M. Januszyk, R. S. Kirsner, G. C. Gurtner, and N. H. Shah. 2016. Rapid identification of slow healing wounds. *Wound Repair and Regeneration* 24(1):181–188.

Ke, C., Y. Jin, H. Evans, B. Lober, X. Qian, J. Liu, and S. Huang. 2017. Prognostics of surgical site infections using dynamic health data. *Journal of Biomedical Informatics* 65:22–33.

Khare, R., L. Utidjian, B. J. Ruth, M. G. Kahn, E. Burrows, K. Marsolo, N. Patibandla, H. Razzaghi, R. Colvin, D. Ranade, and M. Kitzmiller. 2017. A longitudinal analysis of data quality in a large pediatric data research network. *Journal of the American Medical Informatics Association* 24(6):1072–1079.

Kilkenny, M. F., and K. M. Robinson. 2018. Data quality: "Garbage in–garbage out." *Health Information Management* 47(3):103–105.

Komorowski, M., L. A. Celi, O. Badawi, A. C. Gordon, and A. A. Faisal. 2018. The Artificial Intelligence Clinician learns optimal treatment strategies for sepsis in intensive care. *Nature Medicine* 24(11):1716–1720.

Kroll, J. A. 2018. Data science data governance [AI Ethics]. *IEEE Security & Privacy* 16(6):61–70.

Kwong, C., A. Y. Ling, M. H. Crawford, S. X. Zhao, and N. H. Shah. 2017. A clinical score for predicting atrial fibrillation in patients with crytogenic stroke or transient ischemic attack. *Cardiology* 138(3):133–140.

Licitra, L., A. Trama, and H. Hosni. 2017. Benefits and risks of machine learning decision support systems. *JAMA* 318(23):2356.

Lipton, Z. C. 2016. The mythos of model interpretability. *arXiv.org.* https://arxiv.org/abs/1606.03490 (accessed November 13, 2019).

Lorent, M., H. Maalmi, P. Tessier, S. Supiot, E. Dantan, and Y. Foucher. 2019. Meta-analysis of predictive models to assess the clinical validity and utility for patient-centered medical decision making: Application to the Cancer of the Prostate Risk Assessment (CAPRA). *BMC Medical Informatics and Decision Making* 19(1):Art. 2.

Mason, P. K., D. E. Lake, J. P. DiMarco, J. D. Ferguson, J. M. Mangrum, K. Bilchick, L. P. Moorman, and J. R. Moorman. 2012. Impact of the CHA2DS2-VASc score on anticoagulation recommendations for atrial fibrillation. *American Journal of Medicine* 125(6):603.e1–603.e6.

McClish, D. K. 1989. Analyzing a portion of the ROC curve. *Medical Decision Making* 9(3):190–195.

Meskó, B., G. Hetényi, and Z. Győrffy. 2018. Will artificial intelligence solve the human resource crisis in healthcare? *BMC Health Services Research* 18(1):Art. 545.

Molenberghs, G., and M. Kenward. 2007. *Missing data in clinical studies, vol. 61.* Hoboken, NJ: John Wiley & Sons. https://www.wiley.com/en-us/Missing+Data+in+Clinical+Studies-p-9780470849811 (accessed November 13, 2019).

Moons, K. G., A. P. Kengne, D. E. Grobbee, P. Royston, Y. Vergouwe, D. G. Altman, and M. Woodward. 2012. Risk prediction models: II. External validation, model updating, and impact assessment. *Heart* 98(9):691–698.

Nuttall, J., N. Evaniew, P. Thornley, A. Griffin, B. Deheshi, T. O'Shea, J. Wunder, P. Ferguson, R. L. Randall, R. Turcotte, and P. Schneider. 2016. The inter-rater reliability of the diagnosis of surgical site infection in the context of a clinical trial. *Bone & Joint Research* 5(8):347–352.

O'Neil, C. 2017. *Weapons of math destruction: How big data increases inequality and threatens democracy.* New York: Broadway Books.

Panesar, A., 2019. *Machine learning and AI for healthcare: Big data for improved health outcomes.* New York: Apress.

Pearl, J., and D. Mackenzie. 2018. *The book of why: The new science of cause and effect.* New York: Basic Books.

Poursabzi-Sangdeh, F., D. G. Goldstein, J. M. Hofman, J. W. Vaughan, and H. Wallach. 2018. Manipulating and measuring model interpretability. *arXiv.org.* https://arxiv.org/abs/1802.07810 (accessed November 13, 2019).

Rajkomar, A., E. Oren, K. Chen, A. M. Dai, N. Hajaj, M. Hardt, P. J. Liu, X. Liu, J. Marcus, M. Sun, P. Sundberg, H. Yee, K. Zhang, Y. Zhang, G. Flores, G. E. Duggan, J. Irvine, Q. Le, K. Litsch, A. Mossin, J. Tansuwan, D. Wang, J. Wexler, J. Wilson, D. Ludwig, S. L. Volchenboum, K. Chou, M. Pearson, S. Madabushi, N. H. Shah, A. J. Butte, M. D. Howell, C. Cui, G. S. Corrado, and J. Dean. 2018. Scalable and accurate deep learning with electronic health records. *NPJ Digital Medicine* 1(1):18.

Rajpurkar, P., J. Irvin, R. L. Ball, K. Zhu, B. Yang, H. Mehta, T. Duan, D. Ding, A. Bagul, C. P. Langlotz, B. N. Patel, K. W. Yeom, K. Shpanskaya, F. G. Blankenberg, J. Seekins, T. J. Amrhein, D. A. Mong, S. S. Halabi, E. J. Zucker, A. Y. Ng, and M. P. Lungren. 2018. Deep learning for chest radiograph diagnosis: A retrospective comparison of the CheXNeXt algorithm to practicing radiologists. *PLoS Medicine* 15(11):e1002686.

Roski, J., G. Bo-Linn, and T. Andrews. 2014. Creating value in healthcare through big data: Opportunities and policy implications. *Health Affairs* 33(7):1115–1122.

Sachs, K., O. Perez, D. Pe'er, D. A. Lauffenburger, and G. P. Nolan. 2005. Causal protein-signaling networks derived from multiparameter single-cell data. *Science* 308(5721):523–529.

Saria, S. 2018. Individualized sepsis treatment using reinforcement learning. *Nature Medicine* 24(11):1641–1642.

Saria, S., and A. Goldenberg. 2015. Subtyping: What it is and its role in precision medicine. *IEEE Intelligent Systems* 30(4):70–75.

Schulam, P., and S. Saria. 2017. Reliable decision support using counterfactual models. *arXiv.org.* https://arxiv.org/abs/1703.10651 (accessed November 13, 2019).

Schulam, P., and S. Saria. 2018. Discretizing logged interaction data biases learning for decision-making. *arXiv.org.* https://arxiv.org/abs/1810.03025 (accessed November 13, 2019).

Schuler, A. 2018. *Some methods to compare the real-world performance of causal estimators.* Ph.D. dissertation, Stanford University. http://purl.stanford.edu/vg743rx0211 (accessed November 13, 2019).

Shah, N. D., E. W. Steyerberg, and D. M. Kent. 2018. Big data and predictive analytics: Recalibrating expectations. *JAMA* 320(1):27–28.

Shah, N. H., A. Milstein, and S. C. Bagley. 2019. Making machine learning models clinically useful. *JAMA* 322(14):1351–1352. https://doi.org/10.1001/jama.2019.10306.

Shah, S. J., D. H. Katz, S. Selvaraj, M. A. Burke, C. W. Yancy, M. Gheorghiade, R. O. Bonow, C. C. Huang, and R. C. Deo. 2015. Phenomapping for novel classification of heart failure with preserved ejection fraction. *Circulation* 131(3):269–279.

Shortliffe, E. H. 1974. *MYCIN: A rule-based computer program for advising physicians regarding antimicrobial therapy selection.* No. AIM-251. Stanford University. https://searchworks.stanford.edu/view/12291681 (accessed November 13, 2019).

Sohn, S., D. W. Larson, E. B. Habermann, J. M. Naessens, J. Y. Alabbad, and H. Liu. 2017. Detection of clinically important colorectal surgical site infection using Bayesian network. *Journal of Surgical Research* 209:168–173.

Steyerberg, E. W., A. J. Vickers, N. R. Cook, T. Gerds, M. Gonen, N. Obuchowski, M. J. Pencina, and M. W. Kattan. 2010. Assessing the performance of prediction models: A framework for some traditional and novel measures. *Epidemiology* 21(1):128–138.

Subbaswamy, A., P. Schulam, and S. Saria. 2018. Learning predictive models that transport. *arXiv.org.* https://arxiv.org/abs/1812.04597 (accessed November 13, 2019).

Suresh, H., and J. V. Guttag. 2019. A framework for understanding unintended consequences of machine learning. *arXiv.org.* https://arxiv.org/abs/1901.10002 (accessed November 13, 2019).

Vellido, A. 2019. The importance of interpretability and visualization in machine learning for applications in medicine and health care. *Neural Computing and Applications.* https://doi.org/10.1007/s00521-019-04051-w (accessed November 13, 2019).

Verghese, A., N. H. Shah, and R. A. Harrington. 2018. What this computer needs is a physician: Humanism and artificial intelligence. *JAMA* 319(1):19–20.

Voosen, P. 2017. The AI detectives. *Science* 357(6346):22–27. https://science.sciencemag.org/content/357/6346/22.summary (accessed November 13, 2019).

Wang, W., M. Bjarnadottir, and G. G. Gao. 2018. How AI plays its tricks: Interpreting the superior performance of deep learning-based approach in predicting healthcare costs. *SSRN.* https://papers.ssrn.com/sol3/papers.cfm?abstract_id=3274094 (accessed November 13, 2019).

Wiens, J., S. Saria, M. Sendak, M. Ghassemi, V. X. Liu, F. Doshi-Velez, K. Jung, K. Heller, D. Kale, M. Saeed, P. N. Ossocio, S. Thadney-Israni, and A. Goldenberg. 2019. Do no harm: A roadmap for responsible machine learning for health care. *Nature Medicine* 25(9):1337–1340.

Wikipedia. 2019. *Training, validation, and test sets.* https://en.wikipedia.org/wiki/Training,_validation,_and_test_sets (accessed November 13, 2019).

Wilkinson, M. D., M. Dumontier, I. J. Aalbersberg, G. Appleton, M. Axton, A. Baak, N. Blomberg, J. W. Boiten, L. B. da Silva Santos, P. E. Bourne, and J. Bouwman. 2016. The FAIR Guiding Principles for scientific data management and stewardship. *Scientific Data* 3:Art 160018.

Williams, J. B., D. Ghosh, and R. C. Wetzel. 2018. Applying machine learning to pediatric critical care data. *Pediatric Critical Care Medicine* 19(7):599–608.

Wu, A. 2019. Solving healthcare's big epidemic—Physician burnout. *Forbes.* https://www.forbes.com/sites/insights-intelai/2019/02/11/solving-healthcares-big-epidemicphysician-burnout/#64ed37e04483 (accessed November 13, 2019).

Yadlowsky, S., R. A. Hayward, J. B. Sussman, R. L. McClelland, Y. I. Min, and S. Basu. 2018. Clinical implications of revised pooled cohort equations for estimating atherosclerotic cardiovascular disease risk. *Annals of Internal Medicine* 169(1):20–29.

Yu, K. H., A. L. Beam, and I. S. Kohane. 2018. Artificial intelligence in healthcare. *Nature Biomedical Engineering* 2(10):719–731.

Zhan, A., S. Mohan, C. Tarolli, R. B. Schneider, J. L. Adams, S. Sharma, M. J. Elson, K. L. Spear, A. M. Glidden, M. A. Little, and A. Terzis. 2018. Using smartphones and machine learning to quantify Parkinson disease severity: The mobile Parkinson disease score. *JAMA Neurology* 75(7):876–880.

Zhou, Z. H. 2017. A brief introduction to weakly supervised learning. *National Science Review* 5(1):44–53.

Suggested citation for Chapter 5: Liu, H., H. Estiri, J. Wiens, A. Goldenberg, S. Saria, and N. Shah. 2020. Artificial intelligence model development and validation. In *Artificial intelligence in health care: The hope, the hype, the promise, the peril.* Washington, DC: National Academy of Medicine.

6

DEPLOYING ARTIFICIAL INTELLIGENCE IN CLINICAL SETTINGS

Stephan Fihn, University of Washington; Suchi Saria, Johns Hopkins University; Eneida Mendonça, Regenstrief Institute; Seth Hain, Epic; Michael Matheny, Vanderbilt University Medical Center; Nigam Shah, Stanford University; Hongfang Liu, Mayo Clinic; and Andrew Auerbach, University of California, San Francisco

INTRODUCTION

The effective use of artificial intelligence (AI) in clinical settings currently presents an opportunity for thoughtful engagement. There is steady and transformative progress in methods and tools needed to manipulate and transform clinical data, and increasingly mature data resources have supported novel development of accurate and sophisticated AI in some health care domains (although the risk of not being sufficiently representative is real). However, few examples of AI deployment and use within the health care delivery system exist, and there is sparse evidence for improved processes or outcomes when AI tools are deployed (He et al., 2019). For example, within machine learning risk prediction models—a subset of the larger AI domain—the sizable literature on model development and validation is in stark contrast to the scant data describing successful clinical deployment of those models in health care settings (Shortliffe and Sepúlveda, 2018).

This discrepancy between development efforts and successful use of AI reflects the hurdles in deploying decision support systems and tools more broadly (Tcheng et al., 2017). While some impediments are technical, more relate to the complexity of tailoring applications for integration with existing capabilities in electronic health records (EHRs), poor understanding of users' needs and expectations for information, poorly defined clinical processes and objectives, and even concerns about legal liability (Bates, 2012; Miller et al., 2018; Unertl et al., 2007, 2009). These impediments may be balanced by the potential for gain, as one cross-sectional review of closed malpractice claims found that more than one-half of malpractice claims could have been potentially prevented by well-designed clinical decision support (CDS) in the form of alerts (e.g., regarding potential drug–drug interactions and abnormal test results), reminders, or electronic checklists (Zuccotti et al., 2014). Although, in many instances, the deployment of AI tools in health care may be conducted on a relatively small scale, it is important to recognize that an estimated 50 percent of information technology (IT) projects fail in the commercial sector (Florentine, 2016).

Setting aside the challenges of physician-targeted, point-of-care decision support, there is great opportunity for AI to improve domains outside of encounter-based care delivery, such as in the management of patient populations or in administrative tasks for which data and work standards may be more readily defined, as is discussed in more detail in Chapter 3. These future priority areas will likely be accompanied by their own difficulties, related to translating AI applications into effective tools that improve the quality and efficiency of health care.

AI tools will also produce challenges that are entirely related to the novelty of the technology. Even at this early stage of AI implementation in health care, the use of AI tools has raised questions about the expectations of clinicians and health systems regarding transparency of the data models, the clinical plausibility of the underlying data assumptions, whether AI tools are suitable for discovery of new causal links, and the ethics of how, where, when, and under what circumstances AI should be deployed (He et al., 2019). At this time in the development cycle, methods to estimate the requirements, care, and maintenance of these tools and their underlying data needs remain a rudimentary management science.

There are also proposed regulatory rules that will influence the use of AI in health care. On July 27, 2018, the Centers for Medicare & Medicaid Services (CMS) published a proposed rule that aims to increase Medicare beneficiaries' access to physicians' services routinely furnished via "communication technology." The rule defines such clinician services as those that are defined by and inherently involve the use of computers and communication technology; these services will be associated with a set of Virtual Care payment codes (CMS, 2019). These services would not be subject to the limitations on Medicare telehealth services and would instead be paid under the Physician Fee Schedule, as other physicians' services are. CMS's evidentiary standard of clinical benefit for determining coverage under the proposed rule does not include minor or incidental benefits.

This proposed rule is relevant to all clinical AI applications, because they all involve computer and communication technology and aim to deliver substantive clinical benefit consistent with the examples set forth by CMS. If clinical AI applications are deemed by CMS to be instances of reimbursable Virtual Care services, then it is likely that they would be prescribed like other physicians' services and medical products, and it is likely that U.S.-based commercial payors would establish National Coverage Determinations mimicking CMS's policy. If these health finance measures are enacted as proposed, they will greatly accelerate the uptake of clinical AI tools and provide significant financial incentives for health care systems to do so as well.

In this chapter, we describe the key issues, considerations, and best practices relating to the implementation and maintenance of AI within the health care system. This chapter complements the preceding discussion in Chapter 5 that is focused on considerations at the model creation level within the broader scope of AI development. The information presented will likely be of greatest interest to individuals within health care systems that are deploying AI or considering doing so, and we have limited the scope of this chapter to this audience. National policy, regulatory, and legislative considerations for AI are addressed in Chapter 7.

SETTINGS FOR APPLICATION OF AI IN HEALTH CARE

The venues in which health care is delivered, physically or virtually, are expanding rapidly, and AI applications are beginning to surface in many if not all of these venues. Because there is tremendous diversity in individual settings, each of which presents unique requirements, we outline broad categories that are germane to most settings and provide a basic framework for implementing AI.

Traditional Point of Care

Decision support generally refers to the provision of recommendations or explicit guidance relating to diagnosis or prognosis at the point of care, addressing an acknowledged need for assistance in selecting optimal treatments, tests, and plans of care along with facilitating processes to ensure that interventions are safely, efficiently, and effectively applied.

At present, most clinicians regularly encounter point-of-care tools integrated into the EHR. Recent changes in the 21st Century Cures Act have removed restrictions on sharing information between users of a specific EHR vendor or across vendors' users and may (in part) overcome restrictions that limited innovation in this space. Point-of-care tools, when hosted outside the EHR, are termed software as a medical device (SaMD) and may be regulated under the U.S. Food and Drug Administration's (FDA's) Digital Health Software Precertification Program, as is discussed in more detail in Chapter 7 (FDA, 2018; Lee and

Kesselheim, 2018). SaMD provided by EHR vendors will not be regulated under the Precertification Program, but those supported outside those environments and either added to them or provided to patients via separate routes (e.g., apps on phones, services provided as part of pharmacy benefit managers) will be. The nature of regulation is evolving but will need to account for changes in clinical practice, data systems, populations, etc. However, regulated or not, SaMD that incorporates AI methods will require careful testing and retesting, recalibration, and revalidation at the time of implementation as well as periodically afterward. All point-of-care AI applications will need to adhere to best practices for the form, function, and workflow placement of CDS and incorporate best practices in human–computer interaction and human factors design (Phansalkar et al., 2010). This will need to occur in an environment where widely adopted EHRs continue to evolve and where there will likely be opportunities for disruptive technologies.

Clinical Information Processing and Management

Face-to-face interactions with patients are, in a sense, only the tip of the iceberg of health care delivery (Blane et al., 2002; Network for Excellence in Health Innovation, 2015; Tarlov, 2002). A complex array of people and services are necessary to support direct care and they tend to consume and generate massive amounts of data. Diagnostic services such as laboratory, pathology, and radiology procedures are prime examples and are distinguished by the generation of clinical data, including dense imaging, as well as interpretations and care recommendations that must be faithfully transmitted to the provider (and sometimes the patient) in a timely manner.

AI will certainly play a major role with tasks such as automated image (e.g., radiology, ophthalmology, dermatology, and pathology) and signal processing (e.g., electrocardiogram, audiology, and electroencephalography). In addition to interpretation of tests and images, AI will be used to integrate and array results with other clinical data to facilitate clinical workflow (Topol, 2019).

Enterprise Operations

The administrative systems necessary to maintain the clinical enterprise are substantial and are likely to grow as AI tools grow in number and complexity. In the near term, health care investors and innovators are wagering that AI will assume increasing importance in conducting back-office activities in a wide variety of areas (Parma, 2018). Because these tasks tend to be less nuanced than clinical decisions, and usually pose lower risk, it is likely that they may be more tractable targets for AI systems to support in the immediate future. In addition, the data necessary to train models in these settings are often more easily available than in clinical settings. For example, in a hospital, these tasks might include the management of billing, pharmacy, supply chain, staffing, and patient flow. In an outpatient setting, AI-driven applications could assume some of the administrative tasks such as gathering information to assist with decisions about insurance coverage, scheduling, and obtaining preapprovals. Some of these topics are discussed in greater detail in Chapter 3.

Nontraditional Health Care Settings

Although we tend to think of applying AI in health care locations, such as hospital or clinics, there may be greater opportunities in settings where novel care delivery models are emerging. This might include freestanding, urgent care facilities or pharmacies, or our homes, schools, and workplaces. It is readily possible to envision AI deployed in these venues, such as walk-in service in retail vendors, or pharmacies with embedded urgent and primary care clinics. Although some of these may be considered traditional point-of-care environments, the availability of information may be substantially different in these environments. Likewise, information synthesis, decision support, and knowledge search support are systematically different in these nontraditional health care settings, and thus they warrant consideration as a distinct type of environment for AI implementation purposes.

Additionally, it is worth noting that AI applications are already in use in many nonmedical settings for purposes such as anticipating customers' purchases and managing inventory accordingly. However, these types of tools may be used to link health metrics to purchasing recommendations (e.g., suggesting healthier food options for patients with hypertension or diabetes) once the ethical consent and privacy issues related to use of patient data are addressed (Storm, 2015).

Population Health Management

An increasingly important component of high-quality care falls under the rubric of population health management. This poses a challenge for traditional health systems because some research suggests that only a small fraction of overall health can be attributed to health care (McGinnis et al., 2002) (see Figure 6-1).

Nevertheless, other research suggests that health systems have a major role to play in improving population health that can be distinguished from those of

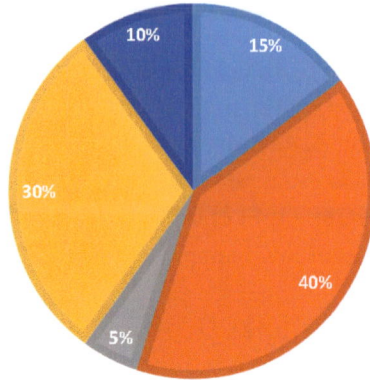

FIGURE 6-1 | Determinants of population health.
SOURCE: Figure created with data from McGinnis et al., 2002.

traditional medical care and public health systems (see Figure 6-2). Although there is no broadly accepted definition of this function within health care delivery systems, one goal is to standardize routine aspects of care, typically in an effort to improve clinical performance metrics across large populations and systems of care with the goal of improving quality and reducing costs.

Promoting healthy behaviors and self-care are major focuses of population health management efforts (Kindig and Stoddart, 2003). Much of the work of

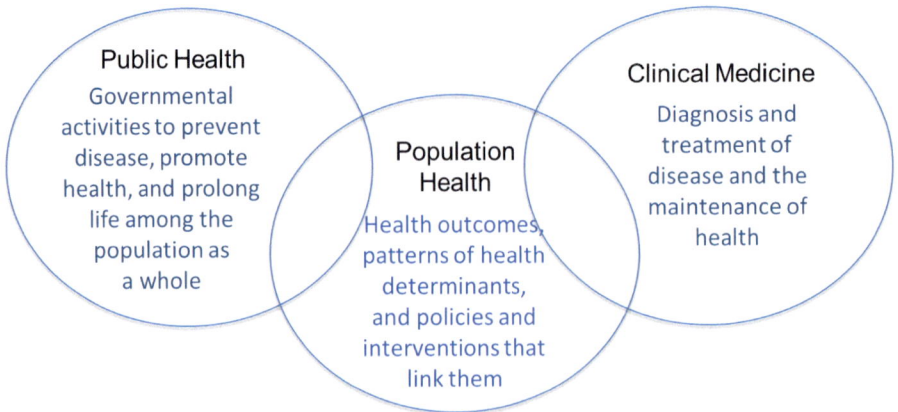

FIGURE 6-2 | Relationship of population health to public health and standard clinical care.
SOURCE: Definition of population health from Kindig, 2007.

health management in this context is conducted outside of regular visits and often involves more than one patient at a time. AI has the potential to assist with prioritization of clinical resources and management of volume and intensity of patient contacts, as well as targeting services to patients most likely to benefit. In addition, an essential component of these initiatives involves contacting large numbers of patients, which can occur through a variety of automated, readily scalable methods, such as text messaging and patient portals (Reed et al., 2019). One such example in a weight loss program among prediabetic patients is the use of Internet-enabled devices with an application to provide educational materials, a communication mechanism to their peer group and health coach, and progress tracking, which showed that completion of lessons and rate of utilization of the tools were strongly correlated with weight loss over multiple years (Sepah et al., 2017). Such communication may be as basic as asynchronous messaging of reminders to obtain a flu shot (Herrett et al., 2016) or to attend a scheduled appointment using secure messaging, automated telephone calls, or postal mail (Schwebel and Larimer, 2018). Higher order activities, such as for psychosocial support or chronic disease management, might entail use of a dedicated app or voice or video modalities, which could also be delivered through encounters using telemedicine, reflecting the fluidity and overlap of technological solutions (Xing et al., 2019) (see Chapter 3 for additional examples).

Because virtual interactions are typically less complex than face-to-face visits, they are likely targets for AI enhancement. Led by efforts in large integrated health delivery systems, there are a variety of examples where statistical models derived from large datasets have been developed and deployed to predict individuals' intermediate and longer term risk of experiencing adverse consequences of chronic conditions including death or hospitalization (Steele et al., 2018). These predictions are starting to be used to prioritize provision of care management within these populations (Rumsfeld et al., 2016). Massive information synthesis is also a key need for this setting, because at-a-glance review of hundreds or thousands of patients at the time is typical, which is a task in which AI excels (Wahl et al., 2018).

Patient- and Caregiver-Facing Applications

The patient- and caregiver-facing application domain merges health care delivery with publicly available consumer hardware and software. It is defined as the space in which applications and tools are directly accessible to patients and their caregivers. Tools and software in this domain enable patients to manage much of their own health care and facilitate interactions between patients and the health care delivery system. In particular, smartphone and mobile applications have transformed the potential for patient contact, active participation in health care behavior modification, and reminders. These applications also hold the potential for health care delivery to access new and important patient data streams to help stratify risk, provide care recommendations, and help prevent complications of chronic diseases. This trend is likely to blur the traditional boundaries of tasks now performed during face-to-face appointments.

Patient- and caregiver-facing tools represent an area of strong potential growth for AI deployment and are expected to empower users to assume greater control over their health and health care (Topol, 2015). Moreover, there is the potential for creating a positive feedback loop where patients' needs and preferences, expressed through their use of AI-support applications, can then be incorporated into other applications throughout the health care delivery system. As growth of online purchasing continues, the role of AI in direct patient interaction—providing wellness, treatment, or diagnostic recommendations via mobile platforms—will grow in parallel to that of brick-and-mortar settings. Proliferation of these applications will continue to amplify and enhance data collected through traditional medical activities (e.g., lab results, pharmacy fill data). Mobile applications are increasingly able to cross-link various sources of data and potentially enhance health care (e.g., through linking grocery purchase data to health metrics to physical steps taken or usage statistics from phones). The collection and presentation of AI recommendations using mobile- or desktop-based platforms is critical because patients are increasingly engaging in self-care activities supported by applications available on multiple platforms. In addition to being used by patients, the technology will likely be heavily used by their family and caregivers.

Unfortunately, the use of technologies intended to support self-management of health by individuals has been lagging as has evaluation of their effectiveness (Abdi et al., 2018). Although there are more than 320,000 health apps currently available, and these apps have been downloaded nearly 4 billion times, little research has been conducted to determine whether they improve health (Liquid State, 2018). In a recent overview of systematic reviews of studies evaluating stand-alone, mobile health apps, only 6 meta-analyses including a total of 23 randomized trials could be identified. In all, 11 of the 23 trials showed a meaningful effect on health or surrogate outcomes attributable to apps, but the overall evidence of effectiveness was deemed to be of very low quality (Byambasuren et al., 2018). In addition, there is a growing concern that many of these apps share personal health data in ways that are opaque and potentially worrisome to users (Loria, 2019).

APPLICATIONS OF AI IN CLINICAL CARE DELIVERY

Both information generated by medical science and clinical data related to patient care have burgeoned to a level at which clinicians are overwhelmed. This is a critically important problem because information overload not only leads to disaffection among providers but also to medical errors (Tawfik et al., 2018).

Although clinical cognitive science has made advances toward understanding how providers routinely access medical knowledge during care delivery and the ways in which this understanding could be transmitted to facilitate workflow, this has occurred in only very limited ways in practice (Elstein et al., 1978; Kilsdonk et al., 2016). However, AI is apt to be integral to platforms that incorporate these advances, transforming not only health care delivery but also clinical training and education through the identification and delivery of relevant clinical knowledge at the point of decision making. Key support tasks would include the intelligent search and retrieval of relevant sources of information and customizable display of data; these hypothetical AI tools would relieve clinicians of doing this manually as is now usually the case (Li et al., 2015). Furthermore, these features would enhance the quality and safety of care because important information would be less likely to be overlooked. Additionally, AI holds promise for providing point-of-care decision support powered by the synthesis of existing published evidence, with the reported experiences of similarly diagnosed or treated patients (Li et al., 2015).

Health care is increasingly delivered by teams that include specialists, nurses, physician assistants, pharmacists, social workers, case managers, and other health care professionals. Each of them brings specialized skills and viewpoints that augment and complement the care a patient receives from individual health care providers. As the volume of data and information available for patient care grows exponentially, innovative solutions empowered by AI techniques will naturally become foundational to the care team, providing task-specific expertise in the data and information space for advancing knowledge at the point of care.

Risk Prediction

Risk prediction is defined as any algorithm that forecasts a future outcome from a set of characteristics existing at a particular time point. It typically entails applying sophisticated statistical processes and/or machine learning to large datasets to generate probabilities for a wide array of outcomes ranging from death or adverse events to hospitalization. These large datasets may include dozens, if not hundreds, of variables gathered from thousands, or even millions, of patients. Overall, the risk prediction class of applications focuses on assessing the likelihood of the outcome to individuals by applying thresholds of risk. These individuals may then be targeted to receive additional or fewer resources in terms of surveillance, review, intervention, or follow-up based on some balance of expected risk, benefit, and cost. Predictions may be generated for individual patients, at a specific point in time (e.g., during a clinical encounter or at hospital admission or discharge), or for populations of patients, which identifies a group of patients at high risk of an adverse clinical event.

Tools to predict an individual's risk of a given event have been available for decades but due largely to limitations of available data (e.g., small samples or claims data without clinical information), the accuracy of the predictions has generally been too low for routine use in clinical practice. The advent of large repositories of data extracted from clinical records, administrative databases, and other sources, coupled with high-performance computing, has enabled relatively accurate predictions for individual patients. Reports of predictive tools that have C-statistics (areas under curve) exceeding 0.85 or higher are now common (Islam et al., 2019). Examples that are currently in use include identifying outpatients, including those with certain conditions who are at high risk of hospital admission or emergency department visits who might benefit from some type of care coordination, or hospitalized patients who are at risk of clinical deterioration for whom more intense observation and management are warranted (Kansagara et al., 2011; Smith et al., 2014, 2018; Wang et al., 2013).

Given the rapidly increasing availability of sophisticated modeling tools and very large clinical datasets, the number of models and prediction targets is growing rapidly. Machine learning procedures can sometimes produce greater accuracy than standard methods such as logistic regression; however, the improvements may be marginal, especially when the number of data elements is limited (Christodoulou et al., 2019). These increments may not necessarily compensate for the expense of the computing infrastructure required to support machine leaning, particularly when the goal is to use techniques in real time. Another issue is that, depending on the methods employed to generate a machine learning model, assessing the model's predictive accuracy may not be straightforward. When a model is trained simply to provide binary classifications, probabilities are not generated and it may be impossible to examine the accuracy of predictions across a range of levels of risk. In such instances, it is difficult to produce calibration curves or stratification tables, which are fundamental to assessing predictive accuracy, although techniques are evolving (Bandos et al., 2009; Kull et al., 2017). Calibration performance has been shown to decline quickly, sometimes within 1 year of model development, on both derivation and external datasets (Davis et al., 2017), and this will affect CDS performance as the sensitivity and specificity of a model value threshold changes with calibration performance changes.

As indicated earlier, it is unlikely that simply making predictive information available to clinicians will be an effective strategy. In one example, estimates for risk of death and/or hospitalization were generated for more than 5 million patients in a very large health care system, using models with C-statistics of 0.85 or higher. These predictions were provided to more than 7,000 primary care clinicians weekly for their entire patient panels in a way that was readily accessible through the EHR. Based on usage statistics, however, only about 15 percent of the clinicians regularly accessed these reports, even though, when surveyed, those who used the reports said that they generally found them accurate (Nelson et al., 2019). Accordingly, even when they are highly accurate, predictive models are unlikely to improve clinical outcomes unless they are tightly linked to effective interventions and the recommendations or actions are integrated into clinical workflow. Thus, it is useful to think in terms of prediction–action pairs.

In summary, while there is great potential for AI tools to improve on existing methods for risk prediction, there are still large challenges in how these tools are implemented, how they are integrated with clinical needs and workflows, and how they are maintained. Moreover, as discussed in Chapter 1, health care professionals will need to understand the clinical, personal, and ethical implications of communicating and addressing information about an individual's risk that may extend far into the future, such as predisposition to cancer, cardiovascular disease, or dementia.

Clinical Decision Support

CDS spans a gamut of applications intended to alert clinicians to important information and provide assistance with various clinical tasks, which in some cases may include prediction. Over the past two decades, CDS has largely been applied as rule-driven alerts (e.g., reminders for vaccinations) or alerts employing relatively simple Boolean logic based on published risk indices that change infrequently over time (e.g., Framingham risk index). More elaborate systems have been based upon extensive, knowledge-based applications that assist with management of chronic conditions such as hypertension (Goldstein et al., 2000). Again, with advances in computer science, including natural language processing, machine learning, and programming tools such as business process modeling notation, case management and notation, and related specifications, it is becoming possible to model and monitor more complex clinical processes (Object Management Group, 2019). Coupled with information about providers and patients, systems will be able to tailor relevant advice to specific decisions and treatment recommendations. Other applications may include advanced search and analytical capabilities that could provide information such as the outcomes of past patients who are similar to those currently receiving various treatments.

For example, in one instance, EHR data from nearly 250 million patients were analyzed using machine learning to determine the most effective second-line hypoglycemic agents (Vashisht et al., 2018).

Image Processing

One of the clinical areas in which AI is beginning to have an important early impact is imaging processing. There were about 100 publications on AI in radiology in 2005, but that increased exponentially to more than 800 in 2016 and 2017, related largely to computed tomography, magnetic resonance imaging, and, in particular, neuroradiology and mammography (Pesapane et al., 2018). Tasks for which current AI technology seems well suited include prioritizing and tracking findings that mandate early attention, comparing current and prior images, and high-throughput screenings that enable radiologists to concentrate on images most likely to be abnormal. Over time, however, it is likely that interpretation of routine imaging will be increasingly performed using AI applications.

Interpretation of other types of images by AI are rapidly emerging in other fields as well, including dermatology, pathology, and ophthalmology, as noted earlier. FDA recently approved the first device for screening for diabetic retinopathy, and at least one academic medical center is currently using it. The device is intended for use in primary care settings to identify patients who should be referred to an ophthalmologist (Lee, 2018). The availability of such devices will certainly increase markedly in the near future.

Diagnostic Support and Phenotyping

For nearly 50 years, there have been efforts to develop computer-aided diagnosis exemplified by systems such as Iliad, QMR, Internist, and DXplain, but none of these programs has been widely adopted. More recent efforts such as those of IBM Watson have not been more successful (Palmer, 2018). In part, this is a result of a relative lack of major investment as compared to AI applications for imaging technology. It also reflects the greater challenges in patient diagnosis compared to imaging interpretation. Data necessary for diagnosis arise from many sources including clinical notes, laboratory tests, pharmacy data, imaging, genomic information, etc. These data sources are often not stored in digital formats and generally lack standardized terminology. Also, unlike imaging studies, there is often a wide range of diagnostic possibilities, making the problem space exponentially larger. Nonetheless, computer-aided diagnosis is likely to evolve rapidly in the future.

Another emerging AI application is the development of phenotyping algorithms using data extracted from the EHR and other relevant sources to identify individuals with certain diseases or conditions and to classify them according to stage, severity, and other characteristics. At present, no common standardized, structured, computable format exists for storing phenotyping algorithms, but semantic approaches are under development and hold the promise of far more accurate characterization of individuals or groups than simply using diagnostic codes, as is often done today (Marx, 2015). When linked to genotypes, accurate phenotypes will greatly enhance AI tools' capability to diagnose and understand the genetic and molecular basis of disease. Over time, these advances may also support the development of novel therapies (Papež et al., 2017).

FRAMEWORK AND CRITERIA FOR AI SELECTION AND IMPLEMENTATION IN CLINICAL CARE

As clinical AI applications become increasingly available, health care delivery systems and hospitals will need to develop expertise in evaluation, selection, and assessment of liability. Marketing of these tools is apt to intensify and be accompanied by claims regarding improved clinical outcomes or improved efficiency of care, which may or may not be well founded. While the technical requirements of algorithm development and validation are covered in Chapter 5, this section describes a framework for evaluation, decision making, and adoption that incorporates considerations regarding organizational governance and post-development technical issues (i.e., maintenance of systems) as well as clinical considerations that are all essential to successful implementation.

AI Implementation and Deployment as a Feature of Learning Health Systems

More than a decade ago, the National Academy of Medicine (NAM) recognized the necessity for health systems to respond effectively to the host of challenges posed by rising expectations for quality and safety in an environment of rapidly evolving technology and accumulating massive amounts of data (IOM, 2011). The health system was reimagined as a dynamic system that does not merely deliver health care in the traditional manner based on clinical guidelines and professional norms, but is continually assessing and improving by harnessing the power of IT systems—that is, a system with ongoing learning hardwired into its operating model. In this conception, the wealth of data generated in the process of providing health care becomes readily available in a secure manner for incorporation into continuous improvement activities within the system and for research to advance health care delivery in general (Friedman et al., 2017). In this manner, the value of the care that is delivered to any individual patient imparts benefit to the larger population of similar patients. To provide context for how the learning health system (LHS) is critical for how to consider AI in health care, we have referenced 10 recommendations from a prior NAM report in this domain, and aligned them with how AI could be considered within the LHS for each of these key recommendation areas (see Table 6-1).

Clearly listed as 1 of the 10 priorities is involvement of patients and families, which should occur in at least two critically important ways. First, they need to be informed, both generally and specifically, about how AI applications are being integrated into the care they receive. Second, AI applications provide an opportunity to enhance engagement of patients in shared decision making. Although interventions to enhance shared decision making have not yet shown consistently beneficial effects, these applications are very early in development and have great potential (Légaré et al., 2018).

The adoption of AI technology provides a sentinel opportunity to advance the notion of LHSs. AI requires the digital infrastructure that enables the LHS to operate and, as described in Table 6-1, AI applications can be fundamentally designed to facilitate evaluation and assessment. One large health system in the United States has proclaimed ambitious plans to incorporate AI into "every patient interaction, workflow challenge and administrative need" to "drive improvements in quality, cost and access," and many other health care delivery organizations and IT companies share this vision, although it is clearly many years off (Monegain, 2017). As AI is increasingly embedded into the infrastructure of health care delivery, it is mandatory that the data generated be available not only to evaluate the performance of AI applications themselves, but also to advance understanding about how our health care systems are functioning and how patients are faring.

Institutional Readiness and Governance

For AI deployment in health care practice to be successful, it is critical that the life cycle of AI use be overseen through effective governance. IT governance is the set of processes that ensure the effective and efficient use of IT in enabling an organization to achieve its goals. At its core, governance defines how an organization manages its IT portfolio (e.g., financial and personnel) by overseeing the effective evaluation, selection, prioritization, and funding of competing IT projects, ensuring their successful implementation, and tracking their performance. In addition, governance is responsible for ensuring that IT systems operate in an effective, efficient, and compliant fashion.

TABLE 6-1 | Leveraging Artificial Intelligence Tools into a Learning Health System

Topic	Institute of Medicine Learning Health System Recommendation	Mapping to Artificial Intelligence in Health Care
Foundational Elements		
Digital infrastructure	Improve the capacity to capture clinical, care delivery process, and financial data for better care, system improvement, and the generation of new knowledge.	Improve the capacity for unbiased, representative data capture with broad coverage for data elements needed to train artificial intelligence (AI).
Data utility	Streamline and revise research regulations to improve care, promote and capture clinical data, and generate knowledge.	Leverage continuous quality improvement (QI) and implement scientific methods to help select when AI tools are the most appropriate choice to optimize clinical operations and harness AI tools to support continuous improvement.
Care Improvement Targets		
Clinical decision support	Accelerate integration of the best clinical knowledge into care decisions.	Accelerate integration of AI tools into clinical decision support applications.
Patient-centered care	Involve patients and families in decisions regarding health and health care, tailored to fit their preferences.	Involve patient and families in how, when, and where AI tools are used to support care in alignment with preferences.
Community links	Promote community–clinical partnerships and services aimed at managing and improving health at the community level.	Promote use of AI tools in community and patient health consumer applications in a responsible, safe manner.
Care continuity	Improve coordination and communication within and across organizations.	Improve AI data inputs and outputs through improved card coordination and data interchange.
Optimized operations	Continuously improve health care operations to reduce waste, streamline care delivery, and focus on activities that improve patient health.	Leverage continuous QI and Implementation Science methods to help select when AI tools are the most appropriate choice to optimize clinical operations.
Policy Environment		
Financial incentives	Structure payment to reward continuous learning and improvement in the provision of best care at lower cost.	Use AI tools in business practices to optimize reimbursement, reduce cost, and (it is hoped) do so at a neutral or positive balance on quality of care.
Performance transparency	Increase transparency on health care system performance.	Make robust performance characteristics for AI tools transparent and assess them in the populations within which they are deployed.
Broad leadership	Expand commitment to the goals of a continuously learning health care system.	Promote broad stakeholder engagement and ownership in governance of AI systems in health care.

NOTE: Recommendations from *Best Care at Lower Cost* (IOM, 2013) for a Learning Health System (LHS) in the first two columns are aligned with how AI tools can be leveraged into the LHS in the third column.
SOURCE: Adapted with permission from IOM, 2013.

Another facet of IT governance that is relevant to AI is data governance, which institutes a methodical process that an organization adopts to manage its data and ensure that the data meet specific standards and business rules before entering them into a data management system. Given the intense data requirements of many AI applications, data governance is crucial and may also expand to data curation and privacy-related issues. Capabilities such as SMART on FHIR (Substitutable Medical Apps, Reusable Technology on Fast Healthcare Interoperability Resource) are emerging boons for the field of AI but may exacerbate problems related to the need for data to be exchanged from EHRs to external systems, which in turn create issues related to the privacy and security of data. Relatedly, organizations will also need to consider other ethical issues associated with data use and data stewardship (Faden, 2013). In recent years, much has been written about patient rights and preferences as well as how the LHS is a moral imperative (Morain et al., 2018). Multiple publications and patient-led organizations have argued that the public is willing to share data for purposes that improve patient health and facilitate collaboration with data and medical expertise (Wicks et al., 2018). In other words, these publications suggest that medical data should be understood as a "public good" (Kraft et al., 2018). It is critical for organizations to build on these publications and develop appropriate data stewardship models that ensure that health data are used in ways that align with patients' interests and preferences. Of particular note is the fact that not all patients and/or family have the same level of literacy, privilege, and understanding of how their data might be used or monetized, and the potential unintended consequences of privacy and confidentiality.

A health care enterprise that seeks to leverage AI should consider, characterize, and adequately resolve a number of key considerations prior to moving forward with the decision to develop and implement an AI solution. These key considerations are listed in Table 6-2 and are expanded further in the following sections.

Organizational Approach to Implementation

After the considerations delineated in the previous section have been resolved and a decision has been made to proceed with the adoption of an AI application, the organization requires a systematic approach to implementation. Frameworks for conceptualizing, designing, and evaluating this process are discussed below, but all implicitly incorporate the most fundamental basic health care improvement model, often referred to as a plan-do-study-act (PDSA) cycle. This approach was introduced more than two decades ago by W. E. Deming, the father of modern quality improvement (Deming, 2000). The PDSA cycle relies on the intimate

TABLE 6-2 | Key Considerations for Institutional Infrastructure and Governance

Consideration	Relevant Governance Questions
Organizational capabilities	Does the organization possess the necessary technological (e.g., information technology [IT] infrastructure, IT personnel) and organizational (knowledgeable and engaged workforce, education, and training) capabilities to adopt, assess, and maintain artificial intelligence (AI)-driven tools?
Data environment	What data are available for AI development? Do current systems possess the adequate capacity for storage, retrieval, and transmission to support AI tools?
Interoperability	Does the organization support and maintain data at rest and in motion according to national and local standards for interoperability (e.g., SMART on FHIR [Substitutable Medical Apps, Reusable Technology on Fast Healthcare Interoperability Resource])?
Personnel capacity	What expertise exists in the health care system to develop and maintain the AI algorithms?
Cost, revenue, and value	What will be the initial and ongoing costs to purchase and install AI algorithms and to train users to maintain underlying data models and to monitor for variance in model performance?
	Is there an anticipated return on investment from the AI deployment?
	What is the perceived value for the institution related to AI deployment?
Safety and efficacy surveillance	Are there governance and processes in place to provide regular assessments of the safety and efficacy of AI tools?
Patient, family, consumer engagement	Does the institution have in place formal mechanisms for patient, family, or consumer, such as a council or advisory board, that can engage and voice concerns on relevant issues related to implementation, evaluation, etc.?
Cybersecurity and privacy	Does the digital infrastructure for health care data in the enterprise have sufficient protections in place to minimize the risk of breaches of privacy if AI is deployed?
Ethics and fairness	Is there an infrastructure in place at the institution to provide oversight and review of AI tools to ensure that the known issues related to ethics and fairness are addressed and that vigilance for unknown issues is in place?
Regulatory issues (see Chapter 7)	Are there specific regulatory issues that must be addressed and, if so, what type of monitoring and compliance programs will be necessary?

participation of employees involved in the work, detailed understanding of workflows, and careful ongoing assessment of implementation that informs iterative adjustments. Newer methods of quality improvement introduced since Deming represent variations or elaborations of this approach. All too often, however, quality improvement efforts frequently fail because they are focused narrowly on a given task or set of tasks using inadequate metrics without due consideration of the larger environment in which change is expected to occur (Muller, 2018).

Such concerns are certainly relevant to AI implementation. New technology promises to substantially alter how medical professionals currently deliver health care at a time when morale in the workforce is generally poor (Shanafelt et al., 2012). One of the challenges of the use of AI in health care is that integrating it within the EHR and improving existing decision and workflow support tools may be viewed as an extension of an already unpopular technology (Sinsky et al., 2016). Moreover, there are a host of concerns that are unique to AI, some well and others poorly founded, which might add to the difficulty of implementing AI applications.

In recognition that basic quality improvement approaches are generally inadequate to produce large-scale change, the field of implementation science has arisen to characterize how organizations can undertake change in a systematic fashion that acknowledges their complexity. Some frameworks are specifically designed for evaluating the effectiveness of implementation, such as the Consolidated Framework for Implementation Research or the Promoting Action on Research Implementation in Health Services (PARiHS). In general, these governance and implementation frameworks emphasize sound change management and methods derived from implementation science that undoubtedly apply to implementation of AI tools (Damschroder et al., 2009; Rycroft-Malone, 2004).

Nearly all approaches integrate concepts of change management and incorporate the basic elements that should be familiar because they are routinely applied in health care improvement activities. These concepts, and how they are adapted to the specific task of AI implementation, are included in Table 6-3.

It must be recognized that even when these steps are taken by competent leadership, the process may not proceed as planned or expected. Health care delivery organizations are typically large and complex. These concepts of how to achieve desired changes successfully continue to evolve and increasingly acknowledge the powerful organizational factors that inhibit or facilitate change (Braithwaite, 2018).

Developmental Life Cycle of AI Applications

As is the case with any health care improvement activity, the nature of the effort is cyclical and iterative, as is summarized in Figure 6-3. As discussed earlier, the process begins with clear identification of the clinical problem or need to be addressed. Often the problem will be one identified by clinicians or administrators as a current barrier or frustration or as an opportunity to improve clinical or operational processes. Even so, it is critical for the governance process to delineate the extent and magnitude of the issue and ensure that it is not idiosyncratic and that there are not simpler approaches to addressing the problem, rather than

TABLE 6-3 | Key Artificial Intelligence (AI) Tool Implementation Concepts, Considerations, and Tasks Translated to AI-Specific Considerations

Implementation Task or Concept	Artificial Intelligence Relevant Aspects
Identifying the clinical or administrative problem to be addressed.	Consideration of the problem to be addressed should precede and be distinct from the selection and implementation of specific technologies, such as AI systems.
Assessing organizational readiness for change, which may entail surveying individuals who are likely to be affected. An example would be the Organizational Readiness to Change Assessment tool based on the Promoting Action on Research Implementation in Health Services framework (Helfrich et al., 2009).	It is important to include clinicians, information technology (IT) professionals, data scientists, and health care system leadership. These stakeholders are essential to effective planning for organizational preparation for implementing an AI solution.
Achieving consensus among stakeholders that the problem is important and relevant and providing persuasive information that the proposed solution is likely to be effective if adopted.	It is important to include clinicians, IT professionals, data scientists, and health care system leadership. These stakeholders are essential to effective planning for organizational preparation for implementing an AI solution.
When possible, applying standard organizational approaches that will be familiar to staff and patients without undue rigidity and determining what degree of customization will be permitted.	For AI technologies, this includes developing and adopting standards for approaches for how data are prepared, models are developed, and performance characteristics are reported. In addition, using standard user interfaces and education surrounding these technologies should be considered.
When possible, defining how adoption will improve workflow, patient outcomes, or organizational efficiency.	When possible, explicitly state and evaluate a value proposition, and, as important, assess the likelihood and magnitude of improvements with and without implementation of AI technologies.
Securing strong commitment from senior organizational leadership.	Typically, this includes organizational, clinical, IT and financial leaders for establishing governance and organizational prioritization strategies and directives.
Identifying strong local leadership, typically in the form of clinical champions and thought leaders.	Each AI system placed into practice needs a clinical owner(s) who will be the superusers of the tools, champion them, and provide early warning when these tools are not performing as expected.
Engaging stakeholders in developing a plan for implementation that is feasible and acceptable to users and working to identify offsets if the solution is likely to require more work on the part of users.	It is critical that AI tools be implemented in an environment incorporating user-centered design principles, and with a goal of decreasing user workload, either time or cognition. This requires detailed implementation plans that address changes in workflow, data streams, adoption or elimination of equipment if necessary, etc.
Providing adequate education and technical support during implementation.	Implementation of AI tools in health care settings should be done in concert with educational initiatives and both clinical champion and informatics/IT support that ideally is available immediately and capable of evaluating and remedying problems that arise.

continued

TABLE 6-3 | Continued

Implementation Task or Concept	Artificial Intelligence Relevant Aspects
Managing the unnecessary complexity that arises from the "choices" in current IT systems.	Identify and implement intuitive interfaces and optimal workflows through a user-centered design process.
Defining clear milestones, metrics, and outcomes to determine whether an implementation is successful.	The desirable target state for an AI application should be clearly stated, defined in a measurable way, and processes, such as automation or analytics, put into place to collect, analyze, and report this information in a timely manner.
Conducting after-action assessments that will inform further implementation efforts.	It is important to leverage the human–computer interaction literature to assess user perceptions, barriers, and lessons learned during implementation of AI tools and systems.

undertaking a major IT project. It is essential to delineate existing workflows, and this usually entails in-depth interviews with staff and direct observation that assist with producing detailed flowcharts (Nelson et al., 2011). It is also important to define the desired outcome state, and all feasible options for achieving that outcome should be considered and compared. In addition, to the greatest extent feasible, at each relevant step in the development process, input should be sought

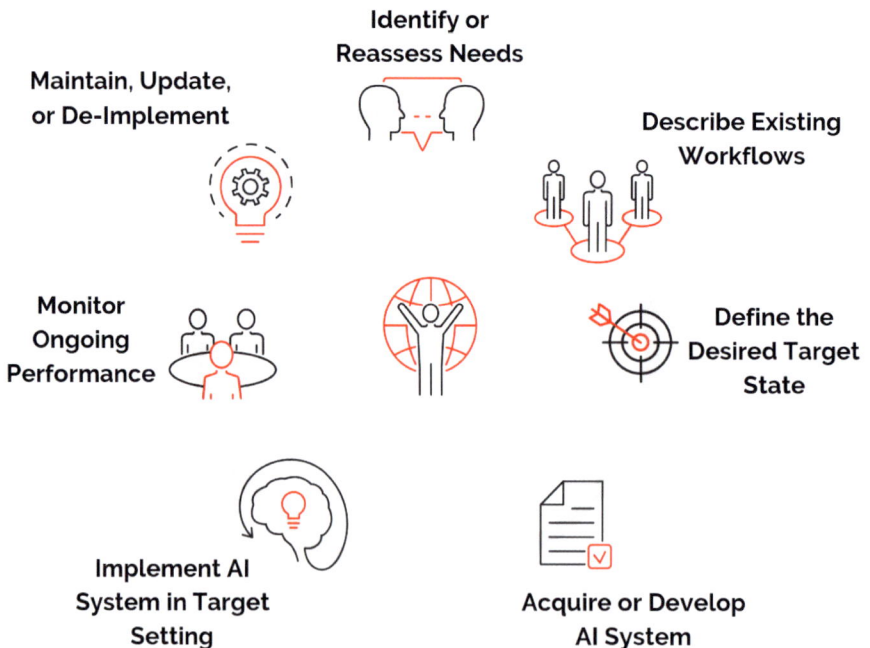

FIGURE 6-3 | Developmental life cycle of artificial intelligence applications.

from other stakeholders such as patients, end users, and members of the public. Although AI applications are currently a popular topic and new products are being touted, it is important to recall that the field is near the peak of the Gartner Hype Cycle (see Chapter 4), and some solutions are at risk for overpromising the achievable benefit. Thus, it is likely that early adopters will spend more and realize less value than organizations that are more strategic and, perhaps, willing to defer investments until products are more mature and have been proven. Ultimately, it will be necessary for organizations to assess the utility of an AI application in terms of the value proposition. For example, in considering adoption of an AI application for prediction, it is possible that in certain situations, given the cost, logistical complexity, and efficacy of the action, there may not be feasible operating zones in which a prediction–action pair, as described below, has clinical utility. Therefore, assessing the value proposition of deploying AI in clinical settings has to include the utility of downstream actions triggered by the system along with the frequency, cost, and logistics of those actions.

Components of a Clinical Validation and Monitoring Program for AI Tools

The clinical validation of AI tools should be viewed as distinct from the technical validation described in Chapter 5. For AI, clinical validation has two key axes:

1. Application of traditional medical hierarchy of evidence to support adoption and continued use of the AI tool. The hierarchy categorizes pilot data as the lowest level of evidence, followed by observational, risk-adjusted assessment results, and places results of clinical trials at the top of the classification scheme.
2. Alignment of the AI target with the desired clinical state. For example, simply demonstrating a high level of predictive accuracy may not ensure improved clinical outcomes if effective interventions are lacking, or if the algorithm is predicting a change in the requirements of a process or workflow that may not have a direct link to downstream outcome achievements. Thus, it is critically important to define prediction–action pairs. Actions should generally not be merely improvements in information knowledge but should be defined by specific interventions that have been shown to improve outcomes.

Given the novelty of AI, the limited evidence of its successful use to date, the limited regulatory frameworks around it, and that most AI tools depend on nuances of local data—and the clinical workflows that generate these data—ongoing monitoring of AI as it is deployed in health care is critical for ensuring its safe and effective use. The basis for ongoing evaluation should be on prediction–action pairs, as discussed earlier in this chapter, and should involve assessment of factors such as

- how often the AI tool is accessed and used in the process of care;
- how often recommendations are accepted and the frequency of overrides (with reasons if available);
- in settings where the data leave the EHR, logs of data access, application programming interface (API) calls, and privacy changes;
- measures of clinical safety and benefit, optimally in the form of agreed-upon outcome or process measures;
- organizational metrics relevant to workflow or back-office AI;
- user-reported issues, such as perceived inaccurate recommendations, untimely or misdirected prompts, or undue distractions;
- records of ongoing maintenance work (e.g., data revision requests); and
- model performance against historical data (e.g., loss of model power due to changes in documentation).

Clinical Outcome Monitoring

The complexity and extent of local evaluation and monitoring may necessarily vary depending on the way AI tools are deployed into the clinical workflow, the clinical situation, and the type of CDS being delivered, as these will in turn define the clinical risk attributable to the AI tool.

The International Medical Device Regulators Forum (IMDRF) framework for assessing risk of SaMD is a potentially useful approach to developing SaMD evaluation monitoring strategies tailored to the level of potential risk posed by the clinical situation where the SaMD is employed. Although the IMRDF framework is currently used to identify SaMD that require regulation, its conceptual model is one that might be helpful in identifying the need for evaluating and monitoring AI tools, both in terms of local governance and larger studies. The IMDRF framework focuses on the clinical acuity of the location of care (e.g., intensive care unit versus general preventive care setting), type of decision being suggested (immediately life-threatening versus clinical reminder), and type of decision support being provided (e.g., interruptive alert versus invisible "nudge"). In general, the potential need for evaluation rises in concert with the clinical setting and decision acuity, and as the visibility of the CDS falls (and the opportunity for providers to identify and catch mistakes becomes lower).

For higher risk AI tools, a focus on clinical safety and effectiveness—from either a noninferiority or superiority perspective—is of paramount importance even as other metrics (e.g., API data calls, user experience information) are considered. High-risk tools will likely require evidence from rigorous studies for regulatory purposes and will certainly require substantial monitoring at the time of and following implementation. For low-risk clinical AI tools used at point of care, or those that focus on administrative tasks, evaluation may rightly focus on process-of-care measures and metrics related to the AI's usage in practice to define its positive and negative effects. We strongly endorse implementing all AI tools using experimental methods (e.g., randomized controlled trials or A/B testing) where possible. Large-scale pragmatic trials at multiple sites will be critical for the field to grow but may be less necessary for local monitoring and for management of an AI formulary. In some instances, due to feasibility, costs, time constraints, or other limitations, a randomized trial may not be practical or feasible. In these circumstances, quasi-experimental approaches such as stepped-wedge designs or even carefully adjusted retrospective cohort studies may provide valuable insights. Monitoring outcomes after implementation will permit careful assessment, in the same manner that systems regularly examine drug usage or order sets and may be able to utilize data that are innately collected by the AI tool itself to provide a monitoring platform. Recent work has revealed that naive evaluation of AI system performance may be overly optimistic, providing a need for more thorough evaluation and validation.

In one such study (Zech et al., 2018), researchers evaluated the ability of a clinical AI application that relied on imaging data to generalize across hospitals. Specifically, they trained a neural network to diagnose pneumonia from patient radiographs in one hospital system and evaluated its diagnostic ability on external radiographs from different hospital systems, with their results showing that performance on external datasets was significantly degraded. The AI application was unable to generalize across hospitals due to differences between the training data and evaluation data, a well-known but often ignored problem termed dataset shift (Quiñonero-Candela et al., 2009; Saria and Subbaswamy, 2019). In this instance, Zech and colleagues (2018) showed that large differences in the prevalence of pneumonia between populations caused performance to suffer. However, even subtle differences between populations can result in significant performance changes (Saria and Subbaswamy, 2019). In the case of radiographs, differences between scanner manufacturers or type of scanner (e.g., portable versus nonportable) result in systematic differences in radiographs (e.g., inverted color schemes or inlaid text on the image). Thus, in the training process, an AI system can be trained to very accurately determine which hospital system (and even which department within the system) a particular radiograph came from (Zech et al., 2018) and to use that information in making its prediction, rather than using more generalizable patient-based data.

Clinical AI performance can also deteriorate within a site when practices, patterns, or demographics change over time. As an example, consider the policy by which physicians order blood lactate measurements. Historically, it may have been the case that, at a particular hospital, lactate measurements were only ordered to confirm suspicion of sepsis. A clinical AI tool for predicting sepsis that was trained using historical data from this hospital would be vulnerable to learning that the act of ordering a lactate measurement is associated with sepsis rather than the elevated value of the lactate. However, if hospital policies change and lactate measurements are more commonly ordered, then the association that had been learned by the clinical AI would no longer be accurate. Alternatively, if the patient population shifts, for example, to include more drug users, then elevated lactate might become more common and the value of lactate being measured would again be diminished. In both the case of changing policy and of patient population, performance of the clinical AI application is likely to deteriorate, resulting in an increase of false-positive sepsis alerts.

More broadly, such examples illustrate the importance of careful validation in evaluating the reliability of clinical AI. A key means for measuring reliability is through validation on multiple datasets. Classical algorithms that are applied natively or used for training AI are prone to learning artifacts specific to the site that produced the training data or specific to the training dataset itself. There are many subtle ways that site-specific or dataset-specific bias can occur in real-world datasets. Validation using external datasets will show reduced performance for models that have learned patterns that do not generalize across sites (Schulam and Saria, 2017). Other factors that could influence AI prediction might include insurance coverage, discriminatory practices, or resource constraints. Overall, when there are varying, imprecise measurements or classifications of outcomes (i.e., labeling cases and controls), machine learning methods may exhibit what is known as causality leakage (Bramley, 2017) and label leakage (Ghassemi et al., 2018). An example of causality leakage in a clinical setting would be when a clinician suspects a problem and orders a test, and the AI uses the test itself to generate an alert, which then causes an action. Label leakage is when information about a targeted task outcome leaks back into the features used to generate the model.

While external validation can reveal potential reliability issues related to clinical AI performance, external validation is reactive in nature because differences between training and evaluation environments are found after the fact due to degraded performance. It is more desirable to detect and prevent problems proactively to avoid failures prior to or during training. Recent work in this direction has produced proactive learning methods that train clinical AI applications to make predictions that are invariant to anticipated shifts in populations or datasets (Schulam and Saria, 2017). For example, in the lactate example, above, the clinical AI application can learn a predictive algorithm that is immune to shifts in practice patterns (Saria and Subbaswamy, 2019). Doing so requires adjusting for confounding, which is only sometimes possible, for instance, when the data meet certain quality requirements. When they can be anticipated, these shifts can be prespecified by model developers and included in documentation associated with the application. By refraining from incorporating learning predictive relationships that are likely to change, performance is more likely to remain robust when deployed at new hospitals or under new policy regimes. Beyond proactive learning, these methods also provide a means for understanding susceptibility to shifts for a given clinical AI model (Subbaswamy and Saria, 2018; Subbaswamy et al., 2019). Such tools have the potential to prevent failures if implemented during the initial phase of approval.

In addition to monitoring overall measures of performance, evaluating performance on key patient subgroups can further expose areas of model vulnerability: High average performance overall is not indicative of high performance across every relevant subpopulation. Careful examination of stratified performance can help expose subpopulations where the clinical AI model performs poorly and therefore poses higher risk. Furthermore, tools that detect individual points where the clinical AI is likely to be uncertain or unreliable can flag anomalous cases. By introducing a manual audit for these individual points, one can improve reliability during use (e.g., Schulam and Saria, 2019; Soleimani et al., 2018). Traditionally, uncertainty assessment was limited to the use of specific classes of algorithms for model development. However, recent approaches have led to wrapper tools that can audit some black box models (Schulam and Saria, 2019). Logging cases flagged as anomalous or unreliable and performing a review of such cases from time to time may be another way to bolster postmarketing surveillance, and FDA requirements for such surveillance could require such techniques.

AI Model Maintenance

As discussed above, there is a large body of work indicating that model performance—whether AI or traditional models—degrades when models are applied to another health care system with systematic differences from the system where it was derived (Koola et al., 2019). Deterioration of model performance can also occur within the same health care system over time, as clinical care environments evolve due to changes in background characteristics of the patients being treated, overall population rates of exposures and outcomes of interest, and clinical practice as new evidence is generated (Davis et al., 2017; Steyerberg et al., 2013). In addition, systematic data shifts can occur if the implementation of AI itself changes clinical care (Lenert et al., 2019).

There are a number of approaches used to account for systematic changes in source data use by AI applications that have largely been adapted from more traditional statistical methods applied to risk models (Moons et al., 2012). These methods range from completely regenerating models on a periodic basis to recalibrating models using a variety of increasingly complex methods. However, there are evolving areas of research into how frequently to update, what volume and types of data are necessary for robust performance maintenance, and how to scale these surveillance and updating activities across what is anticipated to be a high volume of algorithms and models in clinical practice (Davis et al., 2019; Moons et al., 2012). Some of the risks are analogous to those of systems in which Boolean rule–based CDS tools were successfully implemented, but the continual addition of reminders and CDS in an EHR based on guidelines becomes unsustainable (Singh et al., 2013). Without automation and the appropriate scaling and standardization of knowledge, management systems for these types of CDS will face severe challenges.

AI AND INTERPRETABILITY

A lack of transparency and interpretability in AI-derived recommendations is one issue that has received considerable visibility and has often been cited as a limitation for use of AI in clinical applications. Lack of insight into methods and data employed to develop and operate AI models tends to provoke clinicians' questions about the clinical plausibility of the tools, the extent to which the tools can provide clinical justification and reassurance to the patient and provider making care decisions, and potential liability, including implications for insurance coverage. In addition, there is a tendency to question whether observed associations utilized within the model can be used to identify specific clinical or system-level actions that should be taken, or whether they can reveal novel and unsuspected underlying pathophysiologies. These issues are particularly complex as they relate to risk prediction models that can readily be validated in terms of predictive accuracy but for which the inclusion of data elements may not be based on biological relationships.

Requirements for interpretability are likely to be determined by a number of factors, including

- medical liability and federal guidelines and recommendations for how AI is to be used in health care;
- the medical profession's and the public's increasing trust in their reliance on AI to manage clinical information;
- AI tools' effect on current human interactions and design, which may be prepared for to some extent through advance planning for appropriate adoption and implementation into current workflows (Dudding et al., 2018; Hatch et al., 2018; Lynch et al., 2019; Wachter, 2015); and
- Expectations of the general public regarding the safety and efficacy of these systems.

One area of active innovation is the synthesis and display of where and how AI outputs are presented to the end user, in many cases to assist in interpretability. Innovations include establishing new methods, such as parallel models where one is used for core computation and the other for interpretation (Hara and Hayashi, 2018; Krause et al., 2016; Turner, 2016). Others utilize novel graphical displays and data discovery tools that sit alongside the AI to educate and help users in health care settings as they become comfortable using the recommendations.

There remains a paradox, however, because machine learning produces algorithms based upon features that may not be readily interpretable. In the absence of absolute transparency, stringent standards for performance must be monitored and ensured. We may not understand all of the components upon which an algorithm is based, but if the resulting recommendations are highly accurate, and if surveillance of the performance of the AI system over time is maintained, then we might continue to trust it to perform the assigned task. A burgeoning number of applications for AI in the health care system do not assess end users' needs for the level of interpretability. Although the most stringent criteria for transparency are within the point-of-care setting, there are likely circumstances under which accuracy may be desired over transparency. Regardless of the level of interpretability of the outputs of the AI algorithms, considerations for users' requirements should be addressed during development. With this in mind, there are a few key factors related to the use and adoption of AI tools that are algorithmically nontransparent but worthy of consideration by clinicians and health care delivery systems.

Although the need for algorithm transparency at a granular level is probably overstated, descriptors of how data were collected and aggregated are essential, comparable to the inclusion/exclusion criteria of a clinical trial. For models that seek to produce predictions only (i.e., suggest an association between observable data and an outcome), at a minimum we believe that it is important to know the populations for which AI is not applicable. This will make informed decisions about the likely accuracy of use in specific situations possible and help implementers avoid introducing systematic errors related to patient socioeconomic or documentation biases. For example, implementers might consider whether the data were collected in a system similar to their own. The generalizability of data sources is a particularly important consideration when evaluating the suitability of an AI tool, because those that use data or algorithms that have been derived outside the target environment are likely to be misapplied. This applies to potential generalizability limitations among models derived from patient data within one part of a health system and then spread to other parts of that system.

For models that seek to suggest therapeutic targets or treatments—and thus imply a causal link or pathway—a higher level of scrutiny of the data assumptions and model approaches should be required. Closer examination is required because these results are apt to be biased by the socioeconomic and system-related factors mentioned above as well as by well-described issues such as allocation and treatment biases, immortal time biases, and documentation biases. At present, AI tools are incapable of accounting for these biases in an unsupervised fashion. Therefore, for the foreseeable future, this class of AI tools will require robust, prospective study before deployment locally and may require repeated recalibrations and reevaluation when expanded outside their original setting.

Risk of a Digital Divide

It should be evident from this chapter that in this early phase of AI development, adopting this technology requires substantial resources. Because of this barrier, only well-resourced institutions may have access to AI tools and systems, while institutions that serve less affluent and disadvantaged individuals will be forced to forgo the technology. Early on, when clinical AI remains in rudimentary stages, this may not be terribly disadvantageous. However, as the technology improves, the digital divide may widen the significant disparities that already exist between institutions. This would be ironic because AI tools have the potential to improve quality and efficiency where the need is greatest. An additional potential risk is that AI technology may be developed in environments that exclude patients of different socioeconomic, cultural, and ethnic backgrounds, leading to poorer performance in some groups. Early in the process of AI development, it is critical that we ensure that this technology is derived from data gathered from diverse populations and that it be made available to affluent and disadvantaged individuals as it matures.

KEY CONSIDERATIONS

As clinical AI applications become increasingly available, marketing of these tools is apt to intensify and be accompanied by claims regarding improved clinical outcomes or improved efficiency of care, which may or may not be well founded. Health care delivery systems and hospitals will need to take a thoughtful approach in the evaluation, decision making, and adoption of these tools that incorporates considerations regarding organizational governance and postdevelopment technical issues (i.e., maintenance of systems) as well as clinical considerations that are all essential to successful implementation.

Effective IT governance is essential for successful deployment of AI applications. Health systems must create or adapt their general IT governance structures to manage AI implementation.

- The clinical and administrative leadership of health care systems, with input from all relevant stakeholders such as patients, end users, and the general public, must define the near- and far-term states that would be required to measurably improve workflow or clinical outcomes. If these target states are clearly defined, AI is likely to positively affect the health care system through efficient integration into the EHR, population health programs, and ancillary and allied health workflows.

- Before deploying AI, health systems should assess through stakeholder and user engagement, especially patients, consumers, and the general public, the degree to which transparency is required for AI to operate in a particular use case. This includes determining cultural resistance and workflow limitations that may dictate key interpretability and actionability requirements for successful deployment.

- Through IT governance, health systems should establish standard processes for the surveillance and maintenance of AI applications' performance and, if at all possible, automate those processes to enable the scalable addition of AI tools for a variety of use cases.

- IT governance should engage health care system leadership, end users, and target patients to establish a value statement for AI applications. This will include analyses to ascertain the potential cost savings and/or clinical outcome gains from implementation of AI.

- AI development and implementation should follow established best-practice frameworks in implementation science and software development.

- Because it remains in early developmental stages, health systems should maintain a healthy skepticism about the advertised benefits of AI. Systems that do not possess strong research and advanced IT capabilities should likely not be early adopters of this technology.
- Health care delivery systems should strive to adopt and deploy AI applications in the context of a learning health system.
- Efforts to avoid introducing social bias in the development and use of AI applications are critical.

REFERENCES

Abdi, J., A. Al-Hindawi, T. Ng, and M. P. Vizcaychipi. 2018. Scoping review on the use of socially assistive robot technology in elderly care. *BMJ Open* 8(2):e018815.

Bandos, A. I., H. E. Rockette, T. Song, and D. Gur. 2009. Area under the free-response ROC curve (FROC) and a related summary index. *Biometrics* 65(1):247–256.

Bates, D. W. 2012. Clinical decision support and the law: The big picture. *Saint Louis University Journal of Health Law & Policy* 5(2):319–324.

Blane, D., E. Brunner, and R. Wilkinson. 2002. *Health and social organization: Towards a health policy for the 21st century.* New York: Routledge.

Braithwaite, J. 2018. Changing how we think about healthcare improvement. *BMJ* 361:k2014.

Bramley, N. R. 2017. *Constructing the world: Active causal learning in cognition.* Ph.D. thesis, University College London. http://discovery.ucl.ac.uk/1540252/9/Bramley_neil_phd_thesis.pdf (accessed November 13, 2019).

Byambasuren, O., S. Sanders, E. Beller, and P. Glasziou. 2018. Prescribable mHealth apps identified from an overview of systematic reviews. *NPI Digital Medicine* 1(1):Art. 12.

Christodoulou, E., J. Ma, G. S. Collins, E. W. Steyerberg, J. Y. Verbakel, and B. A. Van Calster. 2019. Systematic review shows no performance benefit of machine learning over logistic regression for clinical prediction models. *Journal of Clinical Epidemiology* 110:12–22.

CMS (Centers for Medicare & Medicaid Services). 2019. *Proposed policy, payment, and quality provisions changes to the Medicare physician fee schedule for calendar year 2019.* https://www.cms.gov/newsroom/fact-sheets/proposed-policy-payment-and-quality-provisions-changes-medicare-physician-fee-schedule-calendar-year-3 (accessed November 13, 2019).

Damschroder, L. J., D. C. Aron, R. E. Keith, S. R. Kirsh, J. A. Alexander, and J. C. Lowery. 2009. Fostering implementation of health services research findings into practice: A consolidated framework for advancing implementation science. *Implementation Science* 4(1):50.

Davis, S. E., T. A. Lasko, G. Chen, E. D. Siew, and M. E. Matheny. 2017. Calibration drift in regression and machine learning models for acute kidney injury. *Journal of the American Medical Informatics Association* 24(6):1052–1061.

Davis, S. E., R. A. Greevy, C. Fonnesbeck, T. A. Lasko, C. G. Walsh, and M. E. Matheny. 2019. A nonparametric updating method to correct clinical prediction model drift. *Journal of the American Medical Informatics Association* 26(12):1448–1457. https://doi.org/10.1093/jamia/ocz127.

Deming, W. E. 2000. *The new economics for industry, government, and education.* Cambridge, MA: MIT Press. http://www.ihi.org/resources/Pages/Publications/NewEconomicsforIndustryGovernmentEducation.aspx (accessed November 13, 2019).

Dudding, K. M., S. M. Gephart, and J. M. Carrington. 2018. Neonatal nurses experience unintended consequences and risks to patient safety with electronic health records. *Computers, Informatics, Nursing* 36(4):167–176.

Elstein A. S., L. S. Shulman, and S. A. Sprafka. 1978. *Medical problem solving: An analysis of clinical reasoning.* Boston, MA: Harvard University Press.

Faden, R. R., N. E. Kass, S. N. Goodman, P. Pronovost, S. Tunis, and T. L. Beauchamp. 2013. *An ethics framework for a learning health care system: a departure from traditional research ethics and clinical ethics.* Hastings Center Report; Spec No. S16–S27.

FDA (U.S. Food and Drug Administration). 2018. *Digital Health Software Precertification (Pre-Cert) program.* https://www.fda.gov/medical-devices/digital-health/digital-health-software-precertification-pre-cert-program (accessed November 13, 2019).

Florentine, S. 2016. More than half of IT projects still failing. *CIO.* https://www.cio.com/article/3068502/more-than-half-of-it-projects-still-failing.html (accessed November 13, 2019).

Friedman, C. P., N. J. Allee, B. C. Delaney, A. J. Flynn, J. C. Silverstein, K. Sullivan, and K. A. Young. 2017. The science of learning health systems: Foundations for a new journal. *Learning Health Systems* 1(1):e10020. https://doi.org/10.1002/lrh2.10020.

Ghassemi, M., T. Naumann, P. Schulam, A. L. Beam, and R. Ranganath. 2018. Opportunities in machine learning for healthcare. *arXiv.org.* https://arxiv.org/abs/1806.00388 (accessed November 13, 2019).

Goldstein, M. K., B. B. Hoffman, R. W. Coleman, M. A. Musen, S. W. Tu, A. Advani, R. Shankar, and M. O'Connor. 2000. Implementing clinical practice guidelines while taking account of changing evidence: ATHENA

DSS, an easily modifiable decision-support system for managing hypertension in primary care. In *Proceedings of the AMIA Symposium*. Pp. 300–304.

Hara, S., and K. Hayashi. 2018. Making tree ensembles interpretable: A Bayesian model selection approach. *Proceedings of the Twenty-First International Conference on Artificial Intelligence and Statistics* 84:77–85. http://proceedings.mlr.press/v84/hara18a.html (accessed November 13, 2019).

Hatch, A., J. E. Hoffman, R. Ross, and J. P. Docherty. 2018. Expert consensus survey on digital health tools for patients with serious mental illness: Optimizing for user characteristics and user support. *JMIR Mental Health* 5(2):e46.

He, J., S. L. Baxter, J. Xu, J. Xu, X. Zhou, and K. Zhang. 2019. The practical implementation of artificial intelligence technologies in medicine. *Nature Medicine* 25(1):30.

Helfrich, C. D., Y. F. Li, N. D. Sharp, and A. E. Sales. 2009. Organizational Readiness to Change Assessment (ORCA): Development of an instrument based on the Promoting Action on Research in Health Services (PARIHS) framework. *Implementation Science* 4(1):38.

Herrett, E., E. Wiliamson, T. van Staa, M. Ranopa, C. Free, T. Chadborn, B. Goldacre, and L. Smeeth. 2016. Text messaging reminders for influenza vaccine in primary care: A cluster randomised controlled trial (TXT4FLUJAB). *BMJ Open* 6(2):e010069.

IOM (Institute of Medicine). 2011. *Digital infrastructure for the learning health system: The foundation for continuous improvement in health and health care: Workshop series summary*. Washington, DC: The National Academies Press. https://doi.org/10.17226/12912.

IOM. 2013. *Best care at lower cost: The path to continuously learning health care in America*. Washington, DC: The National Academies Press. https://doi.org/10.17226/13444.

Islam, M. M., T. Nasrin, B. A. Walther, C. C. Wu, H. C. Yang, and Y. C. Li. 2019. Prediction of sepsis patients using machine learning approach: A meta-analysis. *Computer Methods and Programs in Biomedicine* 170:1–9.

Kansagara, D., H. Englander, A. Salanitro, D. Kagen, C. Theobald, M. Freeman, and S. Kripalani. 2011. Risk prediction models for hospital readmission: A systematic review. *JAMA* 306(15):1688–1698.

Kilsdonk, E., L. W. Peute, R. J. Riezebos, L. C. Kremer, and M. W. Jaspers. 2016. Uncovering healthcare practitioners' information processing using the think-aloud method: From paper-based guideline to clinical decision support system. *International Journal of Medical Informatics* 86:10–19. https://doi.org/10.1016/j.ijmedinf.2015.11.011.

Kindig, D. A. 2007. Understanding population health terminology. *Milbank Quarterly* 85(1):139–161.

Kindig, D., and G. Stoddart. 2003. What is population health? *American Journal of Public Health* 93(3):380–323.

Koola, J. D., S. B. Ho, A. Cao, G. Chen, A. M. Perkins, S. E. Davis, and M. E. Matheny. 2019. Predicting 30-day hospital readmission risk in a national cohort of patients with cirrhosis. *Digestive Diseases and Sciences*. https://doi.org/10.1007/s10620-019-05826-w.

Kraft, S. A., M. K. Cho, K. Gillespie, M. Halley, N. Varsava, K. E. Ormond, H. S. Luft, B. S. Wilfond, and S. Soo-Jin Lee. 2018. Beyond consent: Building trusting relationships with diverse populations in precision medicine research. *American Journal of Bioethics* 18:3–20.

Krause, J., A. Perer, and E. Bertini. 2016. Using visual analytics to interpret predictive machine learning models. *arXiv.org*. https://arxiv.org/abs/1606.05685 (accessed November 13, 2019).

Kull, M., T. M. S. Filho, and P. Flach. 2017. Beyond sigmoids: How to obtain well-calibrated probabilities from binary classifiers with beta calibration. *Electronic Journal of Statistics* 11:5052–5080. https://doi.org/10.1214/17-EJS1338SI.

Lee, K. J. 2018. AI device for detecting diabetic retinopathy earns swift FDA approval. *American Academy of Ophthalmology ONE Network*. https://www.aao.org/headline/first-ai-screen-diabetic-retinopathy-approved-by-f (accessed November 13, 2019).

Lee, T. T., and A. S. Kesselheim. 2018. U.S. Food and Drug Administration precertification pilot program for digital health software: Weighing the benefits and risks. *Annals of Internal Medicine* 168(10):730–732. https://doi.org/10.7326/M17-2715.

Légaré, F., R. Adekpedjou, D. Stacey, S. Turcotte, J. Kryworuchko, I. D. Graham, A. Lyddiatt, M. C. Politi, R. Thomson, G. Elwyn, and N. Donner-Banzhoff. 2018. Interventions for increasing the use of shared decision making by healthcare professionals. *Cochrane Database of Systematic Reviews*. https://doi.org/10.1002/14651858.CD006732.pub4.

Lenert, M. C., M. E. Matheny, and C. G. Walsh. 2019. Prognostic models will be victims of their own success, unless. . . . *Journal of the American Medical Informatics Association* 26(10). https://doi.org/10.1093/jamia/ocz145.

Li, P., S. N. Yates, J. K. Lovely, and D. W. Larson. 2015. Patient-like-mine: A real time, visual analytics tool for clinical decision support. In *2015 IEEE International Conference on Big Data*. Pp. 2865–2867.

Liquid State. 2018. *4 digital health app trends to consider for 2018*. https://liquid-state.com/digital-health-app-trends-2018 (accessed November 13, 2019).

Loria, K. 2019. Are health apps putting your privacy at risk? *Consumer Reports*. https://www.consumerreports.org/health-privacy/are-health-apps-putting-your-privacy-at-risk (accessed November 13, 2019).

Lynch, J. K., J. Glasby, and S. Robinson. 2019. If telecare is the answer, what was the question? Storylines, tensions and the unintended consequences of technology-supported care. *Critical Social Policy* 39(1):44–65.

Marx, V. 2015. Human phenotyping on a population scale. *Nature Methods* 12:711–714.

McGinnis, J. M., P. Williams-Russo, and J. R. Knickman. 2002. The case for more active policy attention to health promotion. *Health Affairs* 21(2):78–93.

Miller, A., J. D. Koola, M. E. Matheny, J. H. Ducom, J. M. Slagle, E. J. Groessl, F. F. Minter, J. H. Garvin, M. B. Weinger, and S. B. Ho. 2018. Application of contextual design methods to inform targeted clinical decision support interventions in sub-specialty care environments. *International Journal of Medical Informatics* 117:55–65.

Monegain, B. 2017. Partners HealthCare launches 10-year project to boost AI use. *Healthcare IT News.* https://www.healthcareitnews.com/news/partners-healthcare-launches-10-year-project-boost-ai-use (accessed November 13, 2019).

Moons, K. G., A. P. Kengne, D. E. Grobbee, P. Royston, Y. Vergouwe, D. G. Altman, and M. Woodward. 2012. Risk prediction models: II. External validation, model updating, and impact assessment. *Heart* 98(9):691–698.

Morain, S. R., N. E. Kass, and R. R. Faden. 2018. Learning is not enough: Earning institutional trustworthiness through knowledge translation. *American Journal of Bioethics* 18:31–34.

Muller, J. Z. 2018. *The tyranny of metrics.* Princeton, NJ: Princeton University Press.

Nelson, E. C., P. B. Batalden, and M. M. Godfrey. 2011. *Quality by design: A clinical microsystems approach.* San Francisco, CA: John Wiley & Sons.

Nelson, K. M., E. T. Chang, D. M. Zulman, L. V. Rubenstein, F. D. Kirkland, and S. D. Fihn. 2019. Using predictive analytics to guide patient care and research in a national health system. *Journal of General Internal Medicine* 34(8):1379–1380.

Network for Excellence in Health Innovation. 2015. *Healthy People/Healthy Economy: An initiative to make Massachusetts the national leader in health and wellness.* https://www.nehi.net/publications/65-healthy-people-healthy-economy-a-five-year-review-and-five-priorities-for-the-future/view (accessed November 13, 2019).

Object Management Group. *Case management model and notation, v1.1.* https://www.omg.org/cmmn/index.htm (accessed November 13, 2019).

Palmer, A. 2018. IBM's Watson AI suggested "often inaccurate" and "unsafe" treatment recommendations for cancer patients, internal documents show. *DailyMail.com.* https://www.dailymail.co.uk/sciencetech/article-6001141/IBMs-Watson-suggested-inaccurate-unsafe-treatment-recommendations-cancer-patients.html?ito=email_share_article-top (accessed November 13, 2019).

Papež, V., S. Denaxas, and H. Hemingway. 2017. Evaluation of semantic web technologies for storing computable definitions of electronic health records phenotyping algorithms. In *AMIA Annual Symposium Proceedings*. Pp. 1352–1362.

Parma, A. 2018. Venrock VCs on AI potential: Focus on back office and not on what doctors do. *MedCity News*. https://medcitynews.com/2018/01/venrock-vcs-ai-potential-focus-back-office-not-doctors (accessed November 13, 2019).

Pesapane, F., M. Codari, and F. Sardanelli. 2018. Artificial intelligence in medical imaging: Threat or opportunity? Radiologists again at the forefront of innovation in medicine. *European Radiology Experimental* 2(1):35.

Phansalkar, S., J. Edworthy, E. Hellier, D. L. Seger, A. Schedlbauer, A. J. Avery, and D. W. Bates. 2010. A review of human factors principles for the design and implementation of medication safety alerts in clinical information systems. *Journal of the American Medical Informatics Association* 17(5):493–501. https://doi.org/10.1136/jamia.2010.005264.

Quiñonero-Candela, J., M. Sugiyama, A. Schwaighofer, and N. D. Lawrence. 2009. *Dataset shift in machine learning*. Cambridge, MA: MIT Press. http://www.acad.bg/ebook/ml/The.MIT.Press.Dataset.Shift.in.Machine.Learning.Feb.2009.eBook-DDU.pdf (accessed November 13, 2019).

Reed, M. E., J. Huang, A. Millman, I. Graetz, J. Hsu, R. Brand, D. W. Ballard, and R. Grant. 2019. Portal use among patients with chronic conditions: Patient-reported care experiences. *Medical Care* 57(10):809–814.

Rumsfeld, J. S., K. E. Joynt, and T. M. Maddox. 2016. Big data analytics to improve cardiovascular care: Promise and challenges. *Nature Reviews Cardiology* 13(6):350–359.

Rycroft-Malone, J. 2004. The PARIHS framework—A framework for guiding the implementation of evidence-based practice. *Journal of Nursing Care Quality* 19(4):297–304.

Saria, S., and A. Subbaswamy. 2019. Tutorial: Safe and reliable machine learning. *arXiv.org*. https://arxiv.org/abs/1904.07204 (accessed November 13, 2019).

Schulam, P., and S. Saria. 2017. Reliable decision support using counterfactual models. In *Advances in Neural Information Processing Systems 30* (NIPS 2017). Pp. 1697–1708. https://papers.nips.cc/paper/6767-reliable-decision-support-using-counterfactual-models.pdf (accessed November 13, 2019).

Schulam, P., and S. Saria. 2019. Can you trust this prediction? Auditing pointwise reliability after learning. In *Proceedings of the 22nd International Conference on Artificial Intelligence and Statistics*. Pp. 1022–1031. http://proceedings.mlr.press/v89/schulam19a/schulam19a.pdf (accessed November 13, 2019).

Schwebel, F. J., and M. E. Larimer. 2018. Using text message reminders in health care services: A narrative literature review. *Internet Interventions* 13:82–104.

Sepah, S. C., L. Jiang, R. J. Ellis, K. McDermott, and A. L. Peters. 2017. Engagement and outcomes in a digital Diabetes Prevention Program: 3-year update. *BMJ Open Diabetes Research and Care* 5(1):e000422.

Shanafelt, T. D., S. Boon, L. Tan, L. N. Dyrbye, W. Sotile, D. Satele, C. P. West, J. Sloan, and M. R. Oreskovich. 2012. Burnout and satisfaction with work-life balance among US physicians relative to the general US population. *Archives of Internal Medicine* 172(18):1377–1385.

Shortliffe, E. H., and M. J. Sepúlveda. 2018. Clinical decision support in the era of artificial intelligence. *JAMA* 320(21):2199–2200. https://doi.org/10.1001/jama.2018.17163.

Singh, H., C. Spitzmueller, N. J. Petersen, M. K. Sawhney, and D. F. Sittig. 2013. Information overload and missed test results in electronic health record–based settings. *JAMA Internal Medicine* 173(8):702–704. https://doi.org/10.1001/2013.

Sinsky, C., L. Colligan, L. Li, M. Prgomet, S. Reynolds, L. Goeders, J. Westbrook, M. Tutty, and G. Blike. 2016. Allocation of physician time in ambulatory practice: A time and motion study in 4 specialties. *Annals of Internal Medicine* 165:753–760.

Smith, L. N., A. N. Makam, D. Darden, H. Mayo, S. R. Das, E. A. Halm, and O. K. Nguyen. 2018. Acute myocardial infarction readmission risk prediction models: A systematic review of model performance. *Circulation: Cardiovascular Quality and Outcomes* 11(1):e003885.

Smith, M. E., J. C. Chiovaro, M. O'Neil, D. Kansagara, A. R. Quiñones, M. Freeman, M. L. Motu'apuaka, and C. G. Slatore. 2014. Early warning system scores for clinical deterioration in hospitalized patients: A systematic review. *Annals of the American Thoracic Society* 11(9):1454–1465.

Soleimani, H., J. Hensman, and S. Saria. 2018. Scalable joint models for reliable uncertainty-aware event prediction. *IEEE Transactions on Pattern Analysis and Machine Intelligence* 40(8):1948–1963.

Steele, A. J., S. C. Denaxas, A. D. Shah, H. Hemingway, and N. M. Luscombe. 2018. Machine learning models in electronic health records can outperform conventional survival models for predicting patient mortality in coronary artery disease. *PLoS One* 13(8):e0202344.

Steyerberg, E. W., K. G. Moons, D. A. van der Windt, J. A. Hayden, P. Perel, S. Schroter, R. D. Riley, H. Hemingway, D. G. Altman, and PROGRESS Group. 2013. Prognosis Research Strategy (PROGRESS) 3: Prognostic model research. *PLoS Medicine* 10(2):e1001381.

Storm, D. 2015. ACLU: Orwellian Citizen Score, China's credit score system, is a warning for Americans. *ComputerWorld*. https://www.computerworld.com/article/2990203/aclu-orwellian-citizen-score-chinas-credit-score-system-is-a-warning-for-americans.html (accessed November 13, 2019).

Subbaswamy, A., and S. Saria. 2018. Counterfactual normalization: Proactively addressing dataset shift and improving reliability using causal mechanisms. *arXiv.org*. https://arxiv.org/abs/1808.03253 (accessed November 13, 2019).

Subbaswamy, A., P. Schulam, and S. Saria. 2019. Preventing failures due to dataset shift: Learning predictive models that transport. In *Proceedings of the 22nd International Conference on Artificial Intelligence and Statistics*. Pp. 3118–3127. https://arxiv.org/abs/1812.04597 (accessed November 13, 2019).

Tarlov, A. R. 2002. *Social determinants of health: The sociobiological translation. Health and social organization: Towards a health policy for the 21st century*. New York: Routledge.

Tawfik, D. S., J. Profit, T. I. Morgenthaler, D. V. Satele, C. A. Sinsky, L. N. Dyrbye, M. A. Tutty, C. P. West, and T. D. Shanafelt. 2018. Physician burnout, well-being, and work unit safety grades in relationship to reported medical errors. *Mayo Clinic Proceedings* 93(11):1571–1580. https://doi.org/10.1016/j.mayocp.2018.05.014.

Tcheng, J. E., S. Bakken, D. W. Bates, H. Bonner III, T. K. Gandhi, M. Josephs, K. Kawamoto, E. A. Lomotan, E. Mackay, B. Middleton, J. M. Teich, S. Weingarten, and M. Hamilton Lopez, eds. 2017. *Optimizing strategies for clinical decision support: Summary of a meeting series*. Washington, DC: National Academy of Medicine.

Topol, E. 2015. *The patient will see you now: The future of medicine is in your hands*. New York: Basic Books.

Topol, E. J. 2019. High-performance medicine: The convergence of human and artificial intelligence. *Nature Medicine* 25(1):44–56.

Turner, R. 2016. A model explanation system: Latest updates and extensions. *arXiv.org*. https://arxiv. org/abs/1606.09517 (accessed November 13, 2019).

Unertl, K. M., M. Weinger, and K. Johnson. 2007. Variation in use of informatics tools among providers in a diabetes clinic. In *AMIA Annual Symposium Proceedings*. Pp. 756–760.

Unertl, K. M., M. B. Weinger, K. B. Johnson, and N. M. Lorenzi. 2009. Describing and modeling workflow and information flow in chronic disease care. *Journal of the American Medical Informatics Association* 16(6):826–836.

Vashisht, R., K. Jung, A. Schuler, J. M. Banda, R. W. Park, S. Jin, L. Li, J. T. Dudley, K. W. Johnson, M. M. Shervey, and H. Xu. 2018. Association of hemoglobin A1c levels with use of sulfonylureas, dipeptidyl peptidase 4 inhibitors, and thiazolidinediones in patients with type 2 diabetes treated with metformin: Analysis from the Observational Health Data Sciences and Informatics initiative. *JAMA Network Open* 1(4):e181755.

Wachter, R. 2015. *The digital doctor: Hope, hype and harm at the dawn of medicine's computer age*. New York: McGraw-Hill Education.

Wahl, B., A. Cossy-Gantner, S. Germann, and N. R. Schwalbe. 2018. Artificial intelligence (AI) and global Health: How can AI contribute to health in resource-poor settings? *BMJ Global Health* 3:e000798. doi: 10.1136/bmjgh-2018-000798.

Wang, L., B. Porter, C. Maynard, G. Evans, C. Bryson, H. Sun, I. Gupta, E. Lowy, M. McDonell, K. Frisbee, C. Nielson, F. Kirkland, and S. D. Fihn. 2013. Predicting risk of hospitalization or death among patients receiving primary care in the Veterans Health Administration. *Medical Care* 51(4):368–373.

Wicks, P., T. Richards, S. Denegri, and F. Godlee. 2018. Patients' roles and rights in research. *BMJ* 362:k3193.

Xing, Z., F. Yu, Y. A. M. Qanir, T. Guan, J. Walker, and L. Song. 2019. Intelligent conversational agents in patient self-management: a systematic survey using multi data sources. *Studies in Health Technology and Information* 264:1813–1814.

Zech, J. R., M. A. Badgeley, M. Liu, A. B. Costa, J. J. Titano, and E. K. Oermann. 2018. Variable generalization performance of a deep learning model to detect pneumonia in chest radiographs: A cross-sectional study. *PLoS Medicine* 15(11):e1002683.

Zuccotti, G., F. L. Maloney, J. Feblowitz, L. Samal, L. Sato, and A. Wright. 2014. Reducing risk with clinical decision support. *Applied Clinical Informatics* 5(3):746–756.

Suggested citation for Chapter 6: Fihn, S., S. Saria, E. Mendonça, S. Hain, M. Matheny, N. Shah, H. Liu, and A. Auerbach. 2020. Deploying artificial intelligence in clinical settings. In *Artificial intelligence in health care: The hope, the hype, the promise, the peril.* Washington, DC: National Academy of Medicine.

7

HEALTH CARE ARTIFICIAL INTELLIGENCE: LAW, REGULATION, AND POLICY

Douglas McNair, Bill & Melinda Gates Foundation; and
W. Nicholson Price II, University of Michigan Law School

INTRODUCTION

As discussed in previous chapters, artificial intelligence (AI) has the potential to be involved in almost all aspects of the health care industry. The legal landscape for health care AI is complex; AI systems with different intended uses, audiences, and use environments face different requirements at state, federal, and international levels. A full accounting of these legal requirements, or of the policy questions involved, is far beyond the scope of this chapter. Additionally, the legal and regulatory framework for AI in health care continues to evolve, given the nascent stage of the industry.

In this chapter, we offer an overview of the landscape through early April 2019 and undertake three tasks. First, we lay out a broad overview of laws applicable to different forms of health care AI, including federal statutes, federal regulations, and state tort law liability. Second, we address in considerable depth the regulatory requirements imposed on AI systems that help inform or make decisions about individual patients, such as diagnosis or treatment recommendations; these systems are referred to in this report as clinical AI. Clinical AI faces the closest scrutiny, especially by the U.S. Food and Drug Administration (FDA) and by other regulatory agencies internationally. These systems must demonstrate safety and efficacy. They may also generate liability under state tort law, which performs its own regulatory role and is intimately tied to the way FDA oversees clinical AI systems. Third, we note the legal and policy issues around privacy and patient data that affect clinical AI as well as other health care AI systems. Throughout the chapter, we highlight key challenges, opportunities, and gaps in the current framework. The chapter concludes with key considerations for addressing some of these issues.

OVERVIEW OF HEALTH CARE AI LAWS AND REGULATIONS IN THE UNITED STATES

Developers and users of health care AI systems may encounter many different legal regimes, including federal statutes, federal regulations, and state tort law. Below are a few of the most significant among these laws and regulations:

- **Federal Food, Drug, and Cosmetic Act (FDCA):** FDA enforces the FDCA, which regulates the safety and effectiveness of drugs and medical devices, including certain forms of medical software (21 U.S.C. §§ 301 ff.). The bulk of this chapter describes the application of the FDCA to health care clinical AI systems.

- **Health Insurance Portability and Accountability Act (HIPAA):** In addition to the Privacy Rule (described in more detail below), HIPAA authorizes the U.S. Department of Health and Human Services to enforce the Security Rule (45 C.F.R. Parts 160 and 164). These rules create privacy and security requirements for certain health information. The HIPAA Breach Notification Rule also requires certain entities to provide notifications of health information breaches (45 C.F.R. §§ 164.400–164.414). To the extent that the development or use of health care AI systems involves health information covered by HIPAA, those requirements may apply to developers or users of such systems.

- **Common Rule:** The Common Rule sets requirements for research on human subjects that either is federally funded or, in many instances, takes place at institutions that receive any federal research funding (45 C.F.R. Part 46). Among other things, most human subjects research must be reviewed by an institutional review board (45 C.F.R. § 46.109). These requirements can apply to AI used for research or the research used to create health care AI. The Common Rule is enforced by the Office for Human Research Protections.

- **Federal Trade Commission Act (FTCA):** The FTCA prohibits deceptive and unfair trade practices affecting interstate commerce (15 U.S.C. §§ 41–58). These could include acts relating to false and misleading health claims, representations regarding a piece of software's performance, or claims affecting consumer privacy and data security. Health care AI products may raise any of these types of claims. The Federal Trade Commission (FTC) enforces the requirements of the FTCA.

- **FTC Health Breach Notification Rule:** This FTC rule, separate from HIPAA's Breach Notification Rule, requires certain businesses to provide notifications to consumers after a breach of personal health record information, including information that may be collected to train, validate, or use health care AI systems (16 C.F.R. Part 318). The FTC enforces this rule.

- **State tort law:** When one individual or entity injures another, tort law may allow the injured individual to recover damages. Injury could result from the use of health care AI systems, including when the behavior of developers, providers, hospitals, or other health care actors falls below the standard of care. State law determines the applicable standard of care and when tort liability will exist.

We summarize each of these categories of regulatory and legal oversight by application in Table 7-1, referencing the applicable laws and regulations for different types of AI systems. Liability refers to the legal imposition of responsibility for injury through the state tort law system.

TABLE 7-1 | Typical Applicability of Various Laws and Regulations to U.S. Health Care Artificial Intelligence Systems

Clinical Urgency	Type of health care AI system	Description	Common Rule	HIPAA/ Office of Civil Rights	FTC	FDCA	Liability
	Research	AI intended to assist human subjects research	X	X	X		
	Operations	AI that is used to enhance clinical operations, such as patient management, scheduling, and physician documentation		X	X		
	General health and wellness	AI that is used by consumers for entertainment		X	X		
	Clinical: mobile engagement; health and wellness; medical device data systems	AI that is used by consumers for entertainment AI in certain categories for which FDA has announced that it does not intend to enforce FDCA requirements		X	X	X	X
	Direct-to-consumer	AI that is marketed directly to consumers and constitutes a medical device		X	X	X	X
	Clinical: informing clinical management	AI that assists physicians by informing, enhancing, aggregating, and verifying information		X	X	X	X
	Clinical: driving clinical management	AI that assists physicians by giving treatment, diagnosis, or screening advice, while relying on physician interpretation of said advice to direct patient care		X	X	X	X
	Clinical: treating or diagnosing	Autonomous AI that provides treatment or diagnoses, screens, disease without physician inter-pretation		X	X	X	X

SAFETY AND EFFICACY OF CLINICAL SYSTEMS

A key set of laws work to ensure the safety and efficacy of medical technology, including clinical AI systems. The principal requirements are determined by the FDCA and enforced by FDA. State tort law also plays a role in ensuring quality by managing liability for injuries, including those that may arise from insufficient care in developing or using clinical AI.

The raison d'être of clinical AI systems is to be coupled with and to inform human decision making that bears upon the content and conduct of clinical care, including preventive care, to promote favorable, equitable, and inclusive clinical outcomes and/or mitigate risks or interdict adverse events or nonoptimal outcomes. Regulatory authorities in various countries, including FDA, expect the pharmaceutical, medical device, and biotechnology industries to conduct their development of all diagnostics and therapeutics (including companion and complementary diagnostics and therapeutics) toward the goal of safer, more efficacious, and personalized medicine. This development should result in care that is, at a minimum, not inferior to conventional (non–AI-based) standard-of-care outcomes and safety endpoints. Health services are expected to fund such AI-coupled diagnostics and therapeutics, and prescribers and patients are, over time, likely to adopt and accept them. Increased development of "coupled" products (including clinical AI systems) could result in "safer and improved clinical and cost-effective use of medicines, more efficient patient selection for clinical trials, more cost-effective treatment pathways for health services," and a less risky, more profitable development process for therapeutics and diagnostics developers (Singer and Watkins, 2012).

The right level of regulation requires striking a delicate balance. While the over-regulation or over-legislation of AI-based personalized medical apps may delay the translation of machine learning findings to meaningful, widespread deployment, appropriate regulatory oversight is necessary to ensure adoption, trust, quality, safety, equitable inclusivity, and effectiveness. Regulatory oversight is also needed to minimize false-negative and false-positive errors and misinterpretation of clinical AI algorithms' outputs, actions, and recommendations to clinicians. Recent examination of the ethics of genome-wide association studies for multifactorial diseases found three criteria necessary for identification of genes to be useful: (1) the data in the studies and work products derived from them must be reproducible and applicable to the target population; (2) the data and the derived work products should have significant usefulness and potential beneficial impact to the patients to whom they are applied; and (3) the resulting knowledge should lead to measurable utility for the patient and outweigh associated risks or potential harms (Jordan and Tsai, 2010). Thus, regulatory standards for clinical

AI tools should at least extend to accuracy and relevancy of data inputs and model outputs, marketing of AI systems for specific clinical indications, and transparency or auditability of clinical AI performance.

Medical Device Regulation

Some AI systems, particularly those algorithms that will perform or assist with clinical tasks related to diagnosis, interpretation, or treatment, may be classified as medical devices and fall under applicable FDA regulations. Other AI systems may instead be classified as "services" or as "products," but not medical devices (see Box 7-1). FDA's traditional regulatory processes for medical devices include establishment registration and listing plus premarket submissions for review and approval or clearance by FDA's Center for Devices and Radiological Health Office of Device Evaluation or Office of In Vitro Diagnostics and Radiological Health. In the United States, the Medical Device Amendments of 1976 (P.L. 94-295) to the FDCA (21 U.S.C. § 360c) established a risk-based framework for the regulation of medical devices. The law established a three-tiered risk classification system based on the risk posed to patients should the device fail to perform as intended. The FDCA (21 U.S.C. § 360j) definition of a medical device is summarized in Box 7-1.

BOX 7-1

Federal Food, Drug, and Cosmetic Act (21 U.S.C. § 360j)
Medical Device Definition

[A]n instrument, apparatus, implement, machine, contrivance, implant, in vitro reagent, or other similar or related article, including a component part, or accessory which is:

[One from the following]

Recognized in the official National Formulary, or the United States Pharmacopoeia, or any supplement to them OR intended for use in the diagnosis of disease or other conditions, or in the cure, mitigation, treatment, or prevention of disease, in man or other animals OR intended to affect the structure or any function of the body of man or other animals, and which does not achieve its primary intended purposes through chemical action within or on the body of man or other animals AND which does not achieve its primary intended purposes through chemical action within or on the body of man or other animals and which is not dependent upon being metabolized for the achievement of its primary intended purposes.

The 21st Century Cures Act (Cures Act, P.L. 114-255) was signed into law on December 13, 2016. The significant portion with regard to clinical AI systems is Section 3060 ("Regulation of Medical and Certain Decisions Support Software"), which amends Section 520 of the FDCA so as to provide five important exclusions from the definition of a regulatable medical device. Under Section 3060 of the Act, clinical decision support (CDS) software is nominally exempted from regulation by FDA—that is, it is defined as not a medical device—if it is intended for the purpose of:

(i) displaying, analyzing, or printing medical information about a patient or other medical information (such as peer-reviewed clinical studies and clinical practice guidelines);

(ii) supporting or providing recommendations to a health care professional about prevention, diagnosis, or treatment of a disease or condition; and

(iii) enabling such health care professional to independently review the basis for such recommendations that such software presents so that it is not the intent that such health care professional rely primarily on any of such recommendations to make a clinical diagnosis or treatment decision regarding an individual patient.

This exemption does not apply to software that is "intended to acquire, process, or analyze a medical image or a signal from an in vitro diagnostic device or a pattern or signal from a signal acquisition system" (21st Century Cures Act § 3060). FDA has stated that it would use enforcement discretion to not enforce compliance with medical device regulatory controls for medical device data systems, medical image storage devices, and medical image communications devices (FDA, 2017a). The 21st Century Cures Act codifies some of FDA's prior posture of restraint from enforcement.

Under this system, devices that pose greater risks to patients are subject to more regulatory controls and requirements. Specifically, general controls are sufficient to provide reasonable assurance of a Class I device's safety and effectiveness, while special controls are utilized for Class II devices for which general controls alone are insufficient to provide reasonable assurance of device safety and effectiveness (21 C.F.R. § 860.3). FDA classifies Class III devices as ones intended to be used in supporting or sustaining human life or for a use that is of substantial importance in preventing the impairment of human health, or that may present a potential unreasonable risk of illness or injury, and for which insufficient information exists to determine whether general controls or special controls are sufficient to provide reasonable assurance of the safety and effectiveness of a device (21 C.F.R. § 860.3). This highest risk class of devices is subject to premarket approval to demonstrate a reasonable assurance of safety and effectiveness. Even for this highest risk class of devices, the evidence FDA requires for premarket approval has long been flexible, varying according to the characteristics of the device, its conditions of use, the existence and adequacy of warnings and other restrictions, and other factors. There is generally more flexibility in the amount of clinical evidence needed for medical devices than for drugs and biological products, because they are subject to different statutory criteria and the mechanism of action and modes of failure are generally more predictable and better characterized for devices than for drugs and biological products.

Additionally, the design process for a medical device is more often an iterative process based largely on rational design and non-clinical testing rather than clinical studies. However, this last aspect is not, in general, true for clinical AI systems. The machine learning process is itself a kind of observational research study. In some cases—particularly for medium- and high-risk clinical AIs—the design process may depend on lessons learned as such tools are deployed or on intermediate results that inform ways to improve efficacy (FDA, 2019b). The Clinical Decision Support Coalition and other organizations have recently opined that many types of clinical AI tools should not be regulated or that the industry should instead self-regulate in all application areas that FDA chooses not to enforce on the basis of their review of risks to the public health. Notably, the principles and risk-based classification processes have recently been updated to address requirements for software as a medical device (SaMD) products (see FDA, 2017c § 6.0, p. 11; IMDRF, N12 § 5.1).

It is worth noting the distinction between CDS software tools, including clinical AIs, that replace the health professional's role in making a determination for the patient (i.e., automation) and those that simply provide information to the professional, who can then take it into account and independently evaluate it (i.e., assistance). The former may be deemed by FDA to be a medical device and subject to medical device regulations. Under the 21st Century Cures Act, if a CDS product has multiple functions, where one is excluded from the definition of a medical device and another is not, FDA can assess the safety and effectiveness to determine whether the product should be considered a medical device (21st Century Cures Act § 3060). Also, FDA can still regulate the product as a medical device if it finds that the software "would be reasonably likely to have serious adverse health consequences" or meets the criteria for a Class III medical device. Clinical AI systems that are deemed to be medical devices will generally require either De Novo or premarket approval submissions (FDA, 2018a). In some instances, where a valid pre-1976 predicate exists, a traditional 510(k) submission may be appropriate.

Note, too, that the 21st Century Cures Act's statutory language, while already in force, is subject to implementing regulations to be developed by FDA over time and leaves considerable ambiguity that subjects developers of clinical AI systems to FDA enforcement discretion. For example, uncertainty remains when software is being used in "supporting or providing recommendations," or when it "enables a health care professional to independently review the basis for [its] recommendations." FDA has issued some draft guidance (FDA, 2017b), and more guidance will undoubtedly be forthcoming. But ambiguity will likely be present nonetheless, as will the possibility of enforcement discretion.

Oversight of safety and effectiveness does not just come from regulators, whether domestic or international. In particular, diagnostic testing that is provided by laboratories and other enterprises as services is subject to oversight provided by the Clinical Laboratory Improvements Act of 1988 (CLIA, P.L. 100-578) and the Patient Safety and Quality Improvement Act of 2005 (P.L. 109-41). Certain clinical AI tools that are services rather than products may be appropriate to regulate under CLIA. It is possible that some clinical AIs—especially ones that have aspects similar to diagnostics classified as laboratory-developed tests (LDTs), developed and performed in university-based health facilities or other provider organizations—may be deployed strictly as services for patients in the care of those institutions and not marketed commercially.

FDA's Digital Health Initiative

FDA has expressed interest in actively promoting innovation in the digital health space. FDA's proposed Digital Health Software Precertification (Pre-Cert) Program aims to (1) substantially reduce regulatory burdens for most suppliers and operators of clinical AI systems and (2) improve the health system's rates of responsiveness to emerging unmet health needs, including personalized medicine (FDA, 2018c).

The 21st Century Cures Act and FDA documents reflect an increasing realization that data from real-world operations are necessary for oversight. Health care information technology (IT) systems are so complex and the conditions under which clinical AI systems will operate so diverse that development, validation, and postmarket surveillance must depend on utilizing real-world data and not just clinical trials data or static, curated repositories of historical data. "Real-world data (RWD) are data relating to patient health status and/or the delivery of health care routinely collected from a variety of sources," including electronic health record (EHR) systems (FDA, 2019c). "Real-world evidence (RWE) is the clinical evidence regarding the usage, and potential benefits or risks, of a medical product derived from analysis of RWD" (FDA, 2019c). All of these are subject to applicable HIPAA and other privacy protections such that RWD and RWE must be rigorously de-identified (El Emam, 2013) prior to use for the secondary purposes of clinical AI development and productization. RWE and RWD are discussed in greater detail below.

The goal of FDA's Pre-Cert Program (FDA, 2019a) is to establish voluntary, tailored, pragmatic, and least-burdensome regulatory oversight to assess software developer organizations of all sizes. The Pre-Cert Program simultaneously aims to establish trust that developers have adequate quality management system (QMS) processes in place and a culture of quality and organizational excellence such that those developers can develop and maintain safe, effective, high-quality SaMD products. The Pre-Cert Program leverages the transparency of organizational QMS compliance and product safety as well as quality metrics across the entire life cycle of SaMD. It uses a streamlined premarket review process and leverages postmarket monitoring to verify the continued safety, effectiveness, and quality performance of SaMD in the real world. The premarket review for a precertified organization's SaMD product is informed by the organization's precertification status, precertification level, and the SaMD's risk category. With this program, FDA envisions leveraging the risk-category framework for SaMD developed by the International Medical Device Regulators Forum (IMDRF) to inform the risk category (FDA, 2017c, 2019b). The IMDRF framework describes the spectrum of software functions, some of which may not meet the definition of a device in Section 201(h) of the FDCA and others that may meet the definition of a device, but for which FDA has expressed that it does not intend to enforce compliance. For the purposes of the Pre-Cert Program, the application of FDA's long-established risk category framework would remain consistent with the current definition of device under Section 201(h) of the FDCA and FDA's current enforcement policies. The IMDRF framework establishes types and subtypes of SaMD products based on the state of the health care condition and the significance of the information provided by the products (IMDRF, 2014).

Most clinical AI systems are multielement "ensembles" of a plurality of predictive models with an evidence-combining "supervisor" module that establishes a collective answer or output from the ensemble-member models' execution. Clinical AI involves prediction, classification, or other intelligence-related outputs. These are generated from data supplied as inputs to the model, from fewer than 10 to many hundreds of phenotypic input variables or—in the case of time-series or spectrum-analytic AI systems, image-processing AI systems, or AI systems that include genomics biomarkers—a large number of engineered features that are derived from very high-dimensional raw data inputs. Likewise, present-day genomics-based diagnostics typically involve dozens of input variables, for which there are regulatory policies and procedures that have been established for more than 10 years. These govern existing regulated diagnostics, such as in vitro diagnostic multivariate index assays (IVDMIAs) (FDA, 2007a).

Not all clinical AI systems will manifest hazards or have risk levels comparable to those associated with existing IVDMIA products. However, the methodology, review, and clearance criteria that have been found effective for the regulation of IVDMIAs may form a useful point of reference for the regulatory practice for clinical AI systems.

Clinical AI Systems That May Merit Different Regulatory Approaches

FDA has indicated that it will apply a risk-based assessment framework, where the risk level of different clinical AI systems will be influenced by the different types of on-label clinical indications and contexts in which they are intended to be used, plus the different situations in which their off-label usage might plausibly be anticipated, adopting the IMDRF framework (FDA, 2019b; IMDRF, 2014).

For example, a clinical AI system's intended use might be as a screening test to determine the person's susceptibility to, or propensity in the future to, develop a clinical condition or disease that has not yet materialized; this affords time for longitudinal observation, repeat testing, and vigilance to monitor signs and symptoms of the emergence of the disease and is accordingly lower risk. Similarly, an AI system designed to classify a condition's stage or current severity, or to establish the prognosis or probable clinical course and rate of progression of a condition, functions essentially like a biomarker that characterizes risk and does so in a manner that is amenable to multiple repeat tests and observations over a period of time.

Such situations have low time sensitivity and a plurality of opportunities for the experienced clinicians to review, second-guess, and corroborate the recommendations of the screening clinical AI system. In IMDRF parlance, these are clinical AI systems that "inform" clinical management but do not "drive" clinical management. Indeed, the "informing care" function of some present-day clinical AI tools of this type is to automatically/reflexively order the appropriate standard-of-care confirmatory diagnostic testing and monitoring. These clinical AI systems provide additional evidence or advice (e.g., regarding the likelihood of the condition screened for and/or the cost-effectiveness of pursuing a diagnostic workup for the condition) and promote consistency, relevancy, and quality in diagnostic workups. In general, such screening or informational clinical AI systems will be classified as having low risk. As such, many clinical AI systems are outside the formal scope of medical device regulation and do not require establishment registration and listing or other regulatory filings (21st Century Cures Act § 3060).

By contrast, some classification, forecasting, and prognostic biomarker clinical AI algorithms that instead drive clinical management and/or involve clinical indications may be associated with a medium or high risk; the AI systems could contain faults that cause harm via commissive or omissive errors, either directly or through clinicians' actions or inaction. Perioperative, anesthesiology, critical care, obstetrics, neonatology, and oncology use-cases are examples of medium- or high-risk settings (Therapeutic Monitoring Systems, Inc., 2013). In such situations, there is great time sensitivity and there may be little or no time or opportunity to seek additional testing or perform more observations to assess the accuracy of the AI's recommendation or action. In some instances, such as oncology and surgery, the decision making informed by the AI tool may lead to therapeutic actions that are not reversible and either close other therapeutic avenues or alter the clinical course of the illness and perhaps its responsiveness to subsequent therapy. Such AI tools would, by Section 3060 of the 21st Century Cures Act, be formally within the scope of medical device regulation and would require establishment registration, listing, and other regulatory filings—De Novo, 510(k), premarket approval, or precertification—and associated postmarket surveillance, reporting, and compliance procedures.

Explainability and Transparency from a Regulatory Perspective

AI systems are often criticized for being black boxes (Pasquale, 2016) that are very complex and difficult to explain (Burrell, 2016). Nevertheless, such systems can fundamentally be validated and understood in terms of development and performance (Kroll, 2018; Therapeutic Monitoring Systems, Inc., 2013), even if not in terms of mechanism—and even if they do not conform to preexisting clinician intuitions or conventional wisdom (Selbst and Barocas, 2018). Notably, the degree of "black box" lack of explainability that may be acceptable to regulators validating performance might differ from the amount of explainability clinicians demand, although the latter is an open empirical question. This chapter addresses explainability to clinicians and other nonregulators only to the extent that it interacts with regulatory requirements. Instead, the focus is largely on validation by regulators, which may be satisfied by some current development processes.

While the rest of this section focuses on how explainability and transparency may or may not be required for regulators to oversee safety and efficacy, regulators may also require explainability for independent reasons. For instance, regulators may require clinical AI tools to be explainable to clinicians to whose decision making they are coupled; to quality assurance officers and IT staff in a health provider organization who acquire the clinical AI and have risk-management/legal responsibility for their operation; to developers; to regulators; or to other humans. The European Union's General Data Protection Regulation (GDPR) right to explanation rules, for instance, enacted in 2016 and effective

May 2018, applies to AI systems as well as humans and web services (Kaminski, 2019) and governs European Union citizens worldwide. Similar standards may be implemented in the United States and other jurisdictions. Such standards and regulations are important for public safety and for the benefits of clinical AI systems to be realized through appropriate acceptance and widespread use. However, the notion of explainability is not well defined. There is a lack of agreement about both what constitutes an adequate explanation of clinical AI tools, and to whom the explanation must be provided to conform to applicable right to explanation rules and thus be suitable for regulatory approval.

Current right to explanation regulations and standards fails to acknowledge that human data scientists, clinicians, regulators, courts, and the broader public have limitations in recognizing and interpreting subtle patterns in high-dimensional data. Certain types of AI systems are capable of learning—and certain AI models are capable of intelligently and reliably acting upon—patterns that humans are entirely and forever incapable of noticing or correctly interpreting (Seblst and Barocas, 2019). Correspondingly, humans, unable to grasp the patterns that AI recognizes, may be in a poor position to comprehend the explanations of AI recommendations or actions. As noted, the term "black box" is sometimes pejorative toward AI, especially neural networks, deep learning, and other fundamentally opaque models. They are contrasted to logistic regression; decision-tree; and other older-technology, static, deterministic models—all with low dimensionality but are able to show the inputs that led to the recommendation or action, with variables that are generally well known to the clinician and causally related.

If society, lawmakers, and regulatory agencies were to expect every clinical AI system to provide an explanation of its actions, it could greatly limit the capacity of clinical AI developers' use of the best contemporary AI technologies, which markedly outperform older AI technology but are not able to provide explanations understandable to humans. Regulators do not currently require human-comprehensible explanations for AI in other industries that have potential risks of serious injury or death. For example, autonomous vehicles are not required to provide a running explanation or commentary on their roadway actions.

While requiring explainability may not always be compatible with maximizing capacity and performance, different forms of transparency are available that might enable oversight (see Figure 7-1). For instance, transparency of the initial dataset—including provenance and data-processing procedures—helps to demonstrate replicability. Transparency of algorithm or system architecture is similarly important for regulatory oversight. When AI systems are transparent not just to the regulator but more broadly, such transparency can enable independent validation and oversight by third parties and build trust with users.

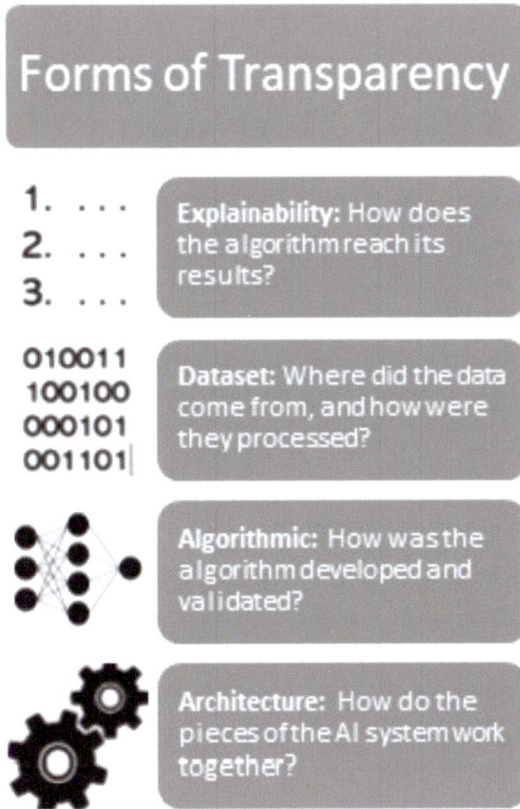

FIGURE 7-1 | Different forms of transparency.

AI Logging and Auditing

Today, developers creating clinical AI systems with their enterprises' risk-management and product liability exposures in mind are engineering and testing their clinical AI deliverables with Agile (Jurney, 2017) or other controlled software development life cycle (SDLC) methods. Defined, well-managed, and controlled SDLC processes produce identifiable and auditable systems and maintain controlled documents of the systems' development processes under the developers' written, reviewed, and approved standard operating procedures. They conform to QMS principles (see ISO-9001, ISO-13485, and 21 C.F.R. Part 820), FDA device master record type, Current Good Manufacturing Practices (CGMPs), and applicable laws and regulations. These include design assurance, design control, hazard analysis, and postmarket surveillance (21 C.F.R. Part 822) provisions. Such industrial-strength developers of clinical AI systems also engineer their systems such that the systems' operation creates (1) a persistent, archived log of each transaction or advisory output that each clinical AI system performs; (2) the versioning of the AI system's elements that performed the transaction, traceable to the data sources; and (3) the validation and software quality-assurance testing that led to the AI systems being authorized for production and subsequent use. These logs enable the examination of the inputs, outputs, and other details in case of anomalies or harms. The logs are open to the clinician-users, employers, organizations who acquire/authorize the AI system's deployment (e.g., health provider organizations, health plans, or public health agencies), regulators, developers, and the courts. The individual release-engineered and version-controlled instances of present-day industrial-strength clinical AI systems are identifiable and rigorously auditable, based on these SDLC controlled-document artifacts, which are maintained by the developer organization that owns the intellectual property.

For this type of clinical AI system, the regulatory agencies' traditional submissions and compliance processes for SaMD are feasible and may not need substantial alteration (e.g., FDA, 2018b). The types of evidence required by plaintiffs, defendants, counsel, and the courts may not need substantial alteration, although the manner of distributed storage, retrieval, and other aspects of provisioning such evidence will change. Moreover, the availability of such evidence will not be significantly altered by the nature of clinical AI systems, provided that developers follow QMS and CGMPs and maintain conformity, including controlled-document artifacts retention.

Some clinical AI tools will be developed using RWD. Because RWD are messy in ways that affect the quality and accuracy of the resulting inferences, as described in Chapter 6, more rigorous requirements for auditing clinical AI systems developed and validated using RWD will need to be established.

AI Performance Surveillance and Maintenance

Several architectural and procedural aspects of machine learning–based clinical AI systems will require significant changes in regulatory compliance and submissions, in terms of scale and scope. In modern AI applications using dynamic data sources—such as clinical data streams stored in EHRs, data collected via sensor-enabled wearable devices and combined with other forms of data, and other RWD—the AI models and algorithms are likely to experience drift over time or as the algorithms are deployed across institutions whose catchment areas and epidemiology differ (dataset shift, see Quiñonero-Candela et al., 2009; Subbaswamy et al., 2019). These longitudinal drifts and shifts entail expanded design control, design assurance, and evidentiary requirements, as discussed in Chapter 6 and below. Therefore, the traditional approach of assessing performance using a static, limited dataset to make assessments about the ongoing safety of a system is inadequate with regard to clinical AI. Continuous machine learning offers one solution for dataset shift and drift by updating with new population-specific data (FDA, 2019b). Not all clinical AI systems aim to do this, and very few clinical AI systems implement continuous learning today. The goals of learning health systems and personalized medicine do create an impetus for more continuous machine learning–based AI systems, as discussed in Chapters 3 and 6 in more detail. However, current regulatory and jurisprudential methods and infrastructure are not prepared for this.

Natural Language Processing and Text Mining AI

Unstructured notes constitute another important source of RWD, and appropriate standards for the extraction, parsing, and curation of unstructured information for clinical AI systems is therefore another open area requiring regulatory oversight. Natural language processing (NLP) algorithms and text mining are important for certain kinds of clinical AI that use unstructured data such as clinical impressions and other remarks, as discussed in Chapter 5.

There will be a need for retention and curation of the unstructured source-text documents as well as the discrete labels or concept codes and values derived by NLP from those documents. Retention of all of these is necessary because NLP algorithms may change over time. The underlying lexical reference data and parameters that govern the parser's operation may likewise change from one release to the next. Thus, release engineering regression testing and validation of successive releases of a clinical AI model that depends on unstructured text must be able to demonstrate that the NLP subsystem continues to meet its specifications and delivers to the clinical AI model inputs that are substantially equivalent to the results it delivered for the same test cases and document content in previous releases. Furthermore, there is natural variability in how different individuals speak. Unlike physiology, factors such as culture and training affect how individuals describe a phenomenon. Clinical AI systems must be robust to these variations.

Clinical Decision Support Systems

Another architectural factor to consider when regulating clinical AI systems is that traditional CDS systems have tended to be embedded in tangible medical devices or in single-site on-premises EHR systems (Evans and Whicher, 2018). The system configurations and dated-signed records of changes in such architectures are readily auditable by users, regulators, and courts. By contrast, many contemporary AI systems are deployed on cloud-based, geographically distributed, nondeterministically parallelized, spatially arbitrary computing architectures that, at any moment, are physically unidentifiable. To create and maintain a full log of each processor that contributed in some part to the execution of a multielement ensemble model AI is possible in principle but would likely be cost-prohibitive and too cumbersome to be practical. Therefore, the limited traceability and fundamental non-recreatability and non-retestability of a patient's or clinician's specific execution of an AI system that may have contained a fault or that produced errors or failures—untoward, unexpected deviations from its specifications, validation testing, and hazard analysis—may pose particular problems for regulators, courts, developers, and the public. These nondeterministic, noncollocation aspects of contemporary cloud-based AI implementations contrast with traditional criteria for tracking product changes (e.g., 510(k) supplements or adverse event reporting systems).

Hazard Identification, Risk Analysis, and Reporting Recommendations for Safe Clinical AI Systems

Identifying hazards is a necessary step to support safe system design and operations. Identifying hazardous situations requires experts to carefully and thoroughly evaluate the system via one of several methods. Successful assurance of public safety rests on (1) identifying and analyzing all significant possible scenarios that could result in accidents of differing severity, and (2) devising and documenting effective means of mitigating the scenarios' likelihood, frequency, and severity. Although hazard identification and quantitative risk assessment are important, risk management also depends on qualitative or subjective judgments (e.g., human observation, intuition, insight regarding processes and mechanisms of causation, creativity in anticipating human actions and psychology, and domain expertise). Each of these judgments introduces biases and chances of omissions. Thus, hazard identification should be a structured process.

Traditional modes of risk assessment and hazard analysis (e.g., hazard and operability study [HAZOP] or process hazard analysis [PHA]) that have been used in regulation of medical devices for decades can also be used for clinical AI systems (ISO, 2009, 2016). However, new hazard types related to geographic dispersity and the dynamic, nondeterministic execution of cloud-based clinical AI systems and machine learning mean that new risks must be evaluated and new mitigations must be devised, tested, and documented. Clinical AI systems may exhibit emergent properties that depend on the whole system as it evolves in time and are not specified or statically defined by the system's parts or subsystems (Johnson, 2002; Louis and Nardi, 2018). This means that the safety of a clinical AI system, like an autonomous vehicle, cannot "solely be analyzed or verified by looking at, for example, a hardware architecture" or only one physical system instantiation (Bagschik et al., 2018). As a result, requirements "must be derived in a top-down development process which incorporates different views on a system at all levels" (Bagschik et al., 2018).

Regulatory agencies should require clinical AI developers to conduct iterative system testing on multiple physical instances of the system and with enough iterations to provide reasonable assurance of detecting faults and hazards from many sources. These could include (1) logic races; (2) nonbinding and nonexecution of worker agents on cloud-based servers; (3) variable or prolonged latencies of data ingestion of accruing clinical information on which an AI depends into noSQL repositories; (4) nonexistent or erroneous mappings of input and output variables utilized by the AI algorithms to do their work; (5) nonreceipt or system-mediated rejection or nonstorage or nondisplay of the AI's output to the relevant user(s); and even (6) potentially automatic software updates (i.e., unsupervised updates of clinical AI systems into "live" production environments, where they immediately begin to affect decisions and might not undergo local review and approval first by the user-clinicians' IT or quality assurance staff). Such an iterative testing requirement is consistent with FDA's recently issued guidance on addressing uncertainty in premarket approval decision making (FDA, 2018a).

For continuous learning and other dynamic, adaptive, and nondeterministic aspects of clinical AI systems and the computing architectures on which they are implemented, developers and regulators could usefully look to risk-assessment and -management methods that have been successfully used for two decades in the chemical process industry and other continuous-process operations such as public utilities (Alley et al., 1998; Allocco, 2010; Baybutt, 2003; Bragatto et al., 2007; Chung and Edwards, 1999; Frank and Whittle, 2001; Hyatt, 2003; Nolan, 2011; Palmer, 2004; Paltrinieri and Khan, 2016; Reniers and Cozzani, 2013; Venkatasubramanian et al., 2000; Villa et al., 2016). Chemical plants, for instance, depend on the availability of public utilities such as water, and chemical plant failure analyses note that dependence. A clinical AI system's developer could similarly list the complete set of utilities (e.g., ongoing access to users' de-identified datasets, on which the AI system's development and validation are based, plus the user's production system and its data on which the AI's runtime operation depends) that might affect a specific node's operation, and assess and manage each of them.

Clinical AI Systems' Prediction/Classification Effectiveness- and Utility-Related Performance

The accuracy, sensitivity, and specificity of clinicians' judgment and of traditional diagnostics are measures against which clinical AI systems' statistical performance must compare favorably. FDA has, for many years, set forth guidance on procedures for assessing noninferiority and superiority of new medical products (FDA, 2016a; Newcombe, 1998a,b). For many applications, the so-called

Number Needed to Treat (NNT) and Number Needed to Harm (NNH) are useful measures of population-level clinical utility of a therapeutic or a diagnostic (Cook and Sackett, 1995; Laupacis et al., 1988). A product (i.e., medication or medical device) or a health service (i.e., clinical intervention, procedure, or care process) that has a very high NNT value (>100) or that has a very low NNH value (<10) is unlikely to meet clinicians' or consumers' expectations of probable clinical benefit and improbable clinical harm.

The international CONsolidated Standards of Reporting Trials (CONSORT, 2010) and STARD (Standards for Reporting of Diagnostic Accuracy Studies; Bossuyt et al., 2003) initiatives pertain to the verification of diagnostic accuracy conforming to existing good clinical practice rules and guidelines (Steyerberg, 2010). While these initiatives are not focused on studies that aim to demonstrate diagnostic device equivalence, many of the reporting concepts involved are nonetheless relevant and applicable to clinical AI. The CONSORT guidelines aim to improve the reporting of randomized controlled trials, enabling reviewers to understand their design, conduct, analysis, and interpretation, and to assess the validity of their results (CONSORT, 2010). However, CONSORT is also applicable to observational, nonrandomized studies and AI derived from machine learning.

According to a 2007 FDA guidance document,

> FDA recognizes two major categories of benchmarks for assessing diagnostic performance of new qualitative [classificatory or binomial/multinomial predictive] diagnostic tests. These categories are (1) comparison to a reference standard (defined below), or (2) comparison to a method or predicate other than a reference standard (non-reference standard).
>
> . . . The diagnostic accuracy of a new test refers to the extent of agreement between the outcome of the new test and the reference standard. We use the term reference standard as defined in STARD. That is, a reference standard is "considered to be the best available method for establishing the presence or absence of the target condition." It divides the intended use population into only two groups (condition present or absent) and does not consider the outcome of the new test under evaluation.
>
> The reference standard can be a single test or method, or a combination of methods and techniques, including clinical follow-up [by appropriately credentialed clinician experts]. If a reference standard is a combination of methods, the algorithm specifying how the different results are combined to make a final positive/negative classification (which may include the choice and ordering of these methods) is part of the standard. (FDA, 2007b)

In addition to the area under the receiver operating characteristic (AUROC) curve, it is also important to evaluate the sensitivity, specificity, positive predictive value (PPV), and negative predictive value (NPV) as part of regulatory assessment of clinical machine learning predictive models and AI. These additional statistical performance metrics take the prevalence of the predicted outcome into account (unlike the AUROC curve, which is independent of prevalence [Cook, 2008]), and therefore have greater clinical relevance. Past studies have shown that PPV and the AUROC curve have minimal correlation for risk prediction models (Goldstein et al., 2017). Conventional statistical measures of accuracy, sensitivity, specificity, PPV, NPV, AUROC and partial AUROC, and so forth are, and will remain, the principal guides for regulatory clearance and enforcement.

Analytical validation involves "establishing that the performance characteristics of a test, tool, or instrument are acceptable" (Scheerens et al., 2017); the relevant performance characteristics are described in Chapter 5 and are important for regulatory oversight as well as internal analytical validation. These characteristics validate the AI's technical performance, but not its usefulness or clinical value. Beyond conventional statistical metrics for diagnostic medical devices and regulatory agencies' de facto norms for these, the objectives of clinical validation testing of an AI tool are to quantitatively evaluate a variety of practical questions:

- How did the AI algorithm outputs inform or obfuscate clinical decision support recommendations?
- How often were AI system recommendations reasonable compared to local licensed peer clinicians addressing similar situations, according to expert clinicians?
- How often did attending clinicians or other staff accept the AI tool's recommendations, and how often did they override or interdict the action or recommendation of the AI tool?
- How often were the AI tool's recommendations or actions unsafe or inefficacious, how often did they lead to errors or harm, and are the AI-associated rates of harm or nonbenefit unacceptably worse (i.e., statistically and clinically inferior) to what competent humans' results are?

Furthermore, clinical utility is an inherent consideration for clinical AIs, as described in Chapter 6. "The conclusion [is] that a given use of a medical product will lead to a net improvement in health outcome or provide useful information about diagnosis, treatment, management, or prevention of a disease. Clinical utility includes the range of possible benefits or risks to individuals and populations" (FDA-NIH Biomarker Working Group, 2016).

Chapter 5 describes bias in sensitivity and specificity estimates in some detail. According to FDA,

> sensitivity and specificity estimates (and other estimates of diagnostic performance) can be subject to bias. Biased estimates are systematically too high or too low. Biased sensitivity and specificity estimates will not equal the true sensitivity and specificity, on average. Often the existence, size (magnitude), and direction of the bias cannot be determined. Bias creates inaccurate estimates.

> [Regulatory agencies hold that] it is important to understand the potential sources of bias to avoid or minimize them [Pepe, 2003]. Simply increasing the overall number of subjects in the study will do nothing to reduce bias. Alternatively, selecting the "right" subjects, changing study conduct, or data analysis procedures may remove or reduce bias. (FDA, 2007b)

These steps are essential to eliminate validation leakage and help to estimate the stability of the model over time.

Two main biases are important to consider: representational bias and information bias (Althubaiti, 2016). Representational bias refers to which individuals or data sources are represented in the data and which are not. Information bias is meant to represent collectively "all the human biases that distort the data on which a decision maker [relies] and that account for the validity of data [that is, the extent these represent what they are supposed to represent accurately]" (Cabitza et al., 2018). These two biases and the related phenomenon of information variability together can degrade the accuracy of the data and, consequently, the accuracy of the clinical AI model derived from them.

Real-World Evidence, Postmarket Surveillance, and Measurement of Clinical AI Systems' Functional Performance

As regulators consider how to set the appropriate balance between regulatory oversight and access to new AI technology, some options include shifting the level of premarket review versus postmarket surveillance for safety and efficacy. Enhanced postmarket surveillance presents an attractive possibility to allow more streamlined premarket review process for AI technology and reflects the likelihood of more frequent product changes over time (FDA, 2019b). Given suitable streams of RWE, clinical AI systems are likely to learn on the fly from an ongoing data stream because population characteristics and underlying models can change. This requires the availability of high-quality labeled RWE as well as continuous oversight via postmarket surveillance, because unlike for a more traditional FDA–approved medical device, many clinical AI systems will change over time with the addition of new data (FDA, 2019b), though for some models and developers the cost of adaptation may exceed the benefits. Especially for lower risk software, allowing market access on the basis of less substantial data on safety and efficacy and then monitoring carefully as the software is deployed in clinical practice may lead to smoother oversight that is still robust. However, prior efforts to rely on increased postmarket surveillance have encountered difficulty in developer compliance and agency enforcement (Woloshin et al., 2017), although the extent of this difficulty is contested (Kashoki et al., 2017).

As part of its Digital Health Innovation Action Plan, FDA is developing the Pre-Cert Program, in which certain developers can apply to be precertified based on a "robust culture of quality and organizational excellence" and commitment to monitoring real-world performance (FDA, 2019c). In the program as envisioned, precertified companies will be able to market lower risk SaMD without premarket review and will receive a streamlined premarket review for higher risk SaMD. FDA will work with developers to collect and interpret real-world information to ensure that the software remains safe and effective in the course of real-world use (FDA, 2019c), including the potential for updates and changes without further review (FDA, 2019b).

Companion Diagnostic Versus Complementary Diagnostic Clinical AIs

Diagnostics that inform the use of drugs, biologics, or therapeutic devices come in several regulatory forms. A companion diagnostic is sometimes required for drug/biologic/device approval (FDA, 2016b); the in vitro diagnostic device (IVD) and the associated therapeutic (i.e., drug, biologic, or other intervention) must be cross-labeled, and the IVD is thereafter used as a "gating" criterion for prescribing the therapeutic product. A complementary diagnostic, in contrast, merely provides additional information relevant to, or supplementary to and corroborative of, decisions guiding care of the patient in regard to the associated therapeutic product. Complementary diagnostics are not required for FDA approval of the associated therapeutic product, and need not be cross labeled. Finally, a combination product is a product composed of two or more regulated components produced and marketed as a single entity (21 C.F.R. § 3.2(e)). It is likely that many clinical AI systems whose hazard analyses indicate that they have medium or high risk could be successfully regulated as complementary diagnostic medical devices.

Two additional types of diagnostics are not regulated as commercially marketed products. An LDT is a type of IVD that is designed, manufactured, and used within a single health services facility for the care of patients for whom named clinicians in that facility have responsibility. Diagnostic tests that are not marketed commercially beyond the therapeutics development process, clinical trials, and regulatory marketing approval are generally referred to by FDA and others as development tools. Such tests are established and overseen similarly to other development tools such as biomarkers.

Liability Under State Tort Law

State tort law also provides a source of risk and of regulatory pressure for the developers and users of clinical AI systems, as well as other AI systems that could cause injury but that are not the focus of this section. Briefly, state tort law may make the developers or users of clinical AI systems liable when patients are injured as a result of using those systems. Such liability could come in the form of malpractice liability—that is, potential lawsuits against health providers, hospitals or other health care systems, and AI system developers for performing below the standard of care (Froomkin et al., 2019). Developers could also face product liability for defects in the design or manufacturing of AI systems or for failure to adequately warn users of the risks of a particular AI system. By imposing liability for injuries caused by AI systems when those injuries could have reasonably been avoided, whether by more careful development or more careful use, tort law exerts pressure on developers.

How exactly tort law will deal with clinical AI systems remains uncertain, because court decisions are retrospective and the technology is nascent. Tort law is principally grounded in state law, and its contours are shaped by courts on a case-by-case basis. This area will continue to develop. Three factors influencing tort liability are of particular note: the interaction of FDA approval and tort liability, liability insurance, and the impact of transparency on tort liability. To be clear, this area of law is still very much developing, and this section only sketches some of the ways different aspects of health care AI systems may interact with the system of tort liability.

Interaction of FDA Approval and Tort Liability

Different regulatory pathways influence the availability of state tort lawsuits against AI developers and, indirectly, the ability of state tort law (and liability insurers reacting to that law) to create independent incentives for the safe and effective development of clinical AI systems. In general, states may not establish statutory requirements that are "different from, or in addition to" FDA requirements regulating devices (21 U.S.C. § 360k). The U.S. Supreme Court has also held that this preempts certain state tort lawsuits alleging negligent design or manufacturing. For devices, including clinical AI apps, that undergo a full premarket approval, state tort lawsuits are generally preempted under the Supreme Court's holding in *Riegel v. Medtronic*, 552 U.S. 312 (2008). Nevertheless, this preemption will not apply to most AI apps, which are likely to be cleared through the 510(k) clearance pathway rather than premarket approval. Clearance under the 510(k) pathway will generally not preempt state tort lawsuits under the reasoning of *Medtronic v. Lohr*, 518 U.S. 470 (1996), because rather than directly determining safety and efficacy, FDA finds the new app to be equivalent to an already approved product. It is unclear what preemptive effect De Novo classification will have on preempting state tort lawsuits, because the Supreme Court emphasized both the thoroughness of premarket review and its determination that the device is safe and effective, rather than equivalent to an approved predicate device.

State tort lawsuits alleging violations of industry-wide requirements, such as CGMP or other validation requirements, are a contestable source of state tort liability. Some courts have found that lawsuits alleging violations of state requirements that parallel industry-wide requirements are preempted by federal law and that such violations may only be addressed by FDA. Other courts disagree, and the matter is currently unsettled (Tarloff, 2011). In at least some jurisdictions, if app developers violate FDA-imposed requirements, courts may find parallel duties under state law and developers may be held liable. Nevertheless, if app developers comply with all FDA-imposed industry-wide requirements, states cannot impose additional requirements.

Liability Insurance

The possibility of liability creates another avenue for regulation through the intermediary of insurance. Developers, providers, and health systems are all likely to carry liability insurance to decrease the risk of a catastrophic tort judgment arising from potential injury. Liability insurers set rules and requirements regarding what information must be provided or what practices and procedures must be followed in order to issue a policy. Although insurers are often not considered regulators, they can exert substantial, if less visible, pressure that may shape the development and use of clinical AI systems (Ben-Shahar and Logue, 2012).

Impact of Transparency on Tort Liability

Transparency and opacity also interact with tort liability. Determining causation can already be difficult in medical tort litigation, because injuries may result from a string of different actions and it is not always obvious which action or combination of actions caused the injury. Opacity in clinical AI systems may further complicate the ability of injured patients, lawyers, or providers or health systems to determine precisely what caused the injury. Explainable algorithms may make it easier to assess tort liability, as could transparency around data provenance, training and validation methods, and ongoing oversight. Perversely, this could create incentives for developers to avoid certain forms of transparency as a way to lessen the likelihood of downstream tort liability. On the other hand, courts— or legislatures—could mandate that due care, in either the development or use of clinical AI tools, requires some form of transparency. To take a hypothetical example, a court might one day hold that when a provider relies on an algorithmic diagnosis, that provider can only exercise due care by assessing how the algorithm was validated. Developers or other intermediaries would then need to provide sufficient information to allow that assessment.

PRIVACY, INFORMATION, AND DATA

Regulation regarding patient privacy and data sharing is also highly relevant to AI development, implementation, and use, whether clinical AI or AI used for other health care purposes ("health care AI"). The United States lacks a general data privacy regime, but HIPAA includes a Privacy Rule that limits the use and disclosure of protected health information (PHI)—essentially any individually identifiable medical information—by covered entities (i.e., almost all providers, health insurers, and health data clearinghouses) and their business associates where the business relationship involves PHI (45 C.F.R. § 160.103). Covered entities and business associates may only use or disclose information with patient authorization, if the entity receives a waiver from an institutional review board or privacy board, or for one of several exceptions (45 C.F.R. § 164.502). These listed exceptions include the use and disclosure of PHI for the purposes of payment, public health, law enforcement, or health care operations, including quality improvement efforts but not including research aimed at creating generalizable knowledge (45 C.F.R. § 164.501). For health systems that intend to use their own internal data to develop in-house AI tools (e.g., to predict readmission rates or the likelihood of complications among their own patients), the quality improvement exception will likely apply. Even when the use or disclosure of information is permitted under HIPAA, the Privacy Rule requires that covered entities take reasonable steps to limit the use or disclosure to the minimum necessary to accomplish the intended purpose. While HIPAA does create protections for patient data, its reach is limited, and health information can come from many sources that HIPAA does not regulate (Price and Cohen, 2019).

A complex set of other laws may also create requirements to protect patient data. HIPAA sets a floor for data privacy, not a ceiling. State laws may be more restrictive; for instance, some states provide stronger protections for especially sensitive information such as HIV status or substance abuse information (e.g., N.Y. Pub. Health Law § 2783). California's Consumer Protection Act creates general protections for consumer information, including health data. And although the European Union's GDPR focuses on actions that directly affect the European Union, it also places limits on the processing of data about EU residents, regardless of where the EU citizen resides globally, and may therefore affect the privacy practices of non-EU entities engaged in medical AI development (Marelli and Testa, 2018). The GDPR generally requires legal and real persons to collect and process only as much personal data as necessary, obtain such data only for a listed legitimate purpose or with consent, notify individuals of the receipt of data, and engage in privacy-centered policy design. Health data are especially protected under the GDPR, and their processing is prohibited unless with explicit consent or in a number of specified exceptions, such as for health operations or scientific research.

Privacy and Patient Consent Issues in Health Care AI

With regard to discrete clinical data, unstructured textual data, imagery data, waveform and time-series data, and hybrid data used in clinical AI models, the development and deployment of AI systems have complex interactions with privacy concerns and privacy law (e.g., Loukides et al., 2010). Adequate oversight of clinical AI systems must address the nature of potential privacy concerns wherever they may arise, approaches to address those concerns, and management of the potential tension between privacy and other governance concerns for clinical AI.

Initial AI Development

Privacy concerns occur in the first instance because training health care AI depends on assembling large collections of health data about patients (Horvitz and Mulligan, 2015). Health data about individuals are typically considered sensitive. Some forms of data are particularly sensitive, such as substance abuse data or sexually transmitted disease information (Ford and Price, 2016). Other forms of data raise privacy concerns about the particular individual, such as genetic data that can reveal information about family members (Ram et al., 2018). Collecting, using, and sharing patient health data raise concerns about the privacy of the affected individuals, whether those concerns are consequentialist (e.g., the possibility of future discrimination based on health status) or not (e.g., dignitary concerns about others knowing embarrassing or personal facts) (Price and Cohen, 2019). The process of collecting and sharing may also make data more vulnerable to interception or inadvertent access by other parties.

External Validation

External validation of clinical AI systems creates other avenues for privacy harms. Some proposals have called for third-party validation of medical AI recommendations and predictions to validate algorithmic quality (Ford and Price, 2016; Price, 2017a). Such an approach would either require making patient data available to those third parties or require the AI developer to have a partnership with a data owner, where data scientists ensure comparable data transformation and algorithm execution to provide external validation without direct data sharing.

Inference Generation

A third form of potential privacy harm that could arise from health care AI is quite different and involves the generation of inferences about individual patients based on their health data. Machine learning makes predictions based on data, and those predictions may themselves be sensitive data, or may at least be viewed that way by patients. In one highly publicized example of such a case, Target identified a teenage woman's pregnancy based on changes in her purchasing habits and then sent her targeted coupons and advertisements, which led to her father learning of her pregnancy from Target before his daughter had shared the news (Duhigg, 2012). The epistemic status of this information is debatable; arguments have been made that inferences cannot themselves be privacy violations, although popular perception may differ (Skopek, 2018).

Some standard privacy-protecting approaches of data collectors and users face difficulties when applied to health care AI. The most privacy-protective approach limits initial data collection to necessarily limit the potential for problematic use or disclosure (Terry, 2017). However, this approach presumes that the data collector knows which data are necessary and which are not, knowledge that is often absent for health care AI.

De-Identification

De-identification, a common privacy-protecting approach, raises several concerns. Under the HIPAA Privacy Rule, patient information is not considered PHI (and thus not subject to the rule's restrictions on use and disclosure) if a set of 17 listed pieces of identifying information have been removed (45 C.F.R. § 164.514(b)(2)(i)). These listed pieces include at least some elements that may be useful to health care AI, such as key dates, zip codes, or photographs of the patient. Thus, de-identification can lead to the loss of relevant data.

De-identification also raises two diametrically opposed concerns about gathering data. On the one hand, de-identification can lead to data fragmentation.

Patient data are gathered in many different contexts, including by different providers and different insurers. This diffuse data collection occurs both laterally, as patients encounter different parts of the medical system at the same time, and longitudinally, as patients shift between different medical environments over the course of time. Identifying information provides the easiest way to reassemble different parts of patient records into more comprehensive datasets that can help drive at least some forms of health care AI (e.g., long-term predictions of efficacy or mortality). When identifying information is removed from patient data, reassembly becomes harder, especially for developers with fewer resources. On the other hand, de-identification is not proof against re-identification (Ohm, 2010). Re-identification can happen at the level of the individual (via targeted efforts) or more broadly across datasets. "Data triangulation" refers to the idea that if data gatherers can collect multiple datasets that include some overlapping information, and if some of those datasets include identifying information, then data users can merge those datasets and identify individuals in the otherwise de-identified datasets (Mello and Cohen, 2018; Terry, 2017). Under current law, covered entities are limited in how they can re-identify data, since once it is re-identified it is again governed by HIPAA restrictions, but this does not govern those that are not covered entities. In addition, data-sharing agreements often include provisions prohibiting efforts at re-identification by the data recipient (Ohmann et al., 2017).

Individual consent and authorization provide the clearest possible path toward ameliorating privacy concerns but raise their own complications. When individuals know the purposes for which their information will be used and can give meaningful informed consent to those uses, privacy concerns can be limited. For machine learning and health care AI, however, future uses may be unpredictable. The revised Common Rule does allow for the provision of broad consent for unspecified future use (45 C.F.R. § 46.116). Nevertheless, systematic differences between those willing to consent to future data use and those unwilling to consent—or unable to consent because they lack that entry into the health data system—means that relying on individual authorization can introduce bias into datasets (Spector-Bagdady, 2016). Furthermore, the more meaningful the individual opportunity to consent, the higher the procedural hurdles created for the assembly of data—and the greater the likelihood of eventual bias. The Office of the National Coordinator for Health Information Technology has developed a Model Privacy Notice to "help developers convey information about their privacy and security policies" (ONC, 2018).

Data Infrastructure

The availability of data is an underlying legal and regulatory challenge for clinical AI system development, which requires large amounts of data for training and validation purposes. Once particular AI systems are deployed in the real world, RWD should be collected to ensure that the AI systems are performing well and, ideally, to improve that performance. However, numerous hurdles exist to the collection of sufficient data (Price, 2016). Various privacy laws, as described above, restrict the collection of identifiable information, and de-identified information can be difficult to assemble to capture either long-term effects or data across different data sources. Informed consent laws, such as the Common Rule for federally funded research or the consent requirements incorporated into the GDPR, create additional barriers to data collection. Even where privacy or informed consent rules do not actually prohibit the collection, use, or sharing of data, some health care actors may limit such actions out of an abundance of caution, creating a penumbra of data limitations. In addition, for those actors who do find ways around these requirements, criticism and outrage may arise if patients feel they are inadequately compensated for their valuable data. On an economic level, holders of data have strong incentives to keep data in proprietary siloes to derive competitive advantage, leading to more fragmentation of data from different sources. For data holders who wish to keep data proprietary for economic reasons, referencing privacy concerns can provide a publicly acceptable reason for these tactics.

At least four possibilities emerge for collection of data, with some evidence of each in current practice:

1. **Large individual data holders:** Some large holders of individual data possess enough data to train AI models on their own, such as health systems (e.g., Partners or Ascension), health care payers (e.g., United Healthcare or Humana), or tech/data companies (e.g., Google or Apple).
2. **Data brokers and collaboration:** The collaboration or collection of data from different sources is possible, but these endeavors often encounter the hurdles described above, which may introduce limitations on data sources or bias in the incorporation process.
3. **Failure to collect data:** In some instances, no actor may have the incentive or ability to collect and gather data. This may be a problem especially for otherwise underserved populations, whose data may be under-represented in AI development and monitoring efforts.
4. **Government data infrastructure:** Governmental agencies can collect health data as part of an effort to support future innovation in clinical AI (among other efforts). The Precision Medicine Initiative's All of Us cohort is an example of such an effort (Frey et al., 2016; NIH, 2019), as is the U.S. Department of Veterans Affairs' Million Veteran Program (Gaziano et al., 2016), although the latter has more restrictive policies for its data use (Price, 2017b).

Of the four models, the first three are the straightforward results of current market dynamics. Each creates challenges, including smaller dataset size, potential bias in collection, access for other developers or for validators, and, in the case of failures to collect data, exclusion of some populations from AI development and validation. Government data infrastructure—that is, data gathered via government efforts for the purposes of fostering innovation, including clinical AI—has the greatest possibility of being representative and available for a variety of downstream AI uses but also faces potential challenges in public will for its collection. Even when the government itself does not collect data, it can usefully promulgate standards for data collection and consolidation (Richesson and Krischer, 2007; Richesson and Nadkarni, 2011); the lack of standards for EHRs, for instance, has led to persistent problems aggregating data across contexts.

Tension Between Privacy and Data Access

In general, there is tension between privacy-protecting approaches and access to big data for the development, validation, and oversight of health care AI. For instance, Google was sued for privacy violations in 2019 as a result of an agreement with the University of Chicago Medical Center to use the system's data in AI and other big data applications (Cohen and Mello, 2019). Higher protections for patient data, whether regarding front-end collection or back-end use, increase the hurdles for the development of health care AI (Ford and Price, 2016). These hurdles may also exacerbate differences in capabilities between large, sophisticated entities—that is, health systems, health insurers, or large technology companies—and smaller developers that may lack the resources to develop AI in a privacy-protective fashion. However, privacy and innovation in health care AI are not in strict opposition. Newer technological approaches such as differential privacy (Malin et al., 2013) and dynamic consent (Kaye et al., 2014) can help enable development while still protecting privacy. In fact, the desire to protect privacy can be its own spur to the development of innovative technologies to collect, manage, and use health data. Nevertheless, resolving this tension presents a substantial ongoing challenge, one familiar in the development of a learning health system more generally. This resolution will not be simple and is beyond the scope of this chapter; it will demand careful policy making and continued engagement by stakeholders at various levels.

KEY CONSIDERATIONS

In summary, clinical AI tools present opportunities for improving patients' and clinicians' point-of-care decision making, and a viable business model is necessary to ensure that safe, effective clinical AI systems are developed, validated, and sustainably deployed, implemented in EHR systems, and curated over time to maintain adequate accuracy and reliability. However, clinical AI systems could potentially pose risks in terms of inappropriate treatment recommendations, privacy breaches, or other harms (Evans and Whicher, 2018), and some types of clinical AI systems will be classified by regulatory agencies as SaMDs, subject to premarket clearance or approval and other requirements that aim to protect the public's health. Other clinical AI tools may be deemed to be LDT-type services, subject to CLIA and similar regulations. Whatever agency is involved in oversight, compliance with regulations should be mandatory rather than voluntary, given the potential for problematic incentives for system developers (Evans and Whicher, 2018). As the law and policy of health care AI systems develop over time, it is both expected and essential that multiple stakeholders—including payers, patients and families, policy makers, diagnostic manufacturers and providers, clinicians, academics, and others—remain involved in helping determine how best to ensure that such systems advance the quintuple aim and improve the health care system more generally.

- The black box nature of a clinical AI system should not disqualify a system from regulatory approval or use, but transparency, where possible, can aid in oversight and adoption and should be encouraged or potentially required. AI systems, including black box systems, should be capable of providing the users with an opportunity to examine quantitative evidence that the recommendation in the current situation is indeed the best recent historical choice, supplying de-identified, aggregated data sufficient for the user to satisfy the user's interest in confirming that this is so, or is at least no worse and no more uncertain than decisions the user would take independently were the AI not involved.
- When possible, machine learning–based predictive models should be evaluated in an independent dataset (i.e., external validation) before they are adopted in the clinical practice. Risk assessment to determine the degree to which dataset-specific biases affect the model should be undertaken. Regulatory agencies should recommend specific statistical methods for evaluating and mitigating bias.
- To the extent that machine learning–based models continuously learn from new data, regulators should adopt postmarket surveillance mechanisms to ensure continuing (and ideally improving) high-quality performance.
- Regulators should engage in collaborative governance efforts with other stakeholders and experts throughout the health system, including data scientists, clinicians, ethicists, and others, to continuously evaluate deployed clinical AI for effectiveness and safety on the basis of RWD.

- Government actors should invest in infrastructure that enables equitable, high-quality data collection, such as technical standards and technological capability building.
- Government actors should continue and increase efforts to develop large, high-quality, voluntary health datasets for clinical AI development (among other purposes), such as the All of Us cohort within the Precision Medicine Initiative, while ensuring adequate measures to address patient notice and potential harms.

REFERENCES

Alley, M., M. Long, D. Walker, and R. Montgomery. 1998. Integrating reliability-centered maintenance studies with process hazard analyses. In *Proceedings of the International Conference and Workshop on Reliability and Risk Management.* American Institute of Chemical Engineers.

Allocco, M. 2010. *Safety analyses of complex systems: Considerations of software, firmware, hardware, human, and the environment.* New York: Wiley.

Althubaiti, A. 2016. Information bias in health research: Definition, pitfalls, and adjustment methods. *Journal of Multidisciplinary Healthcare* 9:211–218.

Bagschik G., M. Nolte, S. Ernst, and M. Maurer. 2018. *A systems perspective towards an architecture framework for safe automated vehicles.* Working paper. Technische Universitat Braunschweig. https://arxiv. org/pdf/1804.07020.pdf (accessed November 14, 2019).

Baybutt, P. 2003. Major hazard analysis: An improved method for process hazard analysis. *Process Safety Progress* 22:21–26.

Ben-Shahar, O., and K. Logue. 2012. Outsourcing regulation: How insurance reduces moral hazard. *Michigan Law Review* 111:197–248.

Bossuyt, P. M., J. B. Reitsma, D. E. Bruns, C. A. Gatsonis, P. P. Glasziou, L. M. Irwig, J. G. Lijmer, D. Moher, D. Rennie, and H. C. De Vet. 2003. Towards complete and accurate reporting of studies of diagnostic accuracy: The STARD initiative. *Clinical Chemistry* 49:1–6.

Bragatto, P., M. Monti, F. Giannini, and S. Ansaldi. 2007. Exploiting process plant digital representation for risk analysis. *Journal of the Loss Prevention Process Industry* 20:69–78.

Burrell, J. 2016. How the machine "thinks": Understanding opacity in machine learning algorithms. *Big Data & Society* 3(1):2053951715622512-9.

Cabitza, F., D. Ciucci, and R. Rasoini. 2018. A giant with feet of clay: On the validity of the data that feed machine learning in medicine. *arXiv.org.* https://arxiv.org/abs/1706.06838 (accessed November 14, 2019).

Chung, P., and D. Edwards. 1999. Hazard identification in batch and continuous computer-controlled plants. *Industrial & Engineering Chemical Research* 38:4359–4371.

Cohen, I., and M. Mello. 2019. Big data, big tech, and protecting patient privacy. *JAMA* 322(12):1141–1142. https://doi.org/10.1001/jama.2019.11365.

CONSORT (CONsolidated Standards of Reporting Trials). 2010. *CONSORT 2010.* http://www.consort-statement.org/consort-2010 (accessed November 14, 2019).

Cook, N. 2008. Statistical evaluation of prognostic versus diagnostic models: Beyond the ROC curve. *Clinical Chemistry* 54:17–23.

Cook, R., and D. Sackett. 1995. The number needed to treat: A clinically useful measure of treatment effect. *BMJ* 310(6977):452–454.

Duhigg, C. 2012. How companies learn your secrets. *The New York Times.* https://www.nytimes.com/2012/02/19/magazine/shopping-habits.html (accessed November 14, 2019).

El Emam, K. 2013. *Guide to the de-identification of personal health information.* New York: CRC Press.

Evans, E., and D. Whicher. 2018. What should oversight of clinical decision support systems look like? *AMA Journal of Ethics* 20:E857–E863.

FDA (U.S. Food and Drug Administration). 2007a. *In vitro diagnostic multivariate index assays—Draft guidance.* https://www.fda.gov/downloads/MedicalDevices/DeviceRegulationandGuidance/GuidanceDocuments/ucm071455.pdf (accessed November 14, 2019).

FDA. 2007b. *Statistical guidance on reporting results from studies evaluating diagnostic tests—Guidance for industry and FDA staff.* https://www.fda.gov/downloads/MedicalDevices/DeviceRegulationandGuidance/GuidanceDocuments/ucm071287.pdf (accessed November 14, 2019).

FDA. 2016a. *Non-inferiority clinical trials to establish effectiveness—Guidance for industry.* https://www.fda.gov/downloads/Drugs/Guidances/UCM202140.pdf (accessed November 14, 2019).

FDA. 2016b. *Principles for co-development of an in vitro companion diagnostic device with a therapeutic product—Draft guidance.* https://www.fda.gov/downloads/MedicalDevices/DeviceRegulationandGuidance/GuidanceDocuments/UCM510824.pdf (accessed November 14, 2019).

FDA. 2017a. *Changes to existing medical software policies resulting from Section 3060 of the 21st Century Cures Act.* https://www.fda.gov/downloads/MedicalDevices/DeviceRegulationandGuidance/GuidanceDocuments/UCM587820.pdf (accessed November 14, 2019).

FDA. 2017b. *Clinical and patient decision support software—Draft guidance.* https://www.fda.gov/downloads/MedicalDevices/DeviceRegulationandGuidance/GuidanceDocuments/UCM587819.pdf (accessed November 14, 2019).

FDA. 2017c. *Software as a Medical Device (SAMD): Clinical evaluation—Guidance for industry and Food and Drug Administration staff.* https://www.fda.gov/downloads/MedicalDevices/DeviceRegulationandGuidance/GuidanceDocuments/UCM524904.pdf (accessed November 14, 2019).

FDA. 2018a. *Consideration of uncertainty in making benefit-risk determinations in medical device premarket approvals, de novo classifications, and humanitarian device exemptions—Draft guidance.* https://www.fda.gov/downloads/MedicalDevices/DeviceRegulationandGuidance/GuidanceDocuments/UCM619220.pdf (accessed November 14, 2019).

FDA. 2018b. *FDA permits marketing of artificial intelligence-based device to detect certain diabetes-related eye problems.* News & Events. https://www.fda.gov/newsevents/newsroom/pressannouncements/ucm604357.htm (accessed November 14, 2019).

FDA. 2018c. *Fostering digital health innovation: Developing the Software Precertification Program—January 30–31, 2018—transcripts.* News & Events. https://www.fda.gov/MedicalDevices/NewsEvents/WorkshopsConferences/ucm587581.htm (accessed November 14, 2019).

FDA. 2019a. *Developing Software Precertification Program: A working model, v1.0.* https://www.fda.gov/downloads/MedicalDevices/DigitalHealth/DigitalHealthPreCertProgram/UCM629276.pdf (accessed November 14, 2019).

FDA. 2019b. *Proposed regulatory framework for modifications to Artificial Intelligence/Machine Learning (AI/ML)-Based Software as a Medical Device (SaMD).* Discussion Paper and Request for Feedback. https://www.fda.gov/downloads/MedicalDevices/DigitalHealth/SoftwareasaMedicalDevice/UCM635052.pdf (accessed November 14, 2019).

FDA. 2019c. *Real world evidence.* Science and Research Special Topics. https://www.fda.gov/scienceresearch/specialtopics/realworldevidence/default.htm (accessed November 14, 2019).

FDA-NIH (National Institutes of Health) Biomarker Working Group. 2016. *BEST (Biomarkers, EndpointS, and other Tools).* https://www.ncbi.nlm.nih.gov/books/NBK326791 (accessed November 14, 2019).

Ford, R., and W. Price. 2016. Privacy and accountability in black–box medicine. *Michigan Telecommunications & Technology Law Review* 23:1–43.

Frank, W., and D. Whittle. 2001. *Revalidating process hazard analyses.* New York: Wiley.

Frey, L., E. Bernstam, and J. Denny. 2016. Precision medicine informatics. *Journal of the American Medical Informatics Association* 23(4):668–670.

Froomkin, M., I. Kerr, and J. Pineau. 2019. When AIs outperform doctors: Confronting the challenges of a tort-induced over-reliance on machine learning. *Arizona Law Review* 61:33–99. https://papers.ssrn.com/sol3/papers.cfm?abstract_id=3114347 (accessed November 14, 2019).

Gaziano, J. M., J. Concato, M. Brophy, L. Fiore, S. Pyarajan, J. Breeling, S. Whitbourne, J. Deen, C. Shannon, D. Humphries, and P. Guarino. 2016. Million Veteran Program: A mega-biobank to study genetic influences on health and disease. *Journal of Clinical Epidemiology* 70:214–223.

Goldstein, B., A. Navar, M. Pencina, and J. Ioannidis. 2017. Opportunities and challenges in developing risk prediction models with electronic health records data: A systematic review. *Journal of the American Medical Informatics Association* 24:198–208.

Horvitz, E., and D. Mulligan. 2015 Data, privacy, and the greater good. *Science* 349(6245):253–255.

Hyatt, N. 2003. *Guidelines for Process Hazards Analysis (PHA, HAZOP), hazards identification, and risk analysis.* New York: CRC Press.

IMDRF (International Medical Device Regulators Forum). 2014. *Software as a Medical Device: Possible framework for risk categorization and corresponding considerations.* http://www.imdrf.org/docs/imdrf/final/technical/imdrf-tech-140918-samd-framework-risk-categorization-141013.pdf (accessed November 14, 2019).

ISO (International Organization for Standardization). 2009. *ISO/IEC-31010:2009: Risk management—Risk assessment techniques.* Geneva, Switzerland: ISO. https://www.iso.org/standard/51073.html (accessed November 14, 2019).

ISO. 2016. *ISO-13485:2016: Medical devices—Quality management systems—Requirements for regulatory purposes.* Geneva, Switzerland: ISO. https://www.iso.org/standard/59752.html (accessed November 14, 2019).

Johnson, S. 2002. *Emergence: The connected lives of ants, brains, cities, and software.* New York: Scribner.

Jordan, B., and D. Tsai. 2010. Whole-genome association studies for multigenic diseases: Ethical dilemmas arising from commercialization—The case of genetic testing for autism. *Journal of Medical Ethics* 36:440–444.

Jurney, R. 2017. *Agile data science 2.0.* Boston, MA: O'Reilly.

Kaminski, M. 2019. The right to an explanation, explained. *Berkeley Technology Law Journal* 34(1). https://papers.ssrn.com/sol3/papers.cfm?abstract_id=3196985 (accessed November 14, 2019).

Kashoki, M., C. Lee, and P. Stein. 2017. FDA oversight of postmarketing studies. *New England Journal of Medicine* 377:1201–1202.

Kaye, J., E. Whitley, D. Lund, M. Morrison, H. Teare, and K. Melham. 2014. Dynamic consent: A patient interface for twenty-first century research networks. *European Journal of Human Genetics* 23:141–146.

Kroll, J. 2018. The fallacy of inscrutability. *Philosophical Transactions of the Royal Society A: Mathematical, Physical and Engineering Sciences* 376(2133). https://doi.org/10.1098/rsta.2018.0084 (accessed November 14, 2019).

Laupacis, A., D. Sackett, and R. Roberts. 1988. An assessment of clinically useful measures of the consequences of treatment. *New England Journal of Medicine* 318:1728–1733.

Louis, P. Y., and F. Nardi. 2018. *Probabilistic cellular automata: Theory, applications and future perspectives.* New York: Springer.

Loukides, G., J. C. Denny, and B. Malin. 2010. The disclosure of diagnosis codes can breach research participants' privacy. *Journal of the American Medical Informatics Association* 17(3):322–327.

Malin, B., K. El Emam, and C. O'Keefe. 2013. Biomedical data privacy: Problems, perspectives, and advances. *Journal of the American Medical Informatics Association* 20:2–6.

Marelli, L., and G. Testa. 2018. Scrutinizing the EU general data protection regulation. *Science* 360:496–498.

Mello, M., and I. Cohen. 2018. HIPAA and protecting health information in the 21st century. *JAMA* 320:231–232.

Newcombe, R. 1998a. Interval estimation for the difference between independent proportions: Comparison of eleven methods. *Statistics in Medicine* 17:873–890.

Newcombe, R. 1998b. Two-sided confidence intervals for the single proportion: Comparison of seven methods. *Statistics in Medicine* 17:857–872.

NIH (National Institutes of Health). 2019. *All of Us research program.* https://allofus.nih.gov (accessed November 14, 2019).

Nolan, D. 2011. *Safety and security review for the process industries: Application of HAZOP, PHA, What-IF, and SVA Reviews.* New York: Gulf.

Ohm, P. 2010. Broken promises of privacy: Responding to the surprising failure of anonymization. *UCLA Law Review* 57:1701.

Ohmann, C., R. Banzi, S. Canham, S. Battaglia, M. Matei, C. Ariyo, L. Becnel, B. Bierer, S. Bowers, L. Clivio, and M. Dias. 2017. Sharing and reuse of individual participant data from clinical trials: Principles and recommendations. *BMJ Open* 7(12):e018647.

ONC (The Office of the National Coordinator for Health Information Technology). 2018. Model Privacy Notice (MPN). *HealthIT.gov.* https://www.healthit.gov/topic/privacy-security-and-hipaa/model-privacy-notice-mpn (accessed November 14, 2019).

Palmer, J. 2004. Evaluating and assessing process hazard analyses. *Journal of Hazardous Materials* 115:181–192.

Paltrinieri, N., and F. Khan. 2016. *Dynamic risk analysis in the chemical and petroleum industry: Evolution and interaction with parallel disciplines in the perspective of industrial application.* New York: Butterworth-Heinemann.

Pasquale, F. 2016. *The black box society: The secret algorithms that control money and information.* Cambridge, MA: Harvard University Press.

Pepe, M. 2003. *The statistical evaluation of medical tests for classification and prediction.* Oxford, UK: Oxford University Press.

Price, W. 2016. Big data, patents, and the future of medicine. *Cardozo Law Review* 37(4):1401–1452.

Price, W. 2017a. Regulating black-box medicine. *Michigan Law Review* 116(3):421–474.

Price, W. 2017b. Risk and resilience in health data infrastructure. *Colorado Technology Law Journal* 16(1):65–85.

Price, W., and I. Cohen. 2019. Privacy in the age of medical big data. *Nature Medicine* 25(1):37–43.

Quiñonero-Candela, J., M. Sugiyama, A. Schwaighofer, and N. Lawrence. 2009. *Dataset shift in machine learning.* Cambridge, MA: MIT Press.

Ram, N., C. Guerrini, and A. McGuire. 2018. Genealogy databases and the future of criminal investigations. *Science* 360(6393):1078–1079.

Reniers, G., and V. Cozzani. 2013. *Domino effects in the process industries: Modelling, prevention and managing.* New York: Elsevier.

Richesson, R., and J. Krischer. 2007. Data standards in clinical research: Gaps, overlaps, challenges and future directions. *Journal of the American Medical Informatics Association* 14(6):687–696.

Richesson, R., and P. Nadkarni. 2011. Data standards for clinical research data collection forms: Current status and challenges. *Journal of the American Medical Informatics Association* 18(3):341–346.

Scheerens, H., A. Malong, K. Bassett, Z. Boyd, V. Gupta, J. Harris, C. Mesick, S. Simnett, H. Stevens, H. Gilbert, and P. Risser. 2017. Current status of companion and complementary diagnostics: Strategic considerations for development and launch. *Clinical and Translational Science* 10(2):84–92.

Seblst, A., and S. Barocas. 2018. The intuitive appeal of explainable machines. *Fordham Law Review* 87:1085–1139.

Singer, D., and J. Watkins. 2012. Using companion and coupled diagnostics within strategy to personalize targeted medicines. *Personalized Medicine* 9(7):751–761.

Skopek, J. 2018. *Big data's epistemology and its implications for precision medicine and privacy.* Cambridge, UK: Cambridge University Press.

Spector-Bagdady, K. 2016. The Google of healthcare: Enabling the privatization of genetic bio/databanking. *Annals of Epidemiology* 26:515–519.

Steyerberg, E. 2010. *Clinical prediction models: A practical approach to development, validation, and updating.* New York: Springer.

Subbaswamy, A., P. Schulam, and S. Saria. 2019. Preventing failures due to dataset shift: Learning predictive models that transport. *arXiv.org*. https://arxiv.org/abs/1812.04597 (accessed November 14, 2019).

Tarloff, E. 2011. Medical devices and preemption: A defense of parallel claims based on violations of non-device specific FDA regulations. *NYU Law Review* 86:1196.

Terry, N. 2017. Regulatory disruption and arbitrage in health-care data protection. *Yale Journal of Health Policy, Law and Ethics* 17:143.

Therapeutic Monitoring Systems, Inc. 2013. *CIMVA universal traditional premarket notification; K123472.* https://www.accessdata.fda.gov/cdrh_docs/pdf12/K123472.pdf (accessed November 14, 2019).

Venkatasubramanian, V., J. Zhao, and S. Viswanathan. 2000. Intelligent systems for HAZOP analysis of complex process plants. *Computers & Chemical Engineering* 24(9–10):2291–2302.

Villa, V., N. Paltrinieri, F. Khan, and V. Cozzani. 2016. Towards dynamic risk analysis: A review of the risk assessment approach and its limitations in the chemical process industry. *Safety Science* 89:77–93.

Woloshin, S., L. Schwartz, B. White, and T. Moore. 2017. The fate of FDA postapproval studies. *New England Journal of Medicine* 377:1114–1117.

Suggested citation for Chapter 7: McNair, D., and W. N. Price II. 2020. Health care artificial intelligence: law, regulation, and policy. In *Artificial intelligence in health care: The hope, the hype, the promise, the peril*. Washington, DC: National Academy of Medicine.

8

ARTIFICIAL INTELLIGENCE IN HEALTH CARE: HOPE NOT HYPE, PROMISE NOT PERIL

*Michael Matheny, Vanderbilt University Medical Center
and U.S. Department of Veterans Affairs; Sonoo Thadaney Israni,
Stanford University; Danielle Whicher, National Academy of Medicine;
and Mahnoor Ahmed, National Academy of Medicine*

INTRODUCTION

Health care delivery in the United States, and globally, continues to face significant challenges from the increasing breadth and depth of data and knowledge generation. This publication focuses on artificial intelligence (AI) designed to improve health and health care, the explosion of electronic health data, the significant advances in data analytics, and mounting pressures to reduce health care costs while improving health care equity, access, and outcomes. AI tools could potentially address known challenges in health care delivery and achieve the vision of a continuously learning health system, accounting for personalized needs and preferences. The ongoing challenge is to ensure the appropriate and equitable development and implementation of health care AI. The term AI is inclusive of machine learning, natural language processing, expert systems, optimization, robotics, speech, and vision (see Chapter 1), and the terms AI tools, AI systems, and AI applications are used interchangeably.

While there have been a number of promising examples of AI applications in health care (see Chapter 3), it is judicious to proceed with caution to avoid another AI winter (see Chapter 2), or further exacerbate health care disparities. AI tools are only as good as the data used to develop and maintain them, and there are many limitations with current data sources (see Chapters 1, 3, 4, and 5). Plus, there is the real risk of increasing current inequities and distrust (see Chapters 1 and 4) if AI tools are developed and deployed without thoughtful preemptive planning, self-governance, trust-building, transparency, appropriate levels of automation and augmentation (see Chapters 3, 4, and 5), and regulatory oversight (see Chapters 4, 5, 6, and 7).

This publication synthesizes the major literature to date, in both the academic and general press, to create a reference document for health care AI model developers, clinical teams, patients, "fRamilies," and regulators and policy makers to:

1. identify the current and near-term uses of AI within and outside the traditional health care systems (see Chapters 2 and 3);
2. highlight the challenges and limitations (see Chapter 4) and the best practices for development, adoption, and maintenance of AI tools (see Chapters 5 and 6);
3. understand the legal and regulatory landscape (see Chapter 7);
4. ensure equity, inclusion, and a human rights lens for this work; and
5. outline priorities for the field.

The authors of the eight chapters are experts convened by the National Academy of Medicine's Digital Health Learning Collaborative to explore the field of AI and its applications in health and health care, consider approaches for addressing existing challenges, and identify future directions and opportunities.

This final chapter synthesizes the challenges and priorities of the previous chapters, highlights current best practices, and identifies key priorities for the field.

SUMMARY OF CHALLENGES AND KEY PRIORITIES

This section summarizes the key findings and priorities of the prior chapters without providing the underlying evidence or more detailed background. Please refer to the referenced chapters for details.

Promote Data Access, Standardization, and Reporting of Data Quality, While Minimizing Data Bias

It is widely accepted that the successful development of an AI system requires high-quality, population-representative, and diverse data (Shrott, 2017; Sun et al., 2017). Figure 8-1 outlines a standardized pathway for the collection and integration of multiple data sources into a common data model, which efficiently feeds the transformation to a feature space for AI algorithm training. However, some of the standardization tools and data quality assessments and methodologies for curating the data do not yet exist. Interoperability is critical at all layers, including across the multivendor electronic health record and ancillary

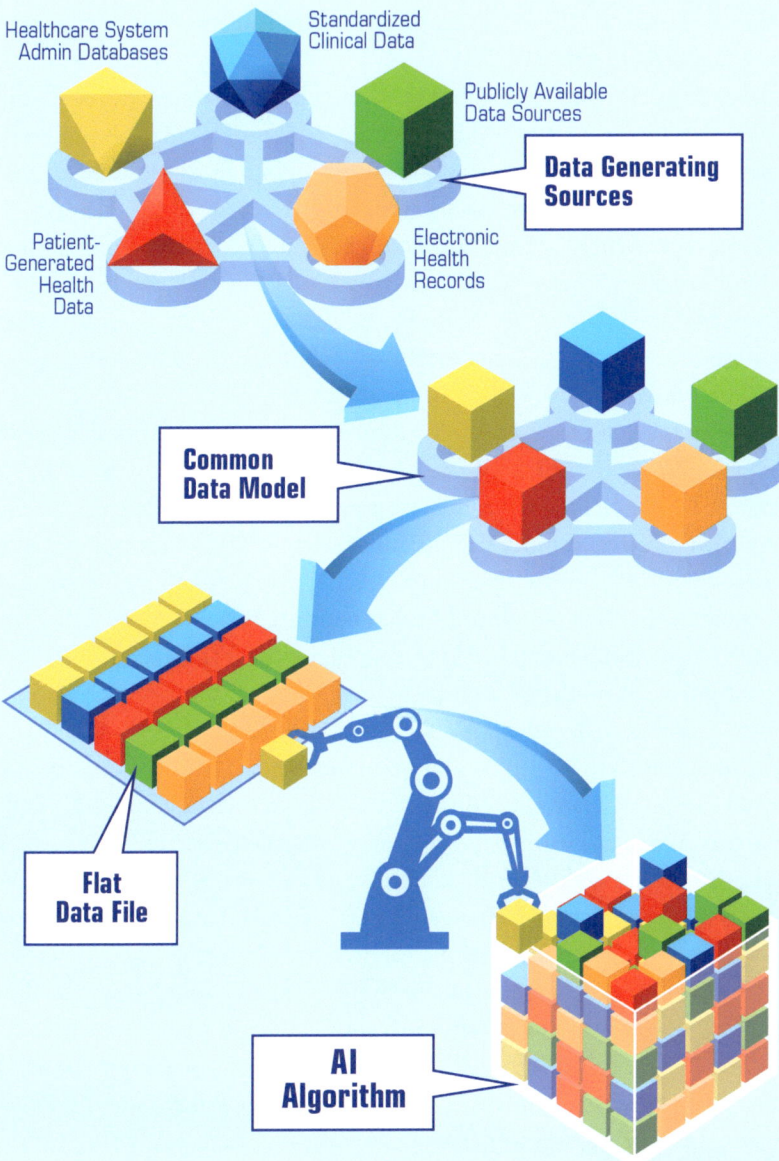

FIGURE 8-1 | Recommended data standardization framework to promote artificial intelligence system development from high-quality, transparent, and interoperable data.
SOURCE: Developed for this publication by Jay Christian Design.

components of a health care system, between different health care systems, and with consumer health applications. We cannot disregard the fact that there are varying data requirements for the training of AI and for the downstream use of AI. Some initiatives do exist and are driving the health care community in the direction of interoperability and data standardization, but they have yet to see widespread use (HL7, 2018; Indiana Health Information Exchange, 2019; NITRD et al., 2019; OHDSI, 2019).

Methods to assess data validity and reproducibility are often ad hoc. Ultimately, for AI models to be trusted, the semantics and provenance of the data used to derive them must be fully transparent, unambiguously communicated, and available, for validation at least, to an independent vetting agent. This is a distinct element of transparency, and the conflation of data transparency with algorithmic transparency complicates the AI ecosystem's discourse. We suggest a clear separation of these topics. One example of a principles declaration that promotes data robustness and quality is the FAIR (findability, accessibility, interoperability, and reusability) Principles (Wilkinson et al., 2016).

These principles, put forth by molecular biology and bioinformatics researchers, are not easily formalized or implemented. However, for health care AI to mature, a similar set of principles should be developed and widely adopted.

The health care community should continue to advocate for policy, regulatory, and legislative mechanisms that improve the ease of data aggregation. These would include (but are not limited to) a national patient health care identifier and mechanisms to responsibly bring together data from multiple sources. The debate should focus on the thoughtful and responsible ability of large-scale health care data resources to serve as a public good and the implications of that ability. Discussions around wider and more representative data access should be carefully balanced by stronger outreach, education, and consensus building with the public and patients in order to address where and how their data can be reused for AI research, data monetization, and other secondary uses; which entities can reuse their data; and what safeguards need to be in place. In a recent commentary, Glenn Cohen and Michelle Mello propose that "it is timely to reexamine the adequacy of the Health Insurance Portability and Accountability Act (HIPAA), the nation's most important legal safeguard against unauthorized disclosure and use of health information. Is HIPAA up to the task of protecting health information in the 21st century?" (Cohen and Mello, 2018).

When entities bring data sources together, they face ethical, business, legislative, and technical hurdles. There is a need for novel solutions that allow for robust data aggregation while promoting transparency and respecting patient privacy and preferences.

Prioritize Equitable and Inclusive Health Care

In addition, these solutions need to be equitable to avoid a potential conundrum (see Chapters 1 and 4) in which patients, especially those who are the least AI-savvy, are unaware of how their data are monetized. "That which is measured, improves," opined Karl Pearson, famed statistician and founder of mathematical statistics. Therefore, prioritizing equity and inclusion should be a clearly stated goal when developing and deploying AI in health care. It is imperative for developers and implementers to consider the data used to develop AI tools and unpack the underlying biases in that data. It is also essential to consider how the tool should be deployed, and whether the range of deployment environments could impact equity and inclusivity. There are widely recognized inequities in health outcomes due to the social determinants of health (BARHII, 2015) and the perverse incentives in existing health care systems (Rosenthal, 2017).

Unfortunately, consumer-facing technologies have often exacerbated historical inequities in other fields, and the digital divide continues to be a reality for wearables deployment and the data-hungry plans they require, even if the initial cost of the device is subsidized. As Cathy O'Neil reported in *Weapons of Math Destruction,* AI and related sciences can exacerbate inequity on a monumental scale. The impact of a single biased human is far less than that of a global or national AI (O'Neil, 2017).

Data transparency is key to ensuring AI adopters can assess the underlying data for biases and to consider whether the data are representative of the population in which the AI tool will be deployed. The United States has some population-representative datasets, such as national claims data, and high levels of data capture in certain markets (such as the Indiana Health Information Exchange). But, in many instances AI is being developed with data that are not population-representative, and while there are efforts to link health care data to the social determinants of health, environmental, and social media data to obtain a comprehensive profile of a person, this is not routine. Nor are there ethical or legal frameworks for doing so. It is imperative that we develop and standardize approaches for evaluating and reporting on data quality and representativeness. It is equally vital that we ensure and report on the diversity of gender, race, age, and other human characteristics of AI development teams to benefit from their much-needed diverse knowledge and life experiences (see Chapters 1 and 5).

Executing and delivering on equity and inclusion will require a new governance framework. Current self-governance efforts by technology companies are plagued with numerous struggles and failures, Google's April 2019 Ethics Board dissolution being one recent example (Piper, 2019). Mark Latonero suggests, "In order for

AI to benefit the common good, at the very least its design and deployment should avoid harms to fundamental human values. International human rights provide a robust and global formulation of those values" (Latonero, 2018).

For objective governance, a new neutral agency or a committee within an existing governmental or nongovernmental entity, supported by a range of stakeholders, could own and manage the review of health care AI products and services while protecting developers' intellectual property rights. One example of this type of solution is the New Model for Industry–Academic Partnerships, which developed a framework for academic access to industry (Facebook) data sources: The group with full access to the data is separate from the group doing the publishing, but both are academic, independent, and trusted. The group with full access executes the analytics and verifies the data, understands the underlying policies and issues, and delivers the analysis to a separate group who publishes the results but does not have open access to the data (Social Science Research Council, 2019). To ensure partisan neutrality, the project is funded by ideologically diverse supporters, including the Laura and John Arnold Foundation, the Democracy Fund, the William and Flora Hewlett Foundation, the John S. and James L. Knight Foundation, the Charles Koch Foundation, the Omidyar Network, and the Alfred P. Sloan Foundation. Research projects use this framework when researchers use Facebook social media data for election impact analysis, and Facebook provides the data required for the research but does not have the right to review or approve the research findings prior to publication.

Perhaps the best way to ensure that equity and inclusion are foundational components of a thriving health care system is to add them as a dimension to the quadruple aim, expanding it to a Quintuple Aim for health and health care: better health, improved care experience, clinician well-being, lower cost, and health equity throughout (see Figure 8-2).

Promote a Spectrum of Transparency-Based Trust, Based on Considerations of Accuracy, Risk, and Liability

A key challenge to the acceptance and widespread use of AI is the tension between data and algorithmic transparency, accuracy, perceived risk, and tort liability. One of the priorities identified in this publication is the need to present each health care AI tool along with the spectrum of transparency related to the potential harms and context of its use. Evaluating and addressing appropriate transparency in each subdomain of data, algorithms, and performance, and systematically reporting it must be a priority. In addition, health system leaders must understand the return on investment and the risks and benefits of adoption,

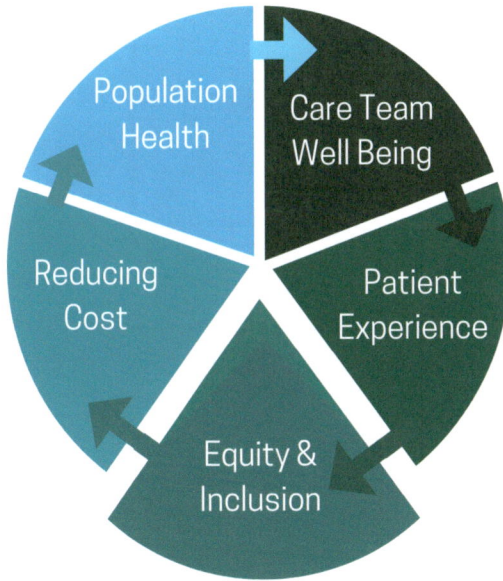

FIGURE 8-2 | The Quintuple Aim to ensure equity and inclusion are stated and measured goals when designing and deploying health care interventions.

including the risks of adverse events post-implementation; and informatics implementers must understand the culture and workflows where AI tools will be used so the algorithms can be adjusted to reflect their needs. All stakeholders should prioritize equity and inclusion, requiring transparency on how AI tools are monitored and updated. Many of these are shared, not siloed, responsibilities.

In all cases, the transparency of the underlying data used for AI model generation should be endorsed. While granular, patient-level data should not be publicly shared, publishing information on the data sources from which they were aggregated; how the data were transformed; data quality issues; inclusion and exclusion criteria that were applied to generate the cohort; summary statistics of demographics; and relevant data features in each source should be conventional practice. This information could be a supporting document and would tremendously improve the current understanding of and trust in AI tools.

The need for algorithmic transparency is largely dependent on the use context. For applications that have immediate clinical impact on patient quality of life or health outcomes, the baseline requirement for transparency is high. However, the level of transparency could be different depending on the (1) known precision accuracy of the AI; (2) clarity of recommended actions to end users; (3) risk to the patient or target; and (4) legal liability. For example, if an AI tool has high-precision accuracy and low risk, provides clear recommendations to the

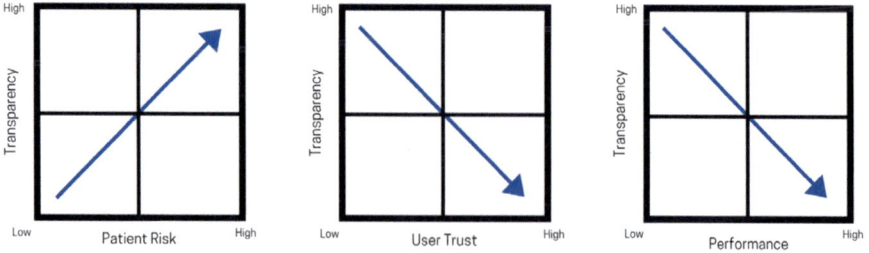

Context-Dependent Transparency Requirements

Example 1: Probabilistic CDS Treatment (High Risk)			
USERS	DATA	MODELING	OUTPUTS
Regulatory	High	Low	High
Clinical	High	Variable	High
Administrative	---	---	---
Patient	Variable	Low	High

Example 2: Population Surveillance for Appointment No-Show Rates			
USERS	DATA	MODELING	OUTPUTS
Regulatory	High	Low	Moderate
Clinical	High	Low	High
Administrative	High	Low	High
Patient	High	Low	High

FIGURE 8-3 | Summary of relationships between requirements for transparency and the three axes of patient risk, user trust, and algorithm performance within three key domains: data transparency, algorithmic transparency, and product/output transparency.

NOTE: While not comprehensive, examples of how different users and use cases require different levels of transparency in each of these three domains.

end user, and is unlikely to impose legal liability on the institution, manufacturer, or end user, then the need for complete algorithmic transparency is likely to be lower. See Figure 8-3 for additional details on the relationships of transparency and these axes within different conceptual domains.

Focus of Near-Term Health Care AI: Augmented Intelligence Versus Full Automation

Although some AI applications for health care business operations are likely to be poised for full automation, most of the near-term dialogue around AI in health care should focus on promoting, developing, and evaluating tools that support human cognition rather than replacing it. Popular culture and marketing have overloaded the term "AI" to the point where it means replacing human labor, and as a result, other terms have emerged to distinguish AI that is used to support human cognition. Augmented intelligence refers to the latter, which is the term the authors of this chapter endorse.

The opportunity for augmenting human cognition is vast, from supporting clinicians with less training in performing tasks currently limited to specialists to filtering out normal or low-acuity clinical cases so specialists can work at the top of their licensure. Additionally, AI could help humans reduce medical error due to cognitive limits, inattention, micro-aggression, or fatigue. In the case of surgery, it might offer capabilities that are not humanly possible.

Opportunities exist for automating some business processes, and greater automation is possible as the field matures in accuracy and trust. But it would not be prudent to deploy fully automated AI tools that could result in inaccuracy when the public has an understandably low tolerance for error, and health care AI lacks needed regulation and legislation. This is most likely to create a third AI Winter or a trough of disillusionment as seen in the Gartner Hype Cycle (see Chapter 4).

Differential levels of automation are even more relevant to consumer health applications because they are likely to have more automation components, but are regulated as entertainment applications, and their standards and quality controls are much more variable. The quandaries here are perhaps even more dire given consumer health applications' widespread use and the difficulties of tracking and surveilling potential harms that could result from their use in the absence of expert oversight.

Develop Appropriate Professional Health Training and Educational Programs to Support Health Care AI

Stanford Univerity's Curt Langlotz, offered the following question and answer: "Will AI ever replace radiologists? I say the answer is no—but radiologists who use AI will replace radiologists who don't" (Stanford University, 2017).

In order to sustain and nurture health care AI, we need a sweeping, comprehensive expansion of relevant professional health education focused on data science, AI, medicine, humanism, ethics, and health care. This expansion must be multidisciplinary and engage AI developers, implementers, health care system leadership, frontline clinical teams, ethicists, humanists, and patients and "fRamilies," because each brings essential expertise and AI progress is contingent on knowledgeable decision makers balancing the conflicting pressures of the relative ease of implementing newly developed AI solutions while understanding their validity and influence on care.

To begin addressing challenges, universities such as the Massachusetts Institute of Technology, Harvard, Stanford, and The University of Texas have added new courses focused on the embedding ethics into their development process.

Mehran Sahami, a Stanford University computer science faculty member who formerly worked at Google as a senior research scientist said, "Technology is not neutral. The choices that get made in building technology then have social ramifications" (Singer, 2018).

Health care professionals have requirements for continuing education as part of their scope of practice; we suggest that new continuing education AI curricula be developed and delivered. Some important topics that should be covered are how to (1) assess the need, validity, and applicability of AI algorithms in clinical care; (2) understand algorithmic performance and the impact on downstream clinical use; (3) navigate medical liability and the ways in which AI tools may impact individual and institutional liability and medical error; (4) advocate for standardization and appropriate transparency for a given use case; (5) discuss emerging AI technologies, their use, and their dependence on patient data with patients and "fRamilies" and the patient–clinician relationship; (6) ensure the Quintuple Aim of equity and inclusion when measuring impact; and (7) know when and how to bring in AI experts for consults. As the field evolves, the nature and emphasis of these topics will change, necessitating periodic review and updating.

Professional health education should incorporate how to critically evaluate the utility and risk of these AI tools in clinical practice. Curricula should provide an understanding of how AI tools are developed, the criteria and considerations for the use of AI tools, how best to engage and use such tools while prioritizing patient needs, and when human oversight is needed.

For health care system leadership and AI implementers, it is important to have training on the importance and lenses of the multiple disciplines that must be brought together to evaluate, deploy, and maintain AI in health care.

Current clinical training programs bear the weight of growing scientific knowledge within a static time window of training. We recognize the impracticality of each clinician or team being an expert on all things health care–AI related. Instead, we propose that each team has a basic and relevant understanding as described and adds an AI consult when and where needed. Such consults could be done virtually, supporting the team effort and group decision making, and costing less than if they were done onsite. Regional or content-expert AI consults could be leveraged across many health care systems. One example of such regional consults is the National Institutes of Health–funded Undiagnosed Diseases Network (UDN), which seeks "to improve and accelerate diagnosis of rare and undiagnosed conditions (NIH, 2019). The UDN uses both basic and clinical research to improve the level of diagnosis and uncover the underlying disease mechanisms associated with these conditions." National (or global) efforts like this can support the building and deployment of responsible AI solutions for health care.

It is necessary to develop retraining programs to target job categories that are likely to be the most susceptible to a shift in desired skill sets with AI deployment. It is unlikely that many health care jobs will be lost, but skill and knowledge mismatches are to be expected (see Chapter 4).

Articulate Success Factors for the Development, Adoption, and Maintenance of AI in Health Care

In order to implement AI tools in health care settings with sustained success, it is important that system leadership, AI developers, AI implementers, regulators, humanists, and patients and "fRamilies" collaboratively build a shared understanding and expectations. The success factors for development, adoption, and maintenance of AI tools will need clarity, acknowledging that practices will differ depending on the physical, psychological, or legal risk to the end user, the adoption setting, the level of augmentation versus automation, and other considerations. Dissonance between levels of success and users' expectations of impact and utility are likely to create harm and disillusionment. Below, we summarize the key components that must be wrangled.

The global health care AI community must develop integrated best-practice frameworks for AI implementation and maintenance, balancing ethical inclusivity, software development, implementation science, and human–computer interaction. These frameworks should be developed within the context of the learning health care system and can be tied to various targets and objectives. Earlier chapters provide summaries and considerations for both technical development (see Chapter 5) and health care system implementation (see Chapter 6). However, the AI implementation and deployment domain is still in a nascent stage, and health systems should maintain appropriate skepticism about the advertised benefits of health care AI.

It is important to approach health care AI as one of many tools for supporting the health and well-being of patients. Thus, AI should be deployed to address real problems that need solving, and only among those problems in which a simpler or more basic solution is inadequate. The complexity of AI has a very real cost to health care delivery environments.

Health care AI could go beyond the current limited, biology-focused research to address individual patient and communal needs. The current medical enterprise is largely focused on the tip of the iceberg (i.e., human biology), lacking meaningful and usable access to relevant patient contexts such as social determinants of health and psychosocial risk factors. AI solutions have the potential (with appropriate consent) to link personal and public data for truly personalized health care.

The April 2019 collaborative effort by UnitedHealthcare and the American Medical Association to create nearly two dozen *International Classification of Diseases, Tenth Revision*, codes to better incorporate social determinants of health into health care delivery is a laudable and responsible step in the right direction (Commins, 2019).

AI should be considered where scale is important and resources are insufficient for current needs. Some of these environments include complex patients with multiple comorbid conditions, such as chronic disease sufferers and the elderly, or low-resource settings. For innovative telehealth—disaster relief and rural areas—when resources are limited and access difficult, triaging or auto-allocating resources can be powered by AI solutions. Current mobile technology allows for critical imaging at the local site, and the U.S. Department of Veterans Affairs has operationalized a robust telehealth program that serves its very diverse population (VA, 2016).

We strongly suggest that a robust and mature underlying information technology governance strategy be in place within health care delivery systems prior to embarking on substantial AI deployment and integration. The needs for on- or offsite hardware infrastructure, change management, inclusive stakeholder engagement, and safety monitoring all require substantial established resources. Systems that do not possess these infrastructure components should develop them before significant AI deployment.

Balancing Regulation and Legislation for Health Care Innovation

The regulatory and legislative considerations for AI use in consumer and professional health care domains are documented in Chapter 7. AI applications have great potential to improve patient health but could also pose significant risks, such as inappropriate patient risk assessment, treatment recommendations, privacy breaches, and other harms (Evans and Whicher, 2018). Overall, the field is advancing rapidly, with a constant evolution of access to data, aggregation of data, new developments in AI methods, and expansions of how and where AI is added to patient health and health care delivery. Regulators should remain flexible, but the potential for lagging legislation remains an issue.

In alignment with recent congressional and U.S. Food and Drug Administration developments and guidance, we suggest a graduated approach to the regulation of AI based on the level of patient risk, the level of AI autonomy, and how static or dynamic certain AI tools are likely to be. To the extent that machine learning–based models continuously learn from new data, regulators should adopt postmarket surveillance mechanisms to ensure continuing (and ideally, improving)

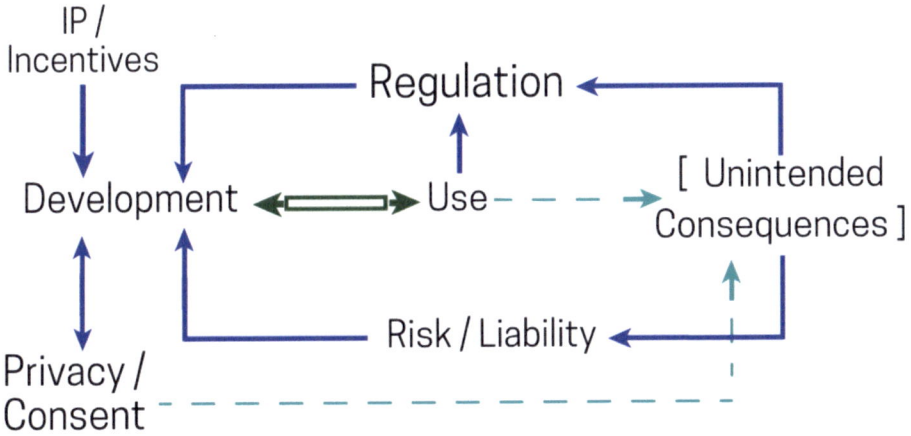

IP /
Incentives

Regulation

Development ⟷ Use

[Unintended
Consequences]

Privacy /
Consent

Risk / Liability

FIGURE 8-4 | Relationship between regulation and risk.

high-quality performance. Liability accrued within the deployment of various contexts of AI will continue to be a developing area as regulators, courts, and the insurance industry weigh in. Understanding regulation and liability is essential to evaluating risks and benefits.

The linkages between innovation, safety, progress, and regulation are complex. Regulators should engage in collaborative efforts with stakeholders and experts to continuously evaluate deployed clinical AI for effectiveness and safety based on real-world data. Throughout that process, transparency can help deliver well-vetted solutions. To enable both AI development and oversight, governmental agencies should invest in infrastructure that promotes wider data collection and access to data resources for building AI solutions, within a framework of equity and data protection (see Figure 8-4).

The Global Conundrum

The United States and many other nations prioritize human rights values and are appropriately measured and thoughtful in supporting data collection, AI development, and AI deployment. Other nations, with China and Russia being prime examples, have different priorities. The current AI arms race in all fields, including and beyond health care, creates a complex and, some argue, untenable geopolitical state of affairs (Apps, 2019). Others point out that it is not an AI arms race because interdependencies and interconnections among nations are needed to support research and innovation. Regardless, Kai Fu Lee outlines China's competitive edge in AI in his 2018 book *AI Superpowers: China, Silicon Valley, and the New World Order* (Lee, 2018). Putin has also outlined a national

AI strategy. And in February 2019, the White House issued an Executive Order on Maintaining American Leadership in Artificial Intelligence (White House, 2019). The downstream implications of this AI arms race in health care raise questions and conundrums this publication does not cover. We acknowledge they are countless and should be investigated.

CONCLUSIONS

AI is poised to make transformative and disruptive advances in health care and could improve the lives of patients, "fRamilies" and health care professionals. However, we cannot start with an AI hammer in our hands and view every problem as the proverbial nail. When balancing the need for thoughtful, inclusive health care AI that plans for and actively manages and reduces potential unintended consequences while not yielding to marketing hype, we should be guided by the adage "haste makes waste" (Sample, 2019). The wisest guidance for AI is to start with real problems in health care that need solving, explore the best solutions for the problem by engaging relevant stakeholders, frontline users, and patients and their "fRamilies"—including AI and non-AI options—and implement and scale the ones that meet the Quintuple Aim.

In *21 Lessons for the 21st Century*, Yuval Noah Harari writes, "Humans were always far better at inventing tools than using them wisely" (Harari, 2018, p. 7).

It is up to us, the stakeholders, experts, and users of these technologies, to ensure that they are used in an equitable and appropriate fashion to uphold the human values that inspired their creation—that is, better health and wellness for all.

REFERENCES

Apps, P. 2019. Are China, Russia winning the AI arms race? *Reuters*. https://www.reuters.com/article/apps-ai/column-are-china-russia-winning-the-ai-arms-race-idINKCN1PA08Y (accessed May 13, 2020).

BARNII (Bay Area Regional Health Inequities Initiative). 2015. *Framework*. http://barhii.org/framework (accessed May 13, 2020).

Cohen, G., and M. Mello. 2018. HIPAA and protecting health information in the 21st century. *JAMA* 320(3):231–232. https://doi.org/10.1001/jama.2018.5630.

Commins, J. 2019. UnitedHealthcare, AMA push new ICS-10 codes for social determinants of health. *HealthLeaders*. https://www.healthleadersmedia.com/clinical-care/unitedhealthcare-ama-push-new-icd-10-codes-social-determinants-health (accessed May 13, 2020).

Evans, E. L., and D. Whicher. 2018. What should oversight of clinical decision support systems look like? *AMA Journal of Ethics* 20(9):857–863.

Harari, Y. N. 2018. *21 Lessons for the 21st century.* New York: Random House.

HL7 (Health Level Seven). 2018. *Fast healthcare interoperability resources.* https://www.hl7.org/fhir (accessed May 13, 2020).

Indiana Health Information Exchange. 2019. https://www.ihie.org (accessed May 13, 2020).

Latonero, M. 2018. Governing artificial intelligence: Upholding human rights & dignity. *Data & Society*, October.

Lee, K. F. 2018. *AI superpowers: China, Silicon Valley, and the new world order.* New York: Houghton Mifflin Harcourt.

NIH (National Institutes of Health). 2019. *Undiagnosed diseases network.* https://commonfund.nih.gov/diseases (accessed May 13, 2020).

NITRD (Networking and Information Technology Research and Development), NCO (National Coordination Office), and NSF (National Science Foundation). 2019. Notice of workshop on artificial intelligence & wireless spectrum: Opportunities and challenges. Notice of workshop. *Federal Register* 84(145):36625–36626.

OHDSI (Observational Health Data Sciences and Informatics). 2019. https://ohdsi.org.

O'Neil, C. 2017. *Weapons of math destruction: How big data increases inequality and threatens democracy.* New York: Broadway Books.

Piper, K. 2019. Exclusive: Google cancels AI ethics board in response to outcry. *Vox.* https://www.vox.com/future-perfect/2019/4/4/18295933/google-cancels-ai-ethics-board?_hsenc=p2ANqtz-81fkloDdAtmNyGvd-pgT9QxeQEtzEGXeQCEi6Kr1BXZ5cLT8AFGx7wh_24vigoA-QP9p0CLTRvbpnI85nEsONPzEvwUQ&_hsmi=71485114 (accessed May 13, 2020).

Rosenthal, E. 2017. *An American sickness: How healthcare became big business and how you can take it back.* London, UK: Penguin Press.

Sample, I. 2019. Scientists call for global moratorium on gene editing of embryos. *The Guardian.* https://www.theguardian.com/science/2019/mar/13/scientists-call-for-global-moratorium-on-crispr-gene-editing?utm_term=RWRpdG9yaWFsX0d1YXJkaWFuVG9kYYlVUy0xOTAzMTQ%3D&utm_source=esp&utm_medium=Email&utm_campaign=GuardianTodayUS&CMP=GTUS_email (accessed May 13, 2020).

Shrott, R. 2017. Deep learning specialization by Andrew Ng—21 lessons learned. *Medium.* https://towardsdatascience.com/deep-learning-specialization-by-andrew-ng-21-lessons-learned-15ffaaef627c (accessed May 13, 2020).

Singer, N. 2018. Tech's ethical "dark side": Harvard, Stanford and others want to address it. *The New York Times.* https://www.nytimes.com/2018/02/12/business/computer-science-ethics-courses.html (accessed May 13, 2020).

Social Science Research Council. 2019. *Social data initiative: Overview: SSRC.* https://www.ssrc.org/ programs/view/social-data-initiative/#overview (accessed May 13, 2020).

Stanford University. 2017. RSNA 2017: Rads who use AI will replace rads who don't. *Center for Artificial Intelligence in Medicine & Imaging.* https://aimi.stanford. edu/about/news/rsna-2017-rads-who-use-ai-will-replace-rads-who-don-t (accessed May 13, 2020).

Sun, C., A. Shrivastava, S. Singh, and A. Gupta. 2017. Revisiting unreasonable effectiveness of data in deep learning era. *arXIV.* https://arxiv.org/pdf/ 1707.02968.pdf (accessed May 13, 2020).

White House. 2019. Executive Order on Maintaining American Leadership in Artificial Intelligence. *Executive orders: Infrastructure & technology.* https://www. whitehouse.gov/presidential-actions/executive-order-maintaining-american-leadership-artificial-intelligence (accessed May 13, 2020).

Wilkinson, M. D., M. Dumontier, I. J. Aalbersberg, G. Appleton, M. Axton, A. Baak, N. Blomberg, J. W. Boiten, L. B. da Silva Santos, P. E. Bourne, and J. Bouwman. 2016. *The FAIR Guiding Principles for scientific data management and stewardship.* Scientific Data 3.

VA (U.S. Department of Veterans Affairs). 2016. *Veteran population projections 2017–2037.* https://www.va.gov/vetdata/docs/Demographics/New_Vetpop_Model/Vetpop_Infographic_Final31.pdf (accessed May 13, 2020).

Suggested citation for Chapter 8: Matheny, M., S. Thadaney Israni, D. Whicher, and M. Ahmed. 2020. Artificial intelligence in health care: Hope not hype, promise not peril. In *Artificial intelligence in health care: The hope, the hype, the promise, the peril.* Washington, DC: National Academy of Medicine.

Appendix A

ADDITIONAL KEY REFERENCE MATERIALS

Author(s)	Title	Content Summary
Jonathan Bush and Stephen Baker	*Where Does It Hurt?*	This book deals with some of the challenges in health care and promotes disruptive technology as a way to improve and transform health care delivery.
Atul Gawande	*Being Mortal: Medicine and What Matters in the End*	This book includes information about geriatric care, assisted living, nursing home care, and hospice care.
Jerome Groopman	*How Doctors Think*	This book describes and discusses the clinical provider's mindset, workflow, and biases they sometimes bring to interactions with patients.
James R. Knickman and Brian Elbel	*Jonas & Kovner's Health Care Delivery in the United States, 12th Edition*	This health care textbook targets postgraduate education and provides a survey of health care in the United States with topics including population health, health care cost, health information technology, and financing.
T. R. Reid	*The Healing of America: A Global Quest for Better, Cheaper, and Fairer Health Care*	This book discusses health care in the global context, with examples of universal health care in other industrialized countries and comparisons made to the U.S. system.
Elizabeth Rosenthal	*An American Sickness: How Healthcare Became Big Business and How You Can Take It Back*	This book describes the for-profit U.S. health care system and the history of how it has evolved into what it is today.
Leiyu Shi and Douglas A. Singh	*Essentials of the U.S. Health Care System*	This book is targeted to post-secondary students interested in or pursuing training in health disciplines and describes the impact of the Patient Protection and Affordable Care Act, implementation of *Healthy People 2020*, and the Health Information Technology for Economic and Clinical Health Act. It also covers clinical provider workforce challenges, health disparities, and access-to-care issues.

continued

Author(s)	Title	Content Summary
Mark D. Shipley	*In Search of Good Medicine: Hospital Marketing Strategies to Engage Healthcare Consumers*	This book includes a discussion of the organization and management of health care organizations and how they market care to the public.
Eric Topol	*The Patient Will See You Now*	This book discusses how technology and the digitization of data can be leveraged to improve care and patient health.
Fred Trotter and David Uhlman	*Hacking Healthcare: A Guide to Standards, Workflows, and Meaningful Use*	This book summarizes some of the key issues in the U.S. health care system with regard to the adoption of electronic health records and other health information technology issues that surround its adoption.

Appendix B

WORKSHOP AGENDA AND PARTICIPANT LIST

National Academy of Medicine Digital Learning Collaborative

November 30, 2017
National Academy of Sciences Building
Room 120
2101 Constitution Avenue, NW
Washington, DC 20418

Meeting Focus: Artificial intelligence and the future of continuous health learning and improvement.

Meeting Objectives:
1. *Aim:* Consider the nature, elements, applications, state of play, and implications of artificial intelligence (AI) and machine learning (ML) in health and health care, and ways the National Academy of Medicine might enhance collaborative progress.
2. *AI/ML opportunities:* Identify and discuss areas within health and health care for which AL and ML have already shown promise. Consider implications for other applications.
3. *Barriers:* Identify and discuss the practical challenges to the advancement and application of AI and ML, including those related to data integration, ethical/regulatory implications, clinician acceptance, workforce development, and business case considerations.

Outcomes Intended: Establishment of a charge and charter for an ongoing NAM Collaborative Working Group for information sharing and facilitating the application of AI and ML for better health.

8:30 a.m.   Coffee and light breakfast available

9:00 a.m.   Welcome, introductions, and meeting overview

Welcome from the National Academy of Medicine
Michael McGinnis, National Academy of Medicine

Opening remarks and meeting overview by Collaborative co-chairs
Jonathan Perlin, Hospital Corporation of America, Inc.
Reed Tuckson, Tuckson Health Connections, LLC

9:30 a.m.   Artificial intelligence and machine learning: Terms and definitions

A "big picture" presentation on the AI/ML field and initial reflections on health applications.
Carla Brodley, Northeastern University
Q&A and *Open Discussion*

10:15 a.m.   Break

10:30 a.m.   Strategies to enhance data integration to advance AI/ML

This session will focus on the role of data integration and sharing in enhancing the capabilities of machine learning algorithms to improve health and health care.
Noel Southall, National Institutes of Health
Douglas McNair, Cerner Corporation
Jonathan Perlin and Edmund Jackson, Hospital Corporation of America, Inc.
James Fackler, Johns Hopkins Medicine
Q&A and Open Discussion

11:45 a.m.   Break

Participants will pick up lunch.

12:00 p.m.   AI/ML opportunities in health and health care

The lunch session will focus on the areas of health care where machine learning has the potential to improve patient outcomes, including opportunities for better, faster, cheaper diagnosis, treatment, prevention, self and family care, service linkages, and etiologic insights.

Paul Bleicher, OptumLabs
Steve Fihn, University of Washington
Daniel Fabbri, Vanderbilt University
Tim Estes, Digital Reasoning
Q&A and Open Discussion

1:15 p.m.   Practical challenges for AI/ML development, spread, and scale

Participants will explore the practical challenges related to AI/ML development, spread, and scale, including developing the business case, addressing regulatory and ethical considerations, and improving clinician acceptance and workforce expertise.

Nigam Shah, Stanford University
Michael Matheny, Vanderbilt University
Seth Hain, Epic Systems
Q&A and Open Discussion

2:30 p.m.   The charge for accelerating progress

The aim of this session is to develop a charge and charter for an ongoing NAM AI/ML Collaborative Working Group. The charge will outline opportunities for the Working Group to address barriers and accelerate progress.

Sean Khozin, U.S. Food and Drug Administration
Javier Jimenez, Sanofi
Leonard D. Avolio, Cyft
Wendy Chapman, University of Utah
Q&A and Open Discussion

3:45 p.m.   Next steps

Comments from the chairs
Jonathan Perlin, Hospital Corporation of America, Inc.
Reed Tuckson, Tuckson Health Connections, LLC

Comments and thanks from the National Academy of Medicine
Michael McGinnis, National Academy of Medicine

4:00 p.m.   Adjourn

WORKSHOP ATTENDEES

Chairs:

Jonathan Perlin, MD, PhD, MSHA,
MACP, FACMI
Chief Medical Officer
Hospital Corporation of America

Reed Tuckson, MD, MD, FACP,
FACP
Managing Director
Tuckson Health Connections

Participants:

Carlos Blanco, MD, PhD
Director
Division of Epidemiology, Services
and Prevention Research (DESPR)
National Institute on Drug Abuse

Paul Bleicher, MD, PhD
Chief Executive Officer
OptumLabs

Carla Brodley, MS, PhD
Dean, College of Computer &
Information Science Professor
Northeastern University

Wendy Chapman, PhD
Chair, Department of Biomedical
Informatics
University of Utah

Jonathan Chen, MD, PhD
Assistant Professor of Biomedical
Informatics Research
Stanford University

Leonard D'Avolio, PhD
Founder and Chief Executive Officer
Cyft

Shahram Ebadollahi, MS, PhD
Vice President, Innovations & Chief
Science Officer
IBM Watson Health Group

Tim Estes
President and Founder
Digital Reasoning

Daniel Fabbri, PhD
Assistant Professor of Biomedical
Informatics
Vanderbilt University Medical Center

James Fackler, MD
Associate Professor
Director of Safety, Quality, &
Logistics in the PICU
John Hopkins Medicine

Steve Fihn, MD, MPH, FACP
Division Head, General Internal
Medicine Professor
University of Washington

Kenneth R. Gersing, MD
Informatics Director
National Center for Advancing
Translational Sciences
National Institutes of Health

Seth Hain, MS
Research & Development Product
    Lead, Machine Learning
Epic Systems

Michael Howell, MD, MPH
Chief Clinical Strategist
Google

Brigham Hyde, PhD
Chief Executive Officer
Precision Health Intelligence

Edmund Jackson, PhD
Chief Data Scientist
Hospital Corporation of America

Javier Jimenez, MD, MPH
Vice President, Global Head Real World
    Evidence & Clinical Outcomes
Sanofi

Sean Khozin, MD, MPH
Acting Associate Director, Oncology
    Center of Excellence
U.S. Food & Drug Administration

Hongfang Liu, MS, PhD
Professor of Biomedical Informatics
Mayo Clinic

Jennifer MacDonald, MD
Director of Clinical Innovations and
    Education
U.S. Department of Veterans Affairs

Michael E. Matheny, MD, MS, MPH
Associate Professor
Vanderbilt University

Douglas McNair, MD, PhD
President, Cerner Math Inc.
Cerner Corporation

Wendy Nilsen, PhD
Program Director
National Science Foundation

Matthew Quinn, MBA
Senior Advisor
Health Information Technology
Health Resources and Services
    Administration

Joachim Roski, PhD, MPH
Principal
Booz Allen Hamilton

Robert E. Samuel, DSc
Senior Director, Technology Strategy
    & Research
Aetna

Noel Southall, PhD
Leader, Informatics Division of Pre-
    Clinical Innovation
National Institutes of Health

Bob Tavares
Vice President, Business
    Development
Emmi Solutions

Sonoo Thadaney-Israni, MBA
Executive Director, Stanford Presence
    Center
Stanford Medicine

Howard Underwood, MD, MBA, MS, FSA
Vice President, Member Management Analytics
Anthem

Shawn Wang, MBA
Vice President, Data Science
Anthem

Daniel Yang, MD
Program Fellow, Patient Care
Moore Foundation

Maryan Zirkle, MD, MS, MA
Senior Program Officer
Patient-Centered Outcomes Research Institute

Observers and Web Participants:
Jia Chen, PhD
Technology Strategy, Watson Health Innovation
IBM Watson Health Group

Catherine Ordun, MPH, MBA
Senior Data Scientist
Booz Allen Hamilton

Nigam H. Shah, MBBS, PhD
Associate Professor of Medicine
Stanford University

Ernest Sohn, MS
Chief Data Scientist
Booz Allen Hamilton

David Sontag, PhD, SM
Principal Investigator, Computer Science & Artificial Intelligence Laboratory
Massachusetts Institute of Technology

National Academy of Medicine Staff:
Urooj Fatima
Senior Program Assistant
National Academy of Medicine

Emma Fine
Senior Program Assistant
National Academy of Medicine

Gwen Hughes
Senior Program Assistant
National Academy of Medicine

Danielle Whicher, PhD, MHS
Senior Program Officer
National Academy of Medicine

Michael McGinnis, MD, MPP
Executive Director, Leadership Consortium for a Value & Science-Driven Health System

Appendix C
AUTHOR BIOGRAPHIES

Mahnoor (Noor) Ahmed, MEng, is an associate program officer for the National Academy of Medicine's (NAM) Leadership Consortium: Collaboration for a Value & Science-Driven Learning Health System. She oversees work in the Leadership Consortium's science and evidence mobilization domains, which are respectively focused on advancing a robust digital infrastructure and promoting the systematic capture and application of real-world evidence in support of a learning health system. Prior to joining the NAM, Ms. Ahmed worked at the Center for Medical Interoperability and Hospital Corporation of America guiding the effective and ethical development and integration of technology in clinical practice. She holds a BA in neuroscience from Vanderbilt University and an ME in biomedical engineering from Duke University.

Andrew Auerbach MD, MPH, is a professor of medicine at the University of California, San Francisco (UCSF), School of Medicine in the Division of Hospital Medicine, where he is the chair of the Clinical Content Oversight Committee for UCSF Health, the operational group responsible for developing and implementing electronic health record tools across the UCSF Health enterprise. Dr. Auerbach is a widely recognized leader in hospital medicine, having authored or co-authored the seminal research describing effects of hospital medicine systems on patient outcomes, costs, and care quality. He leads a 13-hospital research collaborative focused on new discoveries in health care delivery models in acute care settings and continues an active research-mentoring program at UCSF. In addition, Dr. Auerbach serves as editor-in-chief of the *Journal of Hospital Medicine*, the flagship peer-reviewed publication for the field of hospital medicine. Dr. Auerbach's research has been published in prominent journals including the *New England Journal of Medicine, JAMA, Annals of Internal Medicine*, and *Archives of Internal Medicine*. He has received the Mack Lipkin

Award for outstanding research as a fellow and the Western Society for Clinical Investigation Outstanding Investigator award, and is a member of the American Society for Clinical Investigation.

Andrew Beam, PhD, is an assistant professor in the Department of Epidemiology at the Harvard T.H. Chan School of Public Health, with secondary appointments in the Department of Biomedical Informatics at the Harvard Medical School and the Department of Newborn Medicine at Brigham and Women's Hospital. His research develops and applies machine learning methods to extract meaningful insights from clinical and biological datasets, and he is the recipient of a Pioneer Award from the Robert Wood Johnson Foundation for his work on medical artificial intelligence. Previously he was a senior fellow at Flagship Pioneering and the founding head of machine learning at VL56, a Flagship-backed venture that seeks to use machine learning to improve our ability to engineer proteins. He earned his PhD in 2014 from North Carolina State University for work on Bayesian neural networks, and he holds degrees in computer science (BS), computer engineering (BS), electrical engineering (BS), and statistics (MS), also from North Carolina State University. He completed a postdoctoral fellowship in biomedical informatics at the Harvard Medical School and then served as a junior faculty member. Dr. Beam's group is principally concerned with improving, streamlining, and automating decision making in health care through the use of quantitative, data-driven methods. He does this through rigorous methodological research coupled with deep partnerships with physicians and other members of the health care workforce. As part of this vision, he works to see these ideas translated into decision-making tools that doctors can use to better care for their patients.

Paul Bleicher, MD, PhD, is a strategic advisor to OptumLabs. Dr. Bleicher was formerly the chief executive officer of OptumLabs since its inception. Prior to OptumLabs, he was the chief medical officer for Humedica, a next-generation clinical informatics company. He also co-founded and was a leader at Phase Forward, which was instrumental in transforming pharmaceutical clinical trials from paper to the web. Dr. Bleicher has served as a leader in industry organizations such as the National Academy of Medicine's Leadership Consortium for Value & Science-Driven Health Care and the Drug Information Association. He has received numerous awards for his industry leadership. Dr. Bleicher holds a BS from Rensselaer, as well as an MD and a PhD from the University of Rochester School of Medicine and Dentistry. He began his career as a physician/investigator and an assistant professor at the Massachusetts General Hospital and the Harvard Medical School.

Wendy Chapman, PhD, earned her bachelor's degree in linguistics and her PhD in medical informatics from the University of Utah in 2000. From 2000–2010, she was a National Library of Medicine (NLM) postdoctoral fellow and then a faculty member at the University of Pittsburgh. She joined the Division of Biomedical Informatics at the University of California, San Diego, in 2010. In 2013, Dr. Chapman became the chair of the University of Utah's Department of Biomedical Informatics. Dr. Chapman's research focuses on developing and disseminating resources for modeling and understanding information described in narrative clinical reports. She is interested not only in better algorithms for extracting information out of clinical text through natural language processing (NLP) but also in generating resources for improving the NLP development process (such as shareable annotations and open-source toolkits) and in developing user applications to help non–NLP experts apply NLP in informatics-based tasks like clinical research and decision support. She has been a principal investigator on several National Institutes of Health grants from the NLM, National Institute for Dental and Craniofacial Research, and the National Institute for General Medical Sciences. In addition, she has collaborated on multi-center grants, including the ONC SHARP Secondary Use of Clinical Data and the iDASH National Center for Biomedical Computing. Dr. Chapman is a principal investigator and a co-investigator on a number of U.S. Department of Veterans Affairs (VA) Health Services Research and Development grant proposals extending the development and application of NLP within the VA. A tenured professor at the University of Utah, Dr. Chapman continues her research in addition to leading the Department of Biomedical Informatics. Dr. Chapman is an elected fellow of the American College of Medical Informatics and currently serves as treasurer and was the previous chair of the American Medical Informatics Association Natural Language Processing Working Group.

Jonathan Chen, MD, PhD, practices medicine for the concrete rewards of caring for real people and to inspire research focused on discovering and distributing the latent knowledge embedded in clinical data. Dr. Chen co-founded a company to translate his computer science graduate work into an expert system for organic chemistry, with applications from drug discovery to an education tool for students around the world. To gain perspective tackling societal problems in health care, he completed training in internal medicine and a research fellowship in medical informatics. He has published influential work in the *New England Journal of Medicine, JAMA, JAMA Internal Medicine, Bioinformatics, Journal of Chemical Information and Modeling*, and the *Journal of the American Medical Informatics Associations*, with awards and recognition from the National Institutes of Health's Big Data 2 Knowledge initiative, the National Library of Medicine, the American

Medical Informatics Association, the Yearbook of Medical Informatics, and the American College of Physicians, among others. In the face of ever escalating complexity in medicine, informatics solutions are the only credible approach to systematically address challenges in health care. Tapping into real-world clinical data like electronic medical records with machine learning and data analytics will reveal the community's latent knowledge in a reproducible form. Delivering this back to clinicians, patients, and health care systems as clinical decision support will uniquely close the loop on a continuously learning health system. Dr. Chen's group seeks to empower individuals with the collective experience of the many, combining human and artificial intelligence approaches that will deliver better care than either can do alone.

Guilherme Del Fiol, MD, PhD, is currently an associate professor and the vice-chair of research in the University of Utah's Department of Biomedical Informatics. Prior to the University of Utah, Dr. Del Fiol held positions in clinical knowledge management at Intermountain Healthcare and as faculty at the Duke Community and Family Medicine Department. Since 2008, he has served as an elected co-chair of the Clinical Decision Support Work Group at Health Level International (HL7). He is also an elected fellow of the American College of Medical Informatics and a member of the Comprehensive Cancer Center at Huntsman Cancer Institute. Dr. Del Fiol's research interests are in the design, development, evaluation, and dissemination of standards-based clinical decision support interventions. He has been focusing particularly in clinical decision support for cancer prevention. He is the lead author of the HL7 Infobutton Standard and the project lead for OpenInfobutton, an open-source suite of infobutton tools and web services, which is in production use at several health care organizations throughout the United States, including Intermountain Healthcare, Duke University, and the Veterans Health Administration. His research has been funded by various sources including the National Library of Medicine, the National Cancer Institute, the Agency for Healthcare Research and Quality, the Centers for Medicare & Medicaid Services, and the Patient-Centered Outcomes Research Institute. He earned his MD from the University of Sao Paulo, Brazil; his MS in computer science from the Catholic University of Parana, Brazil; and his PhD in biomedical informatics from the University of Utah.

Hossein Estiri, PhD, is a research fellow with the Laboratory of Computer Science (LCS) and an informatics training fellow of the National Library of Medicine. Dr. Estiri's research involves designing data-driven systems for clinical decision making and health care policy. His recent work has focused on designing and developing visual analytics programs (VET, DQe-c, DQe-v, and DQe-p) to explore data quality in electronic health record (EHR) data. His research with LCS is focused on applying statistical learning techniques (Deep Learning and unsupervised clustering) and data science methodologies to design systems that characterize patients and evaluate EHR data quality. Dr. Estiri holds a PhD in urban planning and a PhD track in statistics from University of Washington. Prior to joining LCS, Dr. Estiri completed a 2-year postdoctoral fellowship with the University of Washington's Institute of Translational Health Sciences and Department of Biomedical Informatics.

James Fackler, MD, is an associate professor of anesthesiology and critical care medicine and pediatrics at the Johns Hopkins University School of Medicine. His areas of clinical expertise include acute respiratory distress syndrome, novel respiratory therapies, and signal fusion and monitoring. Dr. Fackler received his undergraduate degree in biology from the University of Illinois and earned his MD from Rush Medical College in Chicago. He completed his residency in anesthesiology and performed a fellowship in pediatric intensive care and pediatric anesthesia at the Johns Hopkins University School of Medicine. Dr. Fackler joined the Johns Hopkins faculty in 2006. He worked for the Cerner Corporation from 2002 to 2006 and left the position of vice president to return to academic medicine. He founded Oak Clinical Informatics Systems and consults for other device and information integration companies. Dr. Fackler's research interests include optimizing patient surgical services by analyzing mathematical models of patient flow through hospitals, on either a scheduled or an emergency basis. He serves as the editor for *Pediatric Critical Care Medicine* and as an ad hoc journal reviewer for many notable publications including *New England Journal of Medicine* and *Critical Care Medicine*. He is a member of the American Association of Artificial Intelligence, the American Medical Informatics Association, and the Society for Critical Care Medicine. Dr. Fackler is a frequent lecturer and panelist on the subject of critical care informatics. He is an expert in data integration.

Stephan Fihn, MD, MPH, attended St. Louis University School of Medicine and completed an internship, residency, and chief residency at the University of Washington (UW). He was a Robert Wood Johnson Foundation Clinical Scholar and earned a master's degree in public health at UW where he is professor of medicine and health services and the head of the Division of General Internal Medicine. During a 36-year career with the U.S. Department of Veterans Affairs (VA), Dr. Fihn held a number of clinical, research, and administrative positions. He directed one of the first primary care clinics in the VA and for 18 years led the Northwest VA Health Services Research & Development Center of Excellence at the Seattle VA. He also served several national roles in the Veterans Health Administration including acting chief research and development officer, chief quality and performance officer, director of analytics and business, and director of clinical system development and evaluation. His own research has addressed strategies for improving the efficiency and quality of primary and specialty medical care and understanding the epidemiology of common medical problems. He received the VA Undersecretary's Award for Outstanding Contributions in Health Services Research in 2002. He has published more than 300 scientific articles and book chapters and two editions of a textbook titled *Outpatient Medicine*. He is deputy editor of *JAMA Network Open*. He is active in several academic organizations including the Society of General Internal Medicine (SGIM) (past-president), the American College of Physicians (fellow), the American Heart Association (fellow), and AcademyHealth. He received the Elnora M. Rhodes Service Award and the Robert J. Glaser Award from SGIM.

Anna Goldenberg, MA, PhD, is a Russian-born computer scientist and an associate professor at the University of Toronto's Department of Computer Science and the Department of Statistics, a senior scientist at the Hospital for Sick Children's Research Institute, and the associate research director for health at the Vector Institute for Artificial Intelligence. She is the first chair in biomedical informatics and artificial intelligence at the Hospital for Sick Children. Dr. Goldenberg completed a master's in knowledge discovery and data mining, followed by a PhD in machine learning at Carnegie Mellon University in Pittsburgh, where her thesis explored scalable graphical models for social networks. Dr. Goldenberg moved to Canada in 2008 as a postdoctoral fellow. She is currently appointed as an associate professor at the University of Toronto's Department of Computer Science and the Department of Statistics and a scientist at the Hospital for Sick Children's Research Institute. Her laboratory explores how machine learning can be used to map the heterogeneity seen in various human diseases, specifically to develop methodologies to identify patterns in collected data and improve patient outcomes. She has more than 50 publications in peer-reviewed journals. Similarity Network Fusion, a networking method devised by her research group is the first data integration method developed to integrate patient data that improved survival outcome predictions in different cancers. She has an h-index of 17, and her research has been cited more than 2,000 times. In 2017, Dr. Goldenberg was appointed as a new Tier 2 CIHR-funded Canada Research Chair in Computational Medicine at the University of Toronto. On January 15, 2019, Dr. Goldenberg was named the first chair in biomedical informatics and artificial intelligence at the Hospital for Sick Children, which is the first of its kind to exist in a Canadian children's hospital.

This position is partially funded by a $1.75 million donation from Amar Varma (a Toronto entrepreneur whose newborn son underwent surgery at the Hospital for Sick Children).

Seth Hain, MS, leads Epic's analytics and machine learning research and development. This includes business intelligence tools, data warehousing software, and a foundational platform for deploying machine learning across Epic applications. Alongside a team of data scientists and engineers, he focuses on a variety of use cases ranging from acute care and population health to operations and improving workflow efficiency.

Jaimee Heffner, PhD, is a clinical psychologist who researches tobacco-cessation interventions for populations who experience health disparities, including people with mental health conditions, low-income veterans, and sexual and gender minorities. Much of her work focuses on new behavioral treatments such as acceptance and commitment therapy and behavioral activation. She develops methods to deliver these interventions—such as websites, smartphone apps, and other forms of technology—to improve the accessibility of treatment for all tobacco users. Her research interests also include implementation of tobacco-cessation interventions in the novel setting of lung cancer screening.

Sonoo Thadaney Israni, MBA, is an intrapreneur at Stanford University. She works with faculty leadership to thought partner and launches new centers, initiatives, academic programs, and more. Currently, she serves as the executive director for Dr. Abraham Verghese's portfolio, including a new center—Presence: The Art and Science of Human Connection in Medicine. She focuses on the intersection of technology, equity, and inclusion. Her intrapreneurial successes at Stanford include the MSc in Community Health and Prevention Research; the Stanford Women and Sex Differences in Medicine Center; the Diversity and First-Gen Office (serving Stanford students who are first in their family to attend college); the Restorative Justice Pilot; and more. She teaches coursework in leveraging conflict for constructive change, leadership skills, and mediation. Ms. Israni co-chairs the National Academy of Medicine's Artificial Intelligence in Healthcare Working Group and co-shepherds its Technology Across the Lifecourse Group. She also serves on the Association of American Medical Colleges Restorative Justice for Academic Medicine Committee teaching curricula to address diversity in health care. She spent more than 25 years in Silicon Valley before coming to Stanford University in 2008. Ms. Israni's academic work includes an MBA, a BA in psychology with minors in sociology and education, and a postbaccalaureate in mass communications. She is also a trained mediator and restorative justice practitioner for the State of California, serving as the co-chair of the Commission on Juvenile Delinquency and Prevention for San Mateo County.

Edmund Jackson, PhD, is the HCA Healthcare chief data scientist and the vice president of data and analytics within the Clinical Services Group. His education is a BscEng and MScEng, both in electronic engineering, followed by a PhD in statistical signal processing from Cambridge University. In that work, Dr. Jackson focused on applications of sequential Markov chain methods in bioinformatics. He pursued a career as a quantitative analyst in the hedge fund industry for several years. More recently, Dr. Jackson has sought more meaningful work and found it at HCA, where his remit is to create algorithms and systems to improve the quality of clinical care, operational efficiency, and financial performance of the firm through better utilization of data.

Jeffrey Klann, PhD, focuses his work with the Laboratory of Computer Science on knowledge discovery for clinical decision support, sharing medical data to improve population health, revolutionizing user interfaces, and making personal health records viable. Dr. Klann holds two degrees in computer science from the Massachusetts Institute of Technology and a PhD from Indiana University in health informatics. He completed a National Library of Medicine Research Training Fellowship concurrently with his PhD. He holds faculty appointments at the Harvard Medical School and Massachusetts General Hospital.

Rita Kukafka, DrPH, MA, FACMI, is a professor of biomedical informatics and sociomedical sciences at the Mailman School of Public Health at Columbia University. Dr. Kukafka received her bachelor's degree in health sciences from Brooklyn College, a master's degree in health education from New York University, and a doctorate in public health with a concentration in sociomedical sciences from the Mailman School of Public Health at Columbia University. Nearly a decade after receiving her doctorate, she returned to Columbia where she completed a National Library of Medicine postdoctoral fellowship, and received a master's degree in biomedical informatics. Having worked at public health agencies and academia, and leading large-scale population health interventions, she was convinced then and remains convinced that public health's "winnable battles" are amenable to informatics solutions. For the duration of her training to the present, Dr. Kukafka has been involved in leadership roles at the national level to influence the growth and direction of public health informatics. At Columbia, Dr. Kukafka holds joint appointments with the Department of Biomedical Informatics and the Mailman School of Public Health (sociomedical sciences). She served as the director of the graduate training program from 2008 to 2013.

She is also the director of the Health Communication and Informatics Laboratory at the Department of Biomedical Informatics and certificate lead for Public Health Informatics at Mailman. Her research interests focus on patient and community engagement technologies, risk communication, decision science, and implementation of health promoting and disease prevention technologies into clinical workflow. Her projects include developing decision aids, portals for community engagement, requirement and usability evaluation, and mixed-method approaches to studying implementation and outcomes. Dr. Kukafka is an elected member of the American College of Medical Informatics and the New York Academy of Medicine. She has been an active contributor to the American Medical Informatics Association (AMIA), and is an AMIA board member. She has chaired the Consumer Health Informatics Working group for AMIA, and served on an Institute of Medicine committee that authored the report *Who Will Keep the Public Healthy?: Educating Public Health Professionals for the 21st Century.* Dr. Kukafka has authored more than 100 articles, chapters, and books in the field of biomedical informatics including a textbook (*Consumer Health Informatics: Informing Consumers and Improving Health Care,* 2005, with D. Lewis, G. Eysenbach, P. Z. Stavri, H. Jimison, and W.V. Slack. New York: Springer).

Hongfang Liu, PhD, is a professor of biomedical informatics in the Mayo Clinic College of Medicine, and is a consultant in the Department of Health Sciences Research at the Mayo Clinic. As a researcher, she is leading the Mayo Clinic's clinical natural language processing (NLP) program with the mission of providing support to access clinical information stored in unstructured text for research and practice. Administratively, Dr. Liu serves as the section head for Medical Informatics in the Division of Biomedical Statistics and Informatics. Dr. Liu's primary research interest is in biomedical NLP and data normalization. She has been developing a suite of open-source NLP systems for accessing clinical information, such as medications or findings from clinical notes. Additionally, she has been conducting collaborative research in the past decade in utilizing existing knowledge bases for high-throughput -omics profiling data analysis and functional interpretation. Dr. Liu's work in informatics has resulted in informatics systems that unlock clinical information stored in clinical narratives. Her work accelerates the pace of knowledge discovery, implementation, and delivery for improved health care.

Michael Matheny, MD, MS, MPH, is a practicing general internist and a medical informatician at Vanderbilt University and the Tennessee Valley Healthcare System of the U.S. Department of Veterans Affairs (VA). He received a BS in chemical engineering and an MD from the University of Kentucky, completed internal medicine residency training at St. Vincent's, Indianapolis, Indiana, and was a National Library of Medicine Biomedical Informatics Fellow at the Decision Systems Group at Brigham & Women's Hospital, Boston, Massachusetts, during which time he completed a master's degree in public health at Harvard University as well as a master's degree of science in biomedical informatics at the Massachusetts Institute of Technology. He has expertise in developing and adapting methods for postmarketing medical device surveillance, and has been involved in the development, evaluation, and validation of automated outcome surveillance statistical methods and computer applications. He is leading the OMOP extract, transform, and load team within VINCI for the national Veterans Health Administration data, and is a co-principal investigator for the pScanner CDRN Phase 2. He also is currently independently funded for two VA HSR&D IIR's in automated surveillance and data visualization techniques for acute kidney injury following cardiac catheterization and patients with cirrhosis. His key focus areas include natural language processing, data mining, and population health analytics as well as health services research in acute kidney injury, diabetes, and device safety in interventional cardiology.

Douglas McNair, MD, PhD, serves as a senior advisor in quantitative sciences—Analytics Innovation in Global Health at the Bill & Melinda Gates Foundation. He assists the foundation's research and development in drug and vaccine development for infectious diseases, childhood diseases, and neglected tropical diseases. Current projects include product development programs in discovery and translational sciences involving Bayesian networks. His activity also includes machine learning and modeling of health economics, collaborating with the Global Development division. Previously, Dr. McNair was the president of Cerner Math Inc., responsible for the artificial intelligence components of Cerner's electronic health record (EHR) solutions, discovering artificial intelligence predictive models from real-world de-identified EHR-derived big data. Dr. McNair is the lead inventor on more than 100 patents and pending patent applications, including several involving Bayesian predictive models for clinical diagnostics.

Eneida Mendonça, MD, PhD, received her MD from the Federal University of Pelotas in Brazil and her PhD in biomedical informatics in 2002 from Columbia University in New York. Dr. Mendonça pioneered the use of natural language processing in both biomedical literature and in electronic medical record narratives in order to identify knowledge relevant to medical decision making in the context of patient care. In addition, she has devoted many years to developing innovative clinical information systems that have been integrated in New York-Presbyterian Hospital, Columbia University Medical Center, and Cornell Medical Center. Most recently, Dr. Mendonça was an associate professor of pediatrics at the University of Chicago. Dr. Mendonça will begin to develop a program in medical/clinical informatics in both research and training under the National Institutes of Health–funded Institute for Clinical and Translational Research (ICTR) in which the Department is a core unit and the College of Engineering is an ICTR partner.

Joni Pierce, MBA, is a principal at J. Pierce and Associates and adjunct faculty at the University of Utah's David Eccles School of Business. Ms. Pierce received her MBA from the University of Utah and is currently pursuing a master's degree in biomedical informatics and clinical decision support.

W. Nicholson Price II, JD, PhD, is an assistant professor of law at the University of Michigan Law School, where he teaches patents and health law and studies life science innovation, including big data and artificial intelligence in medicine. Dr. Price is co-founder of regulation and innovation in the biosciences; co-chair of the Junior IP Scholars Association; co-lead of the Project on Precision Medicine, Artificial Intelligence, and Law at the Harvard Law School's Petrie-Flom Center for Health Law Policy, Biotechnology, and Bioethics; and a core partner at the University of Copenhagen's Center for Advanced Studies in Biomedical Innovation Law.

Joachim Roski, PhD, MPH, delivers solutions in the areas of care transformation, health care business, and outcome analytics; quality/safety; and population health improvement. He supports a range of clients in their health care planning, improvement, strategic measurement, analysis, and evaluation needs. His clients include the Military Health Service, the Veterans Health Administration, the Centers for Medicare & Medicaid Services, The Office of the National Coordinator of Health Information Technology, and others. He is a well-published national expert who speaks frequently on the topics of measuring and improving health care costs, quality/safety, outcomes, and value.

Suchi Saria, PhD, MSc, is a professor of machine learning and health care at Johns Hopkins University, where she uses big data to improve patient outcomes. Her interests span machine learning, computational statistics, and its applications to domains where one has to draw inferences from observing a complex, real-world system evolve over time. The emphasis of her research is on Bayesian and probabilistic graphical modeling approaches for addressing challenges associated with modeling and prediction in real-world temporal systems. In the past 7 years, she has been particularly drawn to computational solutions for problems in health informatics as she sees a tremendous opportunity there for high impact work. Prior to joining Johns Hopkins, she earned her PhD and master's degree at Stanford University in computer science, working with Dr. Daphne Koller. She also spent 1 year at Harvard University collaborating with Dr. Ken Mandl and Dr. Zak Kohane as a National Science Foundation Computing Innovation Fellow. While in the Valley, she also spent time as an early employee at Aster Data Systems, a big data startup acquired by Teradata. She enjoys consulting and advising data-related startups. She is an investor and an informal advisor to Patient Ping.

Nigam Shah, MBBS, PhD, is an associate professor of medicine (biomedical informatics) at Stanford University, an assistant director of the Center for Biomedical Informatics Research, and a core member of the Biomedical Informatics Graduate Program. Dr. Shah's research focuses on combining machine learning and prior knowledge in medical ontologies to enable use cases of the learning health system. Dr. Shah received the American Medical Informatics Association New Investigator Award for 2013 and the Stanford Biosciences Faculty Teaching Award for outstanding teaching in his graduate class on data-driven medicine. Dr. Shah was elected into the American College of Medical Informatics in 2015 and was inducted into the American Society for Clinical Investigation in 2016. He holds an MBBS from Baroda Medical College, India, a PhD from Penn State University, and completed postdoctoral training at Stanford University.

Ranak Trivedi, MA, MS, PhD, is a clinical health psychologist and a health services researcher interested in understanding how families and patients can better work together to improve health outcomes for both. Dr. Trivedi is also interested in identifying barriers and facilitators of chronic illness self-management, and developing family centered self-management programs that address the needs of both patients and their family members. Dr. Trivedi is also interested in improving the assessment and treatment of mental illnesses in primary care settings and evaluating programs that aim to improve these important activities.

Danielle Whicher, PhD, MHS, is a health researcher at Mathematica Policy Research. In this role, she participates in large-scale evaluations of national and state health payment and delivery reform initiatives. She is also engaged in efforts to evaluate health information technologies. Prior to joining Mathematica, Dr. Whicher was a senior program officer for the National Academy of Medicine (NAM) Leadership Consortium for a Value & Science Driven Health System, where she directed policy projects on a variety of topics related to the use of science and technology to inform health and health care. Before her work at the

NAM, Dr. Whicher held positions at the Patient-Centered Outcomes Research Institute, the Johns Hopkins Berman Institute for Bioethics, and the Center for Medical Technology Policy. She has a PhD and an MHS in health policy and management from the Johns Hopkins Bloomberg School of Public Health and currently serves as a co-editor for the journal *Value in Health*. Her work has been published in a variety of reports and peer-reviewed journals, including *Annals of Internal Medicine, Medical Care, PharmacoEconomics, Clinical Trials*, and *The Journal of Law, Medicine, & Ethics*.

Jenna Wiens, PhD, is a Morris Wellman Assistant Professor of Computer Science and Engineering at the University of Michigan in Ann Arbor. She is currently the head of the Machine Learning for Data-Driven Decisions research group. Dr. Wiens's primary research interests lie at the intersection of machine learning and health care. She is particularly interested in time-series analysis, transfer/multitask learning, and causal inference. The overarching goal of her research agenda is to develop the computational methods needed to help organize, process, and transform data into actionable knowledge. Dr. Wiens received her PhD in 2014 from the Massachusetts Institute of Technology (MIT). At MIT, she worked with Professor John Guttag in the Computer Science and Artificial Intelligence Lab. Her PhD research focused on developing accurate patient risk-stratification approaches that leverage spatiotemporal patient data, with the ultimate goal of discovering information that can be used to reduce the incidence of health care–associated infections. In 2015, Dr. Wiens was named one of Forbes' 30 under 30 in Science and Healthcare; she received a National Science Foundation CAREER Award in 2016; and this past year was named to the MIT Tech Review's list of 35 Innovators Under 35.